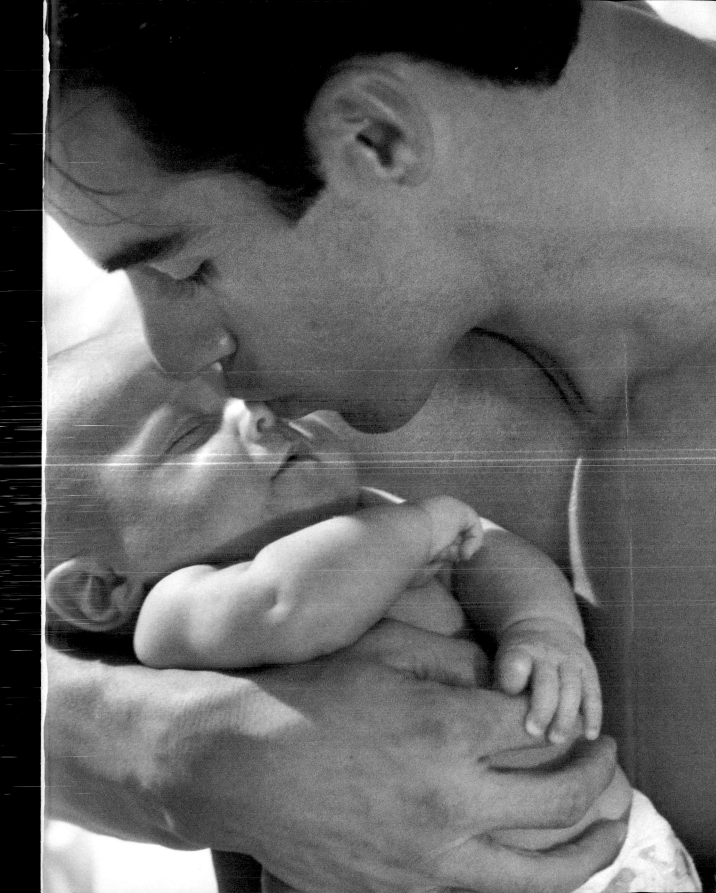

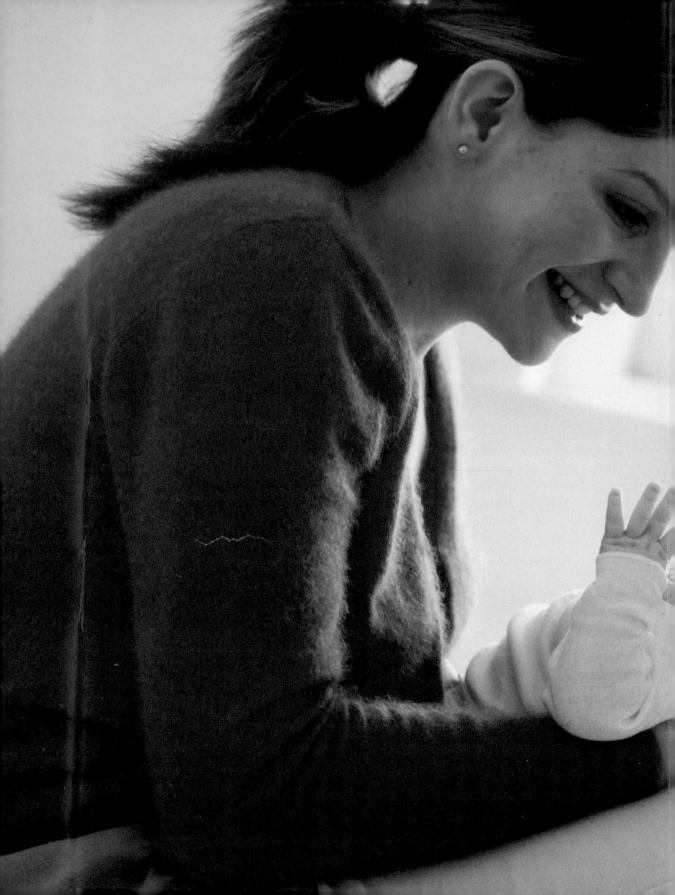

conception
pregnancy
and birth

Dr Miriam Stoppard

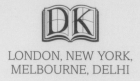

LONDON, NEW YORK,
MELBOURNE, DELHI

For Linzi and Will

Medical consultant
Dr Elizabeth Owen MD FRCOG MHPEd

Managing Editors Penny Warren, Esther Ripley
Managing Art Editor Marianne Markham
Senior Art Editor Glenda Fisher
Editors Jinny Johnson, Andrea Bagg,
Emma Woolf, Diana Vowles
Production Editors Luca Frassinetti,
Ben Marcus
Production Controller Mandy Inness
Special Photography Vanessa Davies
Jacket design Smith and Gilmour

**Produced for Dorling Kindersley
by Cooling Brown**
Creative Director Arthur Brown
Editor Jemima Dunne
Designers Tish Jones, Peter Cooling
Art Direction for Photography Emma Forge

First published by Dorling Kindersley in 1995

This revised edition published
in Great Britain in 2008
by Dorling Kindersley Limited
80 Strand, London WC2R 0RL
A Penguin Company

A CIP catalogue record for this book is available
from the British Library.

ISBN 978-1-4053-2972-9

Reproduced by MDP, Bath, UK
Printed and bound in China by Sheck Wah Tong

Discover more at
www.dk.com

Preface

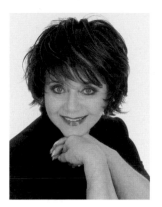

Conception, pregnancy, and birth are the most amazing events in any couple's life. There's so much information to absorb, so many choices to make, and all the time your body's changing in a million marvellous ways. From your first positive pregnancy test to your very last push, I've written what I hope is a practical and accessible guide for you to dip into throughout your pregnancy, helping you and your partner to navigate your way smoothly into parenthood.

With this revised edition of *Conception, Pregnancy and Birth* I've taken the opportunity to give the whole book a refreshingly lighter and more modern feel, with new full-colour pictures wherever possible. Page by page, I've worked with top medical consultants to bring every word right up to date, including all the latest medical research, hospital practices, and new treatments. I've also paid special attention to my real-life casebooks, with material on induced births and on becoming a new dad – a little reassurance for all anxious fathers-to-be!

Although the majority of pregnancies are straightforward, it's true that some can be less so. This book contains lots of information, written with the aim of reassuring you, on specialist fertility treatments, on complications of pregnancy, on special deliveries, and all the special medical interventions on offer in such cases. I always think that forewarned is forearmed – it's better to know about what might happen, and to plan accordingly, than to be taken by surprise.

Notwithstanding all the updating, my overall goal in this book remains the same. That you should have the birth you both want, in the circumstances you both want, helped by carers who have your needs and the needs of your new baby uppermost.

With very best wishes for your pregnancy, and beyond!

Contents

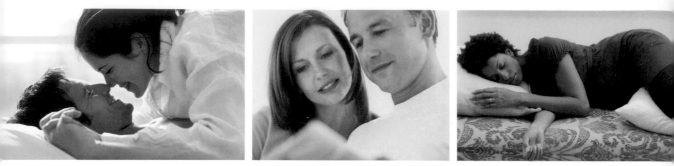

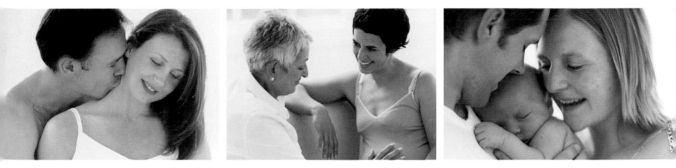

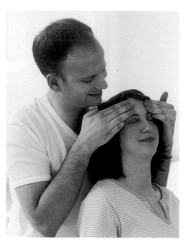

Introduction

Now we're discovering more and more about what can damage eggs and sperm, it's all the more important to prepare for pregnancy with some lifestyle changes. Stopping smoking at least three months before trying for a baby is essential for everyone, and giving up alcohol is important too. A healthy and fit body is the best possible place to conceive and carry a baby to term.

Not everything is always straightforward, of course: chromosomes and genes may be imperfect and fertilization may be difficult, but doctors now know about many of these problems and some of them can be successfully treated.

One in six couples has difficulty conceiving but that doesn't necessarily mean they'll never have a baby. Most couples who think they're infertile are only *subfertile* and with help can manage to conceive. At least half of all problems with conception are due to male fertility problems, something some men have difficulty coming to terms with, but that simple fact means that infertility can only be investigated as a couple. And the first test to be done is semen analysis.

Couples starting on fertility treatment deserve and should get counselling support right from the start – their own doctor can refer them to a counsellor who specializes in dealing with the stress of infertility. There's a bewildering number of treatments available for all kinds of infertility, which is why I've gone into detail on fertility testing and treatment from simple drug therapies to the latest complex assisted reproductive technologies (ART).

Your developing baby

For convenience, the stages of your baby's development can be roughly divided into three different phases: the first, second, and third trimesters. They're divided this way because of the particular changes happening to mother and baby in each of the three stages. In the first trimester your baby's organs form, in the second these organs become complex, and in the third they grow in size.

For you, the first trimester is when your body becomes primed for pregnancy: your breasts grow, your internal organs adapt, and your muscles and ligaments start to slacken in preparation for labour. High levels of pregnancy hormones bring on pregnancy sickness, the desire to go to the lavatory more often, and tenderness in your breasts. During the second trimester the body goes into a phase of consolidation. The third trimester sees your body preparing for delivery and making sure that your baby is growing healthily.

Preparing for fatherhood

Nowadays even the most hardworking dad wants to share childcare and be there for his kids. On the other hand, there are still some men who worry that taking a greater part in child rearing would somehow be feminizing, and that sits uneasily with them. The result is that some men become disillusioned and anxious. Men feel they're on the horns of a dilemma; society, especially mothers, seem to know what sort of chap they want New Dad to be, but often men feel driven into a corner by being pressured into a hitherto unfamiliar role.

Long ago it was established that children can do perfectly well with only one parent of either gender. So even though some children are fine without a father, perhaps we need to encourage New Dads by offering fathers a proper New Deal. For this reason, I've included all aspects of fatherhood and fathering in the hope that, after reading it, more men will feel free to liberate their fathering instincts.

The birth of your choice

Labour and birth can be managed in the way you choose. There are many decisions for you to make and it's important to be aware of all your options. In theory, it's possible to have exactly the kind of birth that you want, but this involves lots of reading, soul searching, and talking with your partner. You'll also have to talk things over with your nursing and medical attendants so that any difficulties that might come up later on can be dealt with.

Home birth is becoming more widely accepted and is something you might want to think seriously about. Alternatively, you can choose a hospital and a team of midwives that provide the facilities, the atmosphere, and the cooperative approach to childbirth that you prefer. It's important to make a birth plan outlining the kind of birth you'd ideally like to have, and by talking this through with your attendants you should be able to have the birth you want unless something unforeseen happens. It's up to women and their partners to take a more assertive role in the way the delivery and birth of their baby will be handled.

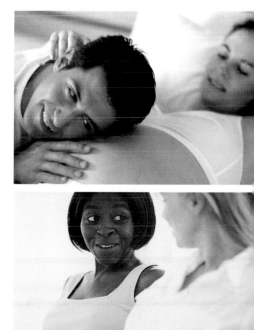

Food in pregnancy

Eating healthily in pregnancy is mainly a question of choosing a wide variety of foods that contain plenty of essential nutrients. Make sure you eat lots of fresh fruit and vegetables, whole grains, and raw food and that you have a healthy intake of protein by eating fish, poultry, and low-fat dairy products, with red meat and eggs now and then. Fish is a good source of vitamin B_{12} and vitamin A, which are also found in green and yellow vegetables.

Your baby uses iron up fast and needs fresh supplies every day, so it's vital for you to eat plenty of iron-rich foods. Food that are rich in iron are apricots, raisins, prunes, red meat, and fish. Ideally a woman should start taking daily folic acid supplements three months ahead of getting pregnant and continue taking them until the twelfth week of pregnancy to avoid neural tube defects like spina bifida. So it makes sense to add folic-acid-rich foods to your diet – green leafy vegetables, nuts, and cereals.

Healthy pregnancy

Regular exercise keeps you mentally and physically in good shape – when you exercise, the body releases tranquillizing chemicals, helping you to relax and soothing away tension. The fast circulation of the blood during exercise means that your body and your baby are well oxygenated. Your labour will probably be easier and more comfortable if your muscles are in tone, and many of the exercises taught in antenatal classes, combined with relaxation and breathing techniques, will help you to be more in touch with what's happening to you during labour and delivery. As well as exercising, learn to save your energy, sleep as much as you can, and catnap whenever possible.

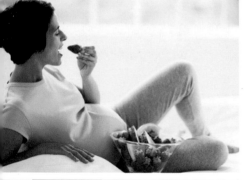

Your antenatal care

Good antenatal care is usually rewarded with healthy mothers and babies. At the antenatal clinic, routine tests are done to spot potential problems, avoid them where possible, and get treatment promptly if needed. Tests such as ultrasound scanning and amniocentesis are carried out for mothers and babies with special needs.

The social and personal aspects of antenatal care are as important as the medical ones. You'll probably find that talking to other mothers, doctors, and midwives reassures you about any worries you might have and helps you feel confident about labour and birth. The clinic gives you the chance to ask questions, explore the different circumstances in which you can have your baby, and plan ahead for the kind of birth that you and your partner want.

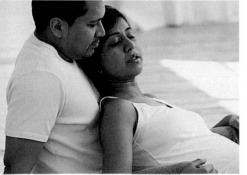

Caring for your unborn baby

You can be in touch with your unborn baby all through your pregnancy. The first time that you really feel you're in touch is when you feel your baby move. Keep talking to your unborn child. Babies have very sensitive hearing and at birth recognize both their mother's and father's voices from simply having heard them as they were growing and developing in the womb. Most parents really enjoy talking and singing songs to their unborn child, and gently massaging him through the abdominal wall. Hearing is one of the first senses to develop and your baby can hear you talking from about 16 weeks after conception.

Not all babies develop normally, but modern techniques are so advanced that we can even care for a developing baby in the womb. Advanced surgery can be carried out while your baby is still inside you so that he has every chance of being born normal and healthy. Not all babies enjoy the perfect conditions for development but, even so, diabetic mothers and mothers with Rhesus incompatibility, for example, can, with careful monitoring and treatment, have healthy pregnancies.

Common complaints

Very few women go through pregnancy without some minor health problems. Most of these are uncomfortable rather than serious. There's a group of complaints particular to pregnancy. Being prepared and knowing about the treatments you can have is half the battle in coping with them. Most are easily dealt with and have no long-term effects.

Medical emergencies

The risk of medical emergencies tends to be concentrated in the first and third trimesters of pregnancy. Nearly all of the classic emergencies are accompanied by classic symptoms, and should you experience any of them, call your doctor immediately. These symptoms include severe abdominal pain, vaginal bleeding, a fever of more than 37.8°C (100°F), severe nausea or vomiting, unremitting headache, blurred vision, swelling of the ankles, fingers, and face, no movement of your baby for more than 24 hours, and rupture of your membranes.

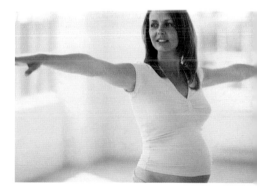

In the first trimester most emergencies are linked with loss of the baby due to haemorrhage or miscarriage, or to the embryo implanting in the wrong place, as in an ectopic pregnancy. Later on, an emergency might be brought on by very high blood pressure leading to pre-eclampsia, by recurrent late abortion, by Rhesus incompatibility, and by abnormalities of the placenta, such as placenta praevia. Nonetheless, the vast majority of babies are delivered safely.

A sensual pregnancy

Most women find that certain parts of the body, such as breasts, nipples, and the genital area, become more sensitive in pregnancy and their sexual organs are more easily aroused. This increased sensuality is due to high levels of pregnancy hormones and means that a woman may find she enjoys all aspects of sex, including sexual intercourse, even more than usual. Making love can be better than ever before, with more heightened sensations, earlier arousal, and intense orgasms. Some women may orgasm for the first time, while others may find they are now able to have multiple orgasms. As your abdomen swells, however, you may find that some positions are uncomfortable.

Getting ready for your baby

In the third trimester, nesting begins in earnest. There's lots to do – getting your baby's room ready, choosing clothes and equipment, deciding what you want to call your baby, working out how long you're going to take off work, and what kind of care you'd like for your child, and for your other children.

If you're going to have your baby at home, you'll need to prepare a room for the birth and have all your equipment carefully chosen and organized. If you're going to give birth in hospital, draw up check lists, go to the hospital, and make yourselves familiar with admission procedures so that you feel in control and free of anxiety.

Managing your labour

Labour is the culmination of your pregnancy and it can be divided into well-defined stages. Pre-labour is a time before labour when you might have a dull backache or pass a "show". Your membranes may also rupture painlessly before your true labour begins.

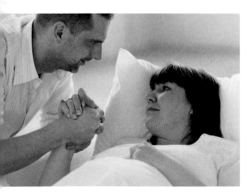

The first stage of labour is predominately taken up with dilatation of your cervix to a size that lets your baby make her way from your uterine cavity into the birth canal. This stage is usually quite straightforward, particularly if you're able to keep moving around and, by staying in an upright position, use the force of gravity to help your cervix to dilate.

Very few labours are pain-free, but there are many methods and types of pain relief from which to choose, including hypnobirthing – a natural and safe state of profound relaxation. And some labours aren't straightforward so I've devoted a whole chapter to "Special deliveries", with information on inductions, breech babies, and sudden births.

Getting to know your newborn baby

Building a relationship with your baby begins the second she's born and you and your partner will want to be left alone with her. We now know that parents who can hold and be with their babies right after the birth tend to be more sympathetic to their children's needs later. Hold your baby next to your skin where she can feel your warmth and your heartbeat. As your baby smells your skin and feels you cuddle her, she starts to get to know you and feel how much you love her.

The first few days will be harder than you think. Feeding can take longer than you expect, as can your baby's daily care. A routine is not always easy to set up, but the guiding and unbreakable rule is to take your lead from your baby.

A new baby can seem so delicate, and some new mums and dads feel nervous about picking up and handling their baby at first. Don't worry – your baby is tougher than she looks. As long as you support her firmly and carefully, there's no need for you to be afraid as you cuddle her, bathe her, and change her nappy.

Parents of special-care babies who need to be nursed in hospital intensive care units don't need to worry about being unable to bond with their babies. As long as parents, under the guidance of the nursing staff, become intimately involved in the day-to-day care of their baby, they shouldn't suffer any disadvantages. The staff will encourage you to stroke, touch, and talk to your baby as much as possible.

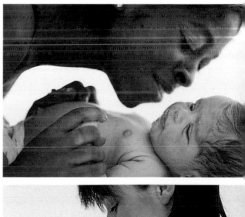

Adjusting to parenthood

Getting to know your newborn baby is a thrilling experience, but don't be surprised if you feel a slight let-down at times. There are so many adjustments to make and few of them are easy. Somehow you have to coax your baby to fit in with your established family routine, maintain a loving relationship with your partner, and attend to your baby's needs and constant demands for attention. Many women get bouts of sadness, and not just the "baby blues", which are so common in the first week after delivery. Much more serious is postnatal depression, which needs immediate attention from your doctor.

The responsibilities of parenthood may weigh heavily upon you, but watching your baby grow and develop should bring more than enough joy to balance any negative feelings that may occasionally creep in. You'll need some time to yourself to recharge your batteries, while time alone with your partner will help you to keep your relationship alive.

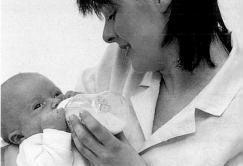

Preparing for pregnancy

As we find out more and more about human eggs and sperm and what makes them healthy, we're realizing how important it is to prepare for pregnancy by looking after ourselves. Not everything, of course, is always straightforward, but more is known about conception problems and some can be treated.

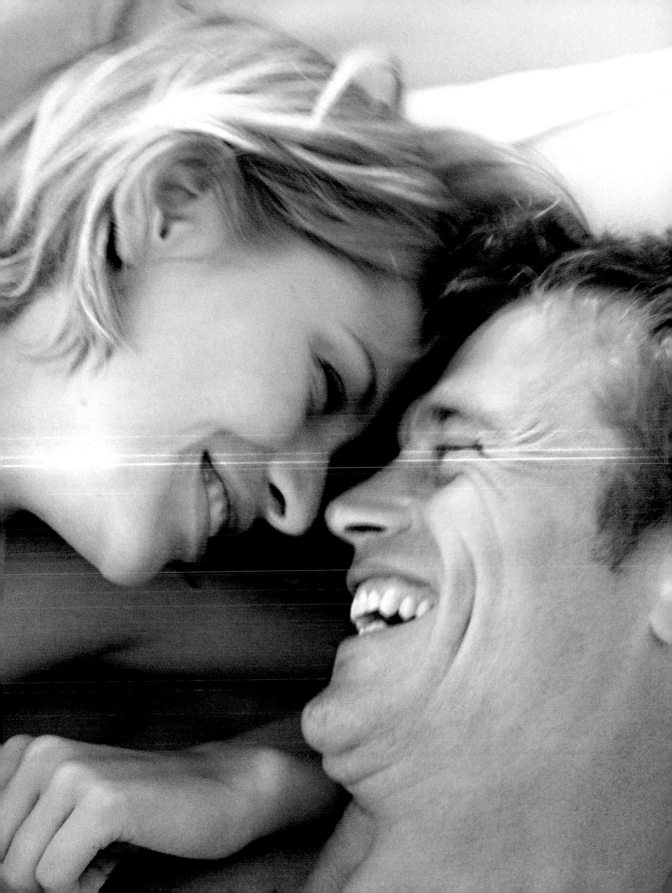

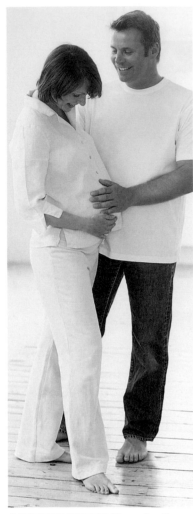

▲ **PREPARED PARENTS** Happy, healthy parents make happy, healthy children, so do your best to make sure you're fit for parenthood before getting pregnant.

Fit for parenthood

Health really does matter when you're conceiving a baby. And your partner's health is just as important as yours. The fitter you both are at the time of conception, the better your chances of having a trouble-free pregnancy and labour, and a healthy baby. Becoming a parent will change your life in lots of ways, so it's a good idea to plan ahead as much as you can.

Your changing lifestyle

All the things you take for granted about your life and what you do will be affected by the arrival of your baby.

Time Most of us live very busy lives and many new parents think that their new baby will just fit in somehow and life will go on as usual. It won't. Babies and children need a lot of time and attention, and as parents you'll have less time to spend with each other – and other people – than you did before.

Costs Whatever you earn, you'll probably need to spend a fair amount of money on things to do with your child, such as clothing and equipment, although you may get some things second hand. Other household costs, such as heating, will rise too, and you may find you want extra items such as a new washing machine or even a larger car.

Relationships Your relationship with your partner will change when you have a baby and so do those with other people. You may start to feel closer to your parents – now they're your baby's grandparents – but you might find you have less in common now with your single and childless friends. It's good to make some new friendships with other parents if you can – they're going through the same experiences as you.

Smoking This is one of the most damaging things you can do as far as the health of your unborn baby is concerned and it's the major cause of avoidable health problems. Risks linked to smoking include miscarriage and stillbirth, damage to the placenta, a low birthweight baby who fails to thrive, and a higher risk of fetal abnormalities. Smoking is one cause of a low sperm count, and a man who smokes while his partner is pregnant may damage his unborn baby's health through passive smoking. And the problems continue. When tested at five, seven, and eleven years old, children of heavy smokers were found to suffer from impaired growth and learning difficulties.

Alcohol This is a poison that can damage the sperm and egg before conception, as well as the developing embryo. The main risks to an unborn baby are developmental delay, growth deficiencies, and damage to the brain and nervous system – well documented as fetal alcohol syndrome. Alcohol can also cause stillbirth. Research suggests that the effect of alcohol on pregnant women varies: some are more affected than others. But one thing is certain: if you don't drink alcohol during your pregnancy you'll avoid any problems.

Drugs Only take over-the-counter medicines if you have to and always check the label. Your pharmacist will advise you about what's safe to take. Don't take recreational drugs if you're planning to conceive. Marijuana interferes with the normal production of sperm in men, and the effects can take three to nine months to wear off. Class A drugs such as cocaine, heroin, and morphine can damage the chromosomes in the sperm and egg, leading to abnormalities. When syringes are shared, there's a high risk of contracting HIV, the virus that leads to AIDS. A mother can pass the HIV virus to her baby during pregnancy and the baby can become HIV positive in his own right (see p.19). Cocaine use can also damage the baby's blood supply, and taking it in pregnancy can lead to the placenta separating from the womb and the risk of a stillbirth.

Diet and exercise Both are vital to your health and the health of your baby. Do your best to eat a sensible balanced diet that's low in animal fat and includes at least five portions of fresh fruit and vegetables a day. Check, too, that you're getting enough folic acid (see p.20) in your diet because it's known to lower the risk of your baby suffering from any neural tube defects, such as spina bifida. It's a very good idea to take regular exercise, too. Pregnancy puts a strain on your body, so the fitter you are beforehand, the better you'll cope.

Age If you're fit and healthy, your pregnancy should not be any more difficult in your 30s or 40s than in your 20s. Whatever your age, you're likely to have a normal pregnancy and birth, although some problems such as infertility and chromosomal defects (for example, Down's syndrome, see p.24) do become more common in older people. Older mothers, and younger women in high-risk groups, are always offered tests for chromosomal abnormalities.

Stopping contraception

When you decide you want to get pregnant you can stop barrier methods, such as the diaphragm and sheath, at once. But if you're on the pill or you're using an intrauterine contraceptive device (IUCD), a little more advance planning is needed.

The pill The usual advice is to stop taking the pill a month before trying to conceive, so that you have at least one normal menstrual period before becoming pregnant. But there's evidence to suggest that some women are more fertile immediately after stopping the pill, so this could be the ideal time to try if you've had fertility problems or you have had a miscarriage.

If you suspect that you're pregnant but you're still on the pill, stop taking it. Conceiving on the pill rarely causes any problems, but go to your doctor as soon as you can.

The intrauterine contraceptive device Known as an IUCD, or coil, this works by preventing the sperm from reaching the egg, or by causing changes in the uterus that prevent fertilized eggs from implanting. A very small number of women do become pregnant while using an IUCD. Even though removing it during pregnancy does increase the risk of miscarriage, it's still generally recommended if at all possible in order to lower the risk of miscarriage and infection later in the pregnancy.

Testing your urine

If tests show that you have sugar in your urine it's possible that you have diabetes. However, it's more likely that some sugar has leaked through your kidneys, as their threshold to sugar is lowered by pregnancy. You'll need more tests to confirm that this is what has happened.

Diabetes results from the pancreas producing insufficient insulin to cope with glucose (sugar) levels in the body. Pregnancy hormones have an anti-insulin effect, which can make diabetes worse, or lead to gestational diabetes (diabetes in pregnancy) in women with an underlying tendency, such as a family background of diabetes.

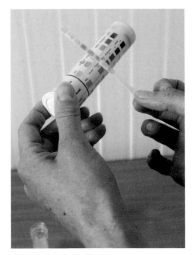

▲ TESTING URINE Urine tests are simple to do. A chemically impregnated strip is dipped into a sample of your urine. If sugar is present the strip changes colour, and the amount can be compared to a chart that shows glucose levels.

Health considerations

If you suffer from a chronic (long-term) condition, such as diabetes mellitus, heart disease, or epilepsy, you can, of course, still have children. It's important, though, to talk things over with your doctor before you become pregnant, so you can get the best possible care and help.

Asthma This is the most common respiratory problem in mums-to-be and is usually controlled by bronchodilator drugs and inhaled steroids. Asthma drugs don't seem to be a risk to the health of the growing baby, although thrush (see p.212), which is often made worse by pregnancy, can be a side effect for the mother, and sometimes labour may start early. If you do suffer from asthma, take extra care of yourself while you're pregnant. Any stress and tension, as well as dust, pollen, and pollution, can cause breathlessness, and strain your already hard-working heart.

Epilepsy This condition affects one in every 200 people. Epilepsy can vary from a momentary loss of consciousness to grand mal seizures. Research has found that the effect of pregnancy on the frequency and intensity of seizures varies – 50 per cent of mothers with epilepsy are unaffected, 40 per cent note slight improvement, and 10 per cent are worse. If you suffer from epileptic seizures, talk to your doctor before you hope to conceive. There's a slightly increased risk of neural tube and other defects linked to anti-epileptic drugs, including sodium valproate, lamatrigine, carbamazepine, and phenytoin. Your doctor can advise you.

Changing the drug treatment can increase the risk of seizures, but women with epilepsy are usually advised to optimize the drugs they take before pregnancy, not during it. While you're pregnant you'll keep on with any drug treatment, but you'll need to be seen frequently by a neurologist or other specialist who can adjust your drug dosage. Anti-epileptic drugs prevent absorption of folic acid, so it's very important to take high doses of folic acid supplements (5mg a day) before you conceive as well as after, to help lower the risk of birth defects (see p.17). All pregnant women on sodium valproate or phenytoin are also advised to take vitamin K supplements from 36 weeks of pregnancy to help mature the baby's liver.

Diabetes mellitus Diabetes can cause the baby to be abnormally large or have heart and respiratory problems, and complications for the mother include chronic thrush and pre-eclampsia (see p.224). It's essential for a woman with pre-existing diabetes to have good glucose (sugar) control at conception as the baby is at a greater risk of abnormalities if sugar levels are high. Anyone at risk of gestational diabetes (diabetes that develops in pregnancy) can have a blood test to check for the condition.

Heart disease If you suffer from any kind of heart condition your doctor will give you specific advice about your pregnancy. Generally you'll be told to get plenty of rest – put your feet up in the afternoon for at least two hours, and spend ten hours in bed at night. Most women with heart disease have easy, spontaneous labours. During labour the extra strain on the heart is intermittent and, in total, is less than that imposed upon it during the third trimester. There's usually no reason why a woman with heart problems should need induction or a Caesarean section.

Kidney disease A woman with kidney disease should be able to have children but will need careful monitoring. Women with kidney disease have a higher than usual risk of hypertension and pre-eclampsia. Urinary tract infection is another common problem, but as long as the kidneys remove waste effectively, the pregnancy can continue. If the fetus isn't growing properly, though, doctors may recommend early induction. (Renal dialysis does pose a risk as a mother's kidneys are unlikely to be able to cope with additional waste from the fetus.)

Sexually transmitted disease There's a risk of infection to your baby if you have a primary herpes infection when your membranes rupture or during labour. Primary herpes simplex II virus infection may slow your baby's growth, and about half the affected infants develop some form of herpetic infection after birth, affecting the eyes, mouth, and skin.

   If you've a history of genital herpes you should be able to have a normal vaginal delivery, even with an active secondary infection. If you have no symptoms, and you're not shedding the virus from your cervix or vagina, the risk that your baby will become infected is less than one in a thousand. But if you have herpes ulcers or a primary infection just before labour commences, you'll be advised to have a Caesarean section to reduce the risk of your baby catching herpes as he descends the birth canal. Doctors will check for signs of infection at the time of delivery.

HIV/AIDS The outlook for babies of mothers who have tested HIV positive is much better than it used to be. The use of oral AZT may protect the developing baby from infection, and the mother will be scanned regularly to check the baby's growth. Doctors may suggest a Caesarean delivery to protect the baby. Although it's not inevitable that the baby of an HIV mother will be HIV positive and develop AIDS, there's a risk that the baby will be born with HIV antibodies; these are usually maternal antibodies and may disappear within 18 months. Because of the risks, an HIV mother will be given counselling and may be offered the chance to terminate her pregnancy if she wishes.

German measles

The German measles (rubella) virus can cause birth defects, particularly if you catch it in the first three months of your pregnancy. Problems may include deafness, blindness, and heart disease. Before trying to conceive, ask your doctor to check you for antibodies to the virus.

Even if you've been vaccinated in the past you can't assume you're immune to the disease – the antibodies lose their efficiency after a period of time. Ask your doctor to check, and if you're not immune you'll need to be vaccinated. After vaccination, you'll need to wait at least three months before trying to conceive, as the vaccine is live.

If you're pregnant and you come into contact with someone who has, or is suspected of having, German measles, you must tell your doctor right away. You'll need to have a blood sample taken that will be sent to a laboratory for antibody testing.

Depending on the result, you might need to have another test ten days later. If the result suggests that you might have German measles, you and your partner will have to decide whether to abort your pregnancy. Some doctors may recommend giving antibodies in the form of gamma globulin to help prevent damage to the fetus.

Miriam's casebook

The importance of folic acid

Julie's first baby, Henry, was born 18 months ago and now she'd like to have a second child. She had a normal delivery with Henry and he was fine, apart from a brown hairy birthmark at the base of his spine. Her doctor explained that this kind of birthmark may be linked to spina bifida, but means nothing by itself. However, Julie is worried that she is at greater risk of having a child with spina bifida because of the birthmark.

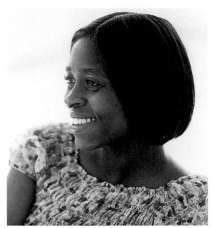

Spina bifida and hydrocephalus

Julie has read about the connection between folic acid deficiency and neural tube defects (spina bifida and hydrocephalus) and knows that she should start taking folic acid supplements now in case she becomes pregnant, but doesn't like taking tablets, even vitamin supplements.

The medical definition of spina bifida is a defect in which part of one or more vertebrae fails to develop completely, leaving part of the spinal cord exposed. Spina bifida can happen anywhere in the spine but it's most common on the lower back. Spina bifida symptoms depend on the severity of the spinal cord exposure; there may be paralysis, incontinence, or hydrocephalus – swelling of the brain.

There are different degrees of spina bifida. In one type the only defect is that the bony arches behind the spinal cord fail to join. When the bone defect is more extensive there may be neural tube defects such as a meningocele with protrusion of the meninges (the membranes surrounding the spinal cord) or, more serious still, a myelocele with deformity of the spinal cord itself. In the developing embryo the skin, brain, the spinal cord, and nerves all arise from the same layer of cells. This is why a birthmark over the end of the embryonic neural tube may be the only sign of late closure

of the fetal neural tube. Parents who've had one child with spina bifida are more at risk, but having a child with a hairy birthmark (sacral naevus) like Henry's does not mean there's any increased risk in the next pregnancy.

The spine and the vertebral column develop from a flat layer of cells whose edges come together to form a tube, which is the hollow cavity inside the spinal cord. The closure of the cord and the bones that surround it, the vertebrae, takes place very early in the development of an embryo, usually within four weeks of conception.

Reducing the risks

Research has shown that a woman needs sufficiently high levels of folic acid in her blood for the neural tube to close normally. Mothers with low blood levels of folic acid have a higher risk of having a spina bifida baby.

There's something else, too: normally folic acid is removed from the blood quite quickly, but when you're pregnant the kidneys filter it out of the blood at four times the normal rate. So if you don't eat folic-acid-rich foods or take folic acid supplements regularly you can become relatively deficient in folic acid, and your levels may drop low enough to put your baby at risk. It's therefore vital for all pregnant women to keep the blood levels of folic acid high.

Taking folic acid

I explained to Julie that her folic acid levels need to be topped up at the very moment she conceives. That means she needs to take folic acid before conception. Experts recommend that all women who're thinking about having a baby start taking 400mcg of folic acid supplements daily three months before trying to conceive. You can get folic acid in several different forms:

■ In green leafy vegetables (the darker green the better), mushrooms, cooked such as kidney beans, nuts (particularly walnuts), peas, and green beans.
■ In fortified cereals and wholewheat bread.
■ As capsules in 400mcg doses, from your pharmacy.
■ In a nutritious folic acid milk drink available from pharmacies. One carton (about a glassful) contains your daily folic acid requirements in liquid rather than tablet form.

Nutritionally vulnerable

All babies are potentially at some risk of spina bifida and other neural tube defects like hydrocephalus whatever their mother's age, even if she's in the best of health herself. But some women should be especially careful about taking folic acid supplements. So I asked Julie if she'd ever been allergic to certain key foods, such as cow's milk or wheat, or been generally run down or underweight through eating a poor, unbalanced diet or putting herself on an overstrict diet that resulted in anorexia nervosa.

I also asked her whether she had had a recent miscarriage or stillbirth, whether she drank or smoked heavily, whether she had been subject to a lot of stress, or had been working particularly hard – all factors that would make it especially important for Julie to make sure her diet was as nutritious as possible during pregnancy. I'm glad to say that Julie decided to start on folic acid immediately, in the form of the milk drink each morning with breakfast.

Miriam's top tips

It's vital for all women to take daily supplements of folic acid before trying to conceive as well as for the first 12 weeks of pregnancy to ensure blood levels of folic acid are high. My advice is to:

■ start taking a folic acid supplement three months before you start trying for a baby

■ make sure you are getting the recommended daily dose of 400mcg of folic acid

■ remember that you can take folic acid in many forms: as tablets or capsules, by eating a selection of foods rich in folic acid, or in a milk drink form that's available from pharmacies.

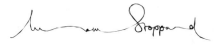

Folic acid in food

Foods high in folic acid (50–100mcg or more per 30g/1oz serving) include cooked black-eyed beans, brussels sprouts, beef extract, yeast extract, parsnips, kale, spinach, granary bread, spring greens, and broccoli.

Foods with medium folic acid (15–50mcg per 30g/1oz serving) include cooked soya and kidney beans, cauliflower, potatoes, iceberg lettuce, oranges, and orange juice, peas, baked beans, wholemeal bread, cabbage, green beans, green papper, courgettes, yogurt, white bread, eggs, brown rice, and wholegrain pasta.

Foods fortified with folic acid include some breads and cereals. Most supermarket chains stock a fortified own-label soft-grain bread. Two slices will provide approximately 90mcg of folic acid. A few leading brands of bread are also fortified; check the label to be certain. Many cereals are also fortified, but to very different levels so always check the label. Some cereals have more than 100mcg per serving.

Inheriting genes

Half of a baby's genes come from his mother, via the egg, and half come from his father, via the sperm.

Each egg and sperm contains a different "mix" of the parents' genes, so each child inherits a different and unique selection of his parents' genetic information.

Most of our individual mix of genes blends together, but some are dominant and others recessive. For example, the gene for brown eyes is dominant and the gene for blue eyes is recessive. So a child with one brown-eyed parent and one blue-eyed parent who receives a gene for each will have brown eyes because the gene for brown eyes prevails over the gene for blue eyes.

What is a gene?

Genes are chemical codes that control the way every cell in the body works. A gene is a minute unit of DNA (deoxyribonucleic acid) carried on a chromosome, which is also made up of DNA. In every body cell, there are at least 50,000 unique genes.

The "blueprint" of the body

Genes influence and direct the growth and function of everything in the human body. They control the pattern for growth, survival, and reproduction, and account for variations in height, hair and eye colour, body shape, and gender. Your genetic inheritance also decides how likely you are to have certain diseases. All cells come from the single egg fertilized by the male's sperm so the same genetic material is duplicated in every cell in your body, except for egg and sperm cells. But not all the genes in an individual cell are active; it's where the cell is and what it does that determines which genes are active. For example, different sets of genes are active in bone cells than blood cells.

Chromosomes Genes are carried in pairs along a chromosome (see opposite) and each gene is either dominant or recessive. A recognizable effect is the result of the dominant gene or genes in each pair; the effect of recessive genes will only be seen when there are two recessive genes.

Every cell in your body, except the egg and sperm cells, normally contains 23 pairs of the thread-like structures called chromosomes. Egg and sperm cells contain only 22 chromosomes plus an X or Y chromosome. Each chromosome contains thousands of genes, which are arranged in single file along its length. Chromosomes arc made up of two chains of DNA, which are arranged together to form a ladder-like structure, the

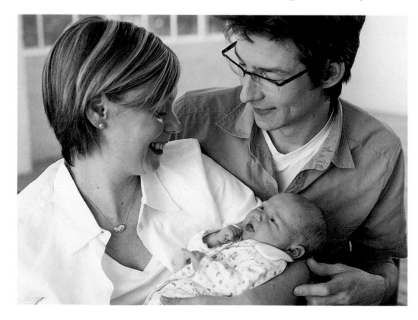

◀ **THE GENETIC MIX** Your baby will have a unique combination of your own and your partner's genes.

sides of which are sugar-phosphate molecules. This spirals around upon itself and is known as a double helix. DNA has four bases – adenine, cytosine, guanine, and thymine – which are arranged in different combinations according to the functions of the genes on the different parts of the chromosome. Each combination of bases provides coded instructions that control and regulate the body's various activities.

Chromosomes, genes, and DNA

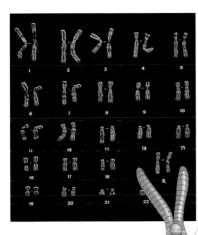

◀ **CHROMOSOMES** There are 23 pairs of chromosomes in the nucleus of every body cell (see left). These thread-like structures consist of 22 general pairs, plus a pair of sex chromosomes (either a pair of X chromosomes, as here, or an X and a Y).

Chromosome

▶ **THE DOUBLE HELIX** The two chains of DNA, which make up each of the 46 chromosomes, are arranged to make a long spiralling ladder.

Each of the four DNA bases – adenine, cytosine, guanine, and thymine – is represented here by a different colour

Sugar-phosphate molecules form the sides of the DNA ladder

Gene

◀ **DNA REPLICATION** When a new cell is about to be formed, the DNA in each of the chromosomes "unzips" along the centre of the rungs of the "ladder", and each half of DNA then duplicates itself. The new DNA chains created are genetically identical to the original chromosomes.

Mutations

Sometimes when a cell divides and duplicates its genetic material the copying process is not perfect, and there's a fault. This leads to a small change, or mutation, in the structure of the genetic material.

Carrying a mutant gene normally has a neutral or harmless effect – most, if not all, of us have a mutant gene as part of our genetic make-up. But sometimes it can have a disadvantageous effect or, more rarely, a beneficial one.

The effects of a mutant gene depend largely upon whether it's carried within the fused egg and sperm, or whether it's a fault in the later copying process of the body cells.

A mutation in the egg or sperm will reproduce itself in all of the body's cells, and can cause genetic disease such as cystic fibrosis (see p.24). A mutated body cell, at worst, will multiply to form a group of abnormal cells in a specific area. These may have only a minor effect in that part of the body, or they could cause deformity or disease. This type of mutation is usually triggered by an outside influence, such as radiation or exposure to cancer-forming agents.

Down's syndrome

This chromosomal disorder is usually the result of a fertilized egg having 47 chromosomes instead of the usual 46 (see column opposite).

In most cases, the egg is defective, because it's formed with the extra chromosome; the sperm may be affected in the same way. This type of Down's syndrome is known as trisomy. Less commonly, one parent may have a chromosomal abnormality, known as translocation, which causes the child to inherit faulty chromosomal material (see column opposite).

The incidence of Down's rises with the age of the mother, particularly over 35, but tests can identify it in a fetus. Chorionic villus sampling (CVS) or nuchal scanning can be carried out at ten to 12 weeks. At around 20 weeks, amniocentesis can be offered to high-risk mothers. (See also pp.184–87.)

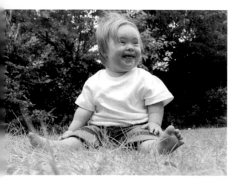

▲ **DOWN'S SYNDROME** Most cases of Down's syndrome occur randomly and aren't passed on. However, one cause – translocation – is inherited, so it's important to explore any family history of Down's syndrome.

Genetic counselling

Inside the nucleus of each cell are the genes and chromosomes that control how the body develops and functions (see also p.22). Genetic disorders happen when genes and chromosomes are abnormal. Genetic diseases can be caused by a single defective gene, several faulty genes, or a fault in the number or shape of chromosomes. There may also be complicating environmental factors. A single defective gene that results in a genetic disorder can be either dominant or recessive, a mutation, or attached to the X chromosome (see column opposite). Abnormal chromosomes that result in genetic disorders are usually new mutations, but may be inherited (see column, left).

If either of you has a history of a genetic disease in your extended family, it's best to ask for genetic counselling (see p.26) before becoming pregnant. The number of tests available for genetic diseases is increasing every year, although they don't tell the potential severity of the condition.

Dominant genetic diseases

Fatal diseases due to dominant genes are rare because those affected normally die before they can pass on the genes. However, some, such as familial hypercholesterolaemia, can be managed.

Familial hypercholesterolaemia This is the most common dominant genetic disease. Sufferers have such high levels of blood cholesterol that they risk heart attacks and other complications caused by narrowing of the arteries. This condition affects one in 500 people and can be detected by a blood test at birth.

Recessive genetic diseases

A defective recessive gene is usually masked by a normal dominant one. But if both parents carry a defective recessive gene, each of their children has a one in four chance of inheriting both recessive genes (and therefore one of several disorders) or neither, and a two in four chance of being a carrier. Thus there are always more carriers than sufferers.

Cystic fibrosis (CF) This is the most common recessive gene disorder. One in 20 of the white population carries the CF gene, and one in 2,000 white babies born is affected by the disease. In non-whites, the incidence is about one in 90,000. This disease mainly affects the lungs and the digestive system. Mucus inside the lungs becomes thick and sticky, and builds up, causing chest infections. The mucus also blocks the ducts of various organs, particularly the pancreas, preventing the normal flow of digestive enzymes. If not treated promptly, CF results in malnutrition.

Rapid and accurate carrier testing involving analysis of blood or mouth cells is possible. Over 60 per cent of sufferers survive into adulthood; some have been helped by heart and/or lung transplant surgery.

Sickle-cell anaemia This is the most common genetic disease among black people (one in 400). It's so called because the red cells are sickle-shaped from defective haemoglobin; this causes them to break down and the small blood vessels to clog, which may result in a stroke. It's usually diagnosed by a blood test, and the mother will be offered chorionic villus sampling (see p.186) if both parents are sufferers. People with sickle-cell anaemia are susceptible to meningitis and other serious infections but can, with care, live a productive life despite some ill health.

Thalassaemia This is common among Asians and people of African and Mediterranean descent. The gene may be dominant or recessive. It causes anaemia and chronic ill health, and sufferers may need blood transfusions. If you're at risk, you can have a blood test to check for the disease and this can show whether your haemoglobin level is reduced. Thalassaemia can be severe, but many cases are mild.

Tay–Sachs disease Common among Ashkenazi Jews, this is a fatal condition causing deterioration of the brain because of a deficiency in enzymes. Few children with the disease live beyond three years, and no adequate treatment is known. Tay–Sachs is diagnosed by a blood test.

Gender-linked diseases

These are conditions caused by defects on the X chromosome and only men are affected. If a second normal X chromosome is present, as in a healthy female, it compensates for the abnormal gene. Therefore, only women carry the disease. Men with the abnormal gene develop the disease because they have only one X chromosome.

Haemophilia This results when the crucial protein involved in blood clotting, Factor VIII, is missing. Sufferers bleed profusely from any injury, external or internal. Effective treatment with Factor VIII derived from normal blood is now available, and haemophiliacs can lead relatively normal lives. Diagnosis can be made from a sample of fetal blood at 18–20 weeks of pregnancy.

Duchenne muscular dystrophy This type of muscular dystrophy affects one boy in 5,000. Symptoms are progressive and children become unable to walk. The disease can be detected before birth.

Chromosomal disorders

These are usually due to some fault that happens when chromosomes are dividing during the formation of the egg or sperm, or when the fertilized egg is first dividing. More rarely, one parent has an abnormal arrangement of chromosomes.

The type of abnormality and how severe it is depends on whether one or both sex chromosomes, or one of the other 44 chromosomes (autosomes) are affected. Autosomal abnormalities are slightly less common than sex chromosomal abnormalities, but can produce more serious effects. If one of the 22 pairs of autosomes has an extra chromosome, this is known as a trisomy (see p.198). The most common trisomy is Down's syndrome (see column opposite).

Occasionally the problem is caused by translocation – there is a normal number of chromosomes, but part of one is joined to another. The parent carrier will be normal, but if a child inherits the translocated chromosomes he may have an abnormality.

Abnormalities of the sex chromosomes can cause defects in sexual development and infertility. Boys may suffer from Klinefelter's syndrome (see p.38), girls from Turner's (they have only one X chromosome instead of two). These abnormalities can be diagnosed by chromosome analysis, which may be offered during genetic counselling.

Can you benefit?

It's important to seek expert advice if you fall into any of the following groups. Not everyone will be referred for genetic counselling, but it's worth checking with your doctor if any of these factors apply to you:

■ if you've had a child with a genetic disorder such as cystic fibrosis, or a chromosomal disorder such as Down's syndrome

■ if you've had a child with a congenital defect – for example, a club foot (see p.199)

■ if there's any history of learning difficulties or abnormal development in your family

■ if there's a blood relationship between you and your partner

■ if you have a history of repeated miscarriages (see pp.218 and 222).

Genetic counselling

Very few couples will need genetic counselling but if you do, the main aim is to discover how great a risk you run of passing on an inheritable disease to your child. Perhaps you're worried because you or your partner have a blood relative (including, perhaps, a previous child) who has suffered from an inheritable disorder. Depending on what you find out, a genetic counsellor will also help you and your partner decide whether or not to go ahead with trying to conceive.

How genetic counselling works

When you first meet a genetic counsellor, you'll be asked lots of questions about your health, and about your family background. Take along as much information as you can and be prepared for the whole project to take some time. The advice you'll be given at the end of it depends on a precise diagnosis of the disease (what it is and why it happened), and on the making of a family tree, with details of all blood relationships and any diseases suffered. Your counsellor will assess the degree of risk in your case and help you make an informed decision. If there's a small risk, you may decide to go ahead and try for a baby. If the risks are very great, you might prefer not to take that chance.

For many genetic disorders, such as sickle-cell anaemia or Tay–Sachs (see p.25), prospective parents can be checked to find out if they are carriers. This can be done by seeing evidence of the disease itself on a blood sample; by looking for the product of the disease, such as the proteins that are present in Tay–Sachs; or by flagging a gene or chromosome. Flagging is a sophisticated technique that's used to find out if a fragment of DNA attaches itself to the patient's chromosome. If it does, the gene, and therefore the disease, is present; if not, it's absent. In most diseases, though, more than one gene is involved, so it can be difficult to check all the elements involved.

If a couple has already had a child with a congenital defect, the counsellor will first rule out any possible causes that aren't inherited, for example rubella (see p.19). Other possible causes such as exposure to radiation, drugs, or injury will also be looked at.

Sometimes it can be difficult to pinpoint the exact cause of any problem, but you'll be given as thorough a diagnosis as possible, and your chances of having another child with the same disorder outlined.

The importance of your family history

A counsellor will examine the medical history of both your families to find out if there's any pattern of disease over several generations. For example, James, when he was six years old, was suffering with painful, swollen joints. During a conversation with James's parents, the counsellor learned that a cousin, and probably a great-uncle as well, suffered from the genetic bleeding disorder known as haemophilia (see family tree, below), which is carried on the X chromosome.

This information pointed almost immediately to the probable diagnosis – James, too, was suffering from haemophilia. The pain and the swelling that he was experiencing was caused by the blood that was leaking into his joints.

▶ **HOW GENES ARE INHERITED** James's mother and some other female relatives are carriers of haemophilia. They don't suffer from the disease themselves, but they do pass on the gene to some of their sons, who develop haemophilia, and to some of their daughters, who become carriers.

- ● Males with haemophilia
- ○ Unaffected males
- ● Probable female carriers of haemophilia gene
- Possible female carriers of haemophilia gene

▶ **TESTING FOR HAEMOPHILIA** Blood tests can show if a man has haemophilia and what type, or whether a woman is a carrier.

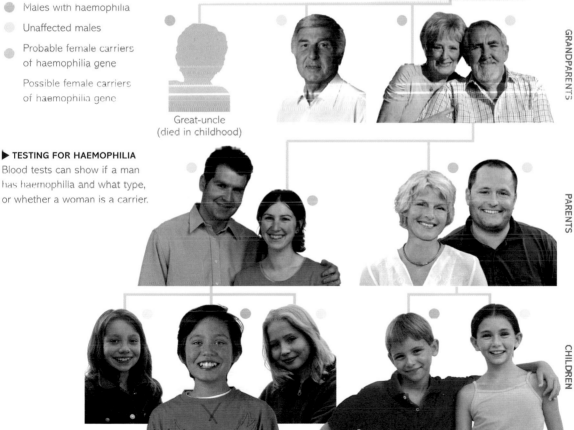

Great-uncle (died in childhood)

James

Cousin

Fertility facts

Fertility varies from person to person and at different stages of life. The following facts are true for most people:

■ the fertility of both men and women reaches its peak at about the age of 24

■ among couples who have regular intercourse without contraception, 25 per cent of women conceive in the first month, 60 per cent within six months, 75 per cent within nine months, 80 per cent within a year, and 90 per cent within 18 months

■ after ovulation, an egg can only be fertilized during the next 12–24 hours or so.

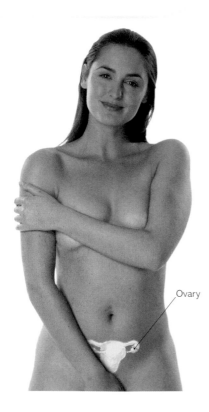

Ovary

Conceiving a baby

The miracle of birth begins when one of your partner's sperm fuses with one of your eggs to form a single cell. This cell contains its own unique genetic blueprint, which is a mix of genetic material from both parents. The cell then divides and divides again until eventually a new human being is made. The vast majority of couples with normal fertility manage to conceive within the first two years of trying for a baby.

A woman's entire stock of eggs is made in her two ovaries before her birth. By the fifth month of development, a baby girl's ovaries contain about seven million eggs. Many of these eggs will die before she's born, leaving her with about two million eggs at birth. Eggs continue to die until at puberty most women have between 200,000 and 500,000 eggs. Of these, only 400–500 mature and they're released by the ovaries during a woman's fertile years at the rate of roughly one a month.

The ovaries are located in the pelvis, close to the trumpet-like endings (fimbriae) of the Fallopian tubes. The germ cells that eventually develop into a woman's eggs form in the yolk sac that sustains the embryo in the first weeks of development. If the embryo is male, these cells are reabsorbed as the placenta develops. If the embryo is female, about 100 germ cells move from the yolk sac, along the umbilical cord, and into the tiny female embryo. Once inside the embryo, the cells migrate to the tissues that will later develop into the ovaries, and begin to multiply.

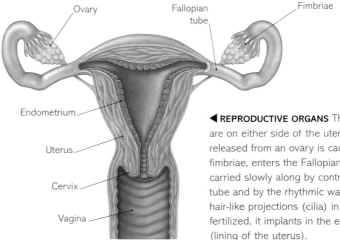

Ovary Fallopian tube Fimbriae

Endometrium

Uterus

Cervix

Vagina

◀ **REPRODUCTIVE ORGANS** The ovaries are on either side of the uterus. An egg released from an ovary is caught in the fimbriae, enters the Fallopian tube, and is carried slowly along by contractions of the tube and by the rhythmic waving of tiny, hair-like projections (cilia) in its lining. If fertilized, it implants in the endometrium (lining of the uterus).

The monthly cycle

Ovulation usually occurs about 14 days after your period, but if your cycle is longer or shorter than 28 days your fertile period will be later or earlier accordingly. During your monthly cycle the body goes through various changes to prepare for conception.

The cycle is mostly controlled by the hormones oestrogen, progesterone, follicle-stimulating hormone (FSH), and luteinizing hormone (LH). A peak in LH triggers ovulation.

Your body temperature drops and then rises just before ovulation. You are fertile for one day before the temperature drops, as well as for one day after it remains elevated.

Your cervical secretions go through a cycle of changes too. As you approach your fertile period, the secretions increase and become clearer, stretchy, and slippery, ready to receive sperm.

At ovulation one follicle ruptures, releases its egg, then becomes a structure called the corpus luteum. This produces the hormone progesterone, which is essential for the development of an embryo. If the egg is not fertilized, however, the corpus luteum shrinks.

After ovulation, under the influence of oestrogen and progesterone, the endometrium (lining of the uterus) becomes thick and spongy to receive a fertilized egg. If the egg isn't fertilized, the corpus lutem dies and the endometrium is shed at your next menstrual period.

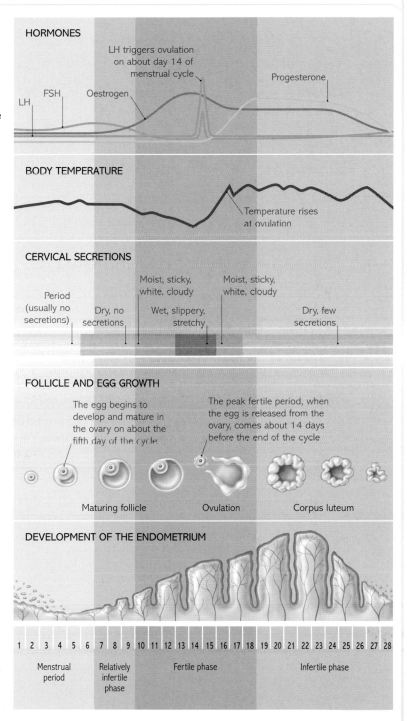

HORMONES

LH triggers ovulation on about day 14 of menstrual cycle

Progesterone

LH FSH Oestrogen

BODY TEMPERATURE

Temperature rises at ovulation

CERVICAL SECRETIONS

Moist, sticky, white, cloudy

Moist, sticky, white, cloudy

Period (usually no secretions)

Dry, no secretions

Wet, slippery, stretchy

Dry, few secretions

FOLLICLE AND EGG GROWTH

The egg begins to develop and mature in the ovary on about the fifth day of the cycle

The peak fertile period, when the egg is released from the ovary, comes about 14 days before the end of the cycle

Maturing follicle Ovulation Corpus luteum

DEVELOPMENT OF THE ENDOMETRIUM

1 2 3 4 5 6 7 8 9 10 11 12 13 14 15 16 17 18 19 20 21 22 23 24 25 26 27 28

Menstrual period

Relatively infertile phase

Fertile phase

Infertile phase

Making sperm

The process of making sperm takes place inside a man's testes and is known as spermatogenesis.

After puberty the testicles make sperm continuously at the rate of about 125 million sperm a day. The whole process, from the initial generation of a sperm to its maturing and ejaculation, takes about seven weeks.

Although the numbers and quality of sperm produced decline from the age of 40, men in their 90s have fathered children.

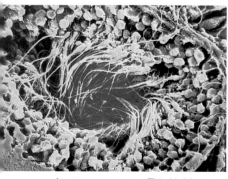

▲ **INSIDE THE TESTIS** This highly magnified image shows a cross-section of the inside of a testis, where a complex network of tiny tubes produce vast numbers of spermatids, the forerunners of sperm.

The man's role

Sperm, a man's contribution to the conception of his child, are made in his testes (testicles). A man begins making sperm at puberty under the influence of testosterone from the testes, and luteinizing hormone (LH) and follicle-stimulating hormone (FSH) from his pituitary gland. LH and FSH act on the testes as they do on the ovaries. A man goes on making sperm throughout his life.

The testes

Inside each testis is a network of minute tubes that contain the cells from which spermatids are created. These tubes connect with about eight larger tubes; these are the efferent ducts that carry the developing sperm into the epididymis where they mature and grow their tails. The sperm travel from the epididymis through a tube called the vas deferens before ejaculation. On this journey sperm are mixed with secretions from other glands to form semen. The semen acts as a vehicle for the sperm to carry them to the female reproductive tract.

The testes also produce hormones, the most important being the male sex hormone testosterone, which is the most powerful of the androgens. These hormones are responsible for male secondary sexual characteristics such as facial hair and deepening of the voice, and for male and female sex drives.

The mature sperm

Each individual sperm is only about one-twentieth of a millimetre long, so cannot be seen by the naked eye. It's shaped like a tadpole and has a strong tail, five or six times longer than its head, which it uses to move itself along. The tail is attached to the head by a short middle section or body. This contains special cell components called mitochondria, which are its energy-producing apparatus. A sperm's head is dark in colour because it contains so much genetic material.

The newly formed sperm pass into the epididymis at the rear of each testis, where they mature. From the epididymis, matured sperm travel up a tube called the vas deferens, which leads to the seminal vesicle, a small, sac-like structure near the bladder. When a man ejaculates, seminal fluid (semen) is discharged from the penis via the urethra. Semen is made up of sperm, mixed with fluid produced by the seminal vesicle and fluids secreted by the prostate and other glands.

Ejaculation

Most men ejaculate about 3.5ml (that's about two-thirds of a teaspoonful) of semen when they make love, but the range is 2–5ml (½–1tsp). Each millilitre contains 20–150 million sperm, of which a high proportion are abnormal in shape. Only about three-quarters of the sperm are motile (able to wriggle). A man's sperm production does speed up at times of sexual activity, but if ejaculation is very frequent, sperm numbers do decrease, which lowers his fertility.

Reaching the egg Although sperm can move 2–3mm per minute, their actual speed varies with the acidity of their environment – the higher the acidity, the slower their movement. Vaginal secretions are slightly acidic; so sperm ejaculated into the vagina probably move quite slowly until they reach the more friendly alkaline environment of the uterine cavity. Having got through the hostile acidic conditions of the vagina, they then face a longer and more dangerous journey before they reach the egg way down a fallopian tube. Of about 300 million sperm in an ejaculation, only a few hundred will actually reach the egg. Most of the rest trickle out of the vagina, or are destroyed by vaginal acidity. Others may be destroyed by cleansing cells within the uterus, enter the wrong Fallopian tube, or go into the correct tube but miss the egg altogether.

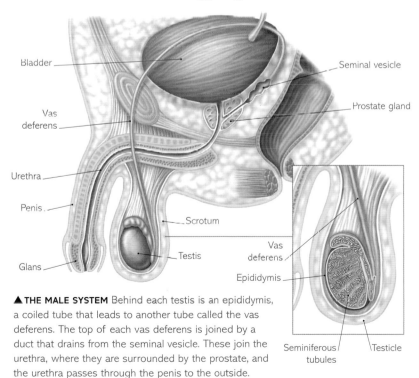

▲ **THE MALE SYSTEM** Behind each testis is an epididymis, a coiled tube that leads to another tube called the vas deferens. The top of each vas deferens is joined by a duct that drains from the seminal vesicle. These join the urethra, where they are surrounded by the prostate, and the urethra passes through the penis to the outside.

Labels: Bladder, Vas deferens, Urethra, Penis, Glans, Seminal vesicle, Prostate gland, Scrotum, Testis, Vas deferens, Epididymis, Seminiferous tubules, Testicle

Your baby's sex

The sex of your child depends on whether the fertilizing sperm contains an X chromosome (female) or a Y chromosome (male). The woman's egg always contains an X chromosome (female).

The X and the Y sperm have different properties. The X sperm (female) are larger, slower, and longer-lived than the Y sperm (male). The X sperm also appears to be favoured by the slightly acidic conditions in the vagina.

Some people believe that you can increase your chances of having a male or female baby by when and how often you make love. There's very little scientific evidence to support these ideas, but you may like to try them if you're keen to choose the gender of your baby.

When to make love For a female baby, make love up to two or three days before ovulation as only female sperm survive this long. For a male baby, make love on the day of, or just after, ovulation, as the faster Y sperm (male) will reach the egg before the X sperm.

How often For a female baby, make love fairly frequently, as this lowers the proportion of Y sperm (male) in the semen. For a male baby, make love less often, as this will increase the proportion of Y sperm (male).

Penetrating the egg

This sequence of pictures, taken with an electron microscope, shows fertilization taking place. A sperm that has travelled along the Fallopian tube, with millions of others, reaches the egg and penetrates its tough outer membrane and the inner part.

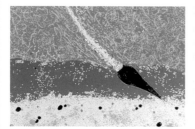

▲ **MEMBRANE PENETRATION** The sperm penetrates the membrane of the egg by releasing enzymes that create a hole in it.

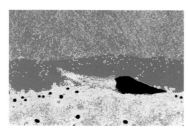

▲ **OOCYTE PENETRATION** The sperm prepares to penetrate the oocyte, the innermost part of the egg.

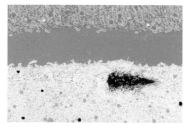

▲ **CHROMOSOME TRANSFER** Before joining its chromosomes with those of the egg, the sperm sheds its body and tail.

Fertilization

Fertilization happens when a sperm meets and then penetrates an egg. Most human cells contain 46 chromosomes – thread-like structures that carry their genetic information. But the sperm cells and egg cells each have only 23 chromosomes. When a sperm and an egg meet and fuse, the resulting fertilized cell has the full 46 chromosomes.

The new cell, which is called a zygote, splits first into two identical cells, each with 46 chromosomes. It continues to divide slowly as it travels down the Fallopian tube, until it reaches the uterus. By the time it reaches the uterus it is a hollow clump of about 100 cells called a blastocyst.

Conception and implantation

▶ **EGG MEETS SPERM** The egg is released from its follicle. It travels one-third of the way along the Fallopian tube, where it is fertilized.

The fertilized egg keeps on dividing as it travels down the Fallopian tube

At the second division, each cell divides into two, creating a four-cell zygote

The third division doubles the cells from four to eight

In its first division, the single-cell zygote divides into two identical cells

▲ **CELL DIVISION** The fertilized egg, now called a zygote, divides repeatedly and eventually forms a solid bundle of cells known as a morula. These cells continue to divide and become a hollow ball of about 100 cells called a blastocyst.

Implantation A week after fertilization has taken place, the blastocyst produces a hormone that helps it to burrow its way into the lining of the uterus, where it is bathed in the mother's blood, allowing food and waste to pass to and fro. Implantation is usually in the upper one-third of the uterus. The pregnancy is now established and the placenta starts to form.

Twins When a woman releases more than one egg at a time, non-identical (fraternal) twins may develop from two separate eggs, fertilized by two separate sperm. Each embryo then has its own placenta inside the mother's uterus.

Identical twins come from a single egg, fertilized by a single sperm. This egg divides into two, and each develops independently into a genetically identical twin sharing a single placenta. Other multiple pregnancies, such as triplets, start in the same ways as twins and, similarly, the siblings may be fraternal or identical.

Boy or girl?

Of the 46 chromosomes that carry the complete human genetic blueprint, the sex of a child is determined by just two, the X and the Y.

The sex chromosomes
A woman's eggs each contain a single X chromosome, while a man's individual sperm carry either an X or a Y chromosome. If an egg is fertilized by an X chromosome sperm, the baby will be a girl (XX). If the sperm has a Y chromosome, the child will be a boy (XY).

Seven days after fertilization, the egg, now called a blastocyst, implants itself in the lining of the uterus

This embryo is about four weeks old

Uterus

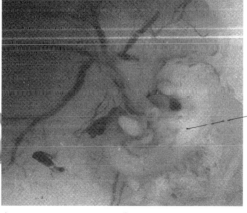

▲ **EMBRYO DEVELOPMENT** Once implanted in the uterine lining, the blastocyst then develops into an embryo. It also forms the placenta that's the vital link between a baby and its mother.

◄ **THE FULLY FORMED BABY** By the time a baby is born, repeated cell divisions will have made a highly complex being with several trillion cells from a single cell.

Points to consider

The older you are, the longer it can take to conceive, so bear this in mind when you're deciding if you should talk to your doctor about any possible problems. Then again, the older you are the less time you have, so you might want to get advice early.

- The number of infertile women increases with age: one in ten women between the ages of 20 and 24 are infertile, but this increases to nearly 30 per cent of women aged 40 to 44.

- All treatments for infertility are significantly more successful in couples under 30.

- The overall quality of a woman's eggs diminishes with age, as does the number of healthy eggs produced at any one time.

- A woman's uterus gets less receptive to a fertilized egg as she gets older, so successful implantation is less likely.

- In women, incorrect amounts of luteinizing hormone (LH) and follicle-stimulating hormone (FSH) can affect ovulation (see p.28). In men, these same two hormones, LH and FSH, stimulate the testes to produce sperm. So, if a man's pituitary gland does not release enough FSH and LH, his ability to produce sperm will be impaired.

- In men and women, if the thyroid and adrenal glands are not functioning properly sperm production and ovulation respectively will be affected.

Having problems?

If you're having difficulty getting pregnant it doesn't necessarily mean you're infertile. Infertility means different things to different people; it certainly means something different to doctors and to couples. Most couples who think they are infertile are only subfertile, and with help do manage to conceive successfully.

What is infertility?

Fertility isn't always a straightforward case of being able, or unable, to conceive. A couple may have no difficulty in conceiving their first child, but find they cannot get pregnant a second time; this is called secondary infertility. Another couple, who have both had children with previous partners, may now find that they cannot conceive together.

The fertility of a couple is the sum of their individual fertilities. If both partners have fertility problems, it may be hard for them to conceive. But if one partner's fertility is strong, it may still be possible for the couple to conceive. Most couples do conceive within four to six months of trying. If a couple don't manage to get pregnant after six months and go to their doctor for advice, they're likely to be told to go away, keep on trying, and come back after a year if nothing happens.

Age is a factor for women (see column, left). As a woman gets older the quality of her eggs declines. Statistics show that about 90 per cent of women in their 20s will become pregnant within a year of trying, and the rest still have a good chance of becoming pregnant naturally within another year or so. But, women in their 30s have a much lower statistical probability of becoming pregnant after a year of trying. They shouldn't wait any longer to get advice.

Ways in which a couple can be helped to conceive a child range from simple advice on sexual technique to drug treatment, surgery, and ultimately to the new assisted reproductive technology (ART) (see p.48). The help is there, but the investigation of infertility can try your patience and resolve. Whichever partner has the fertility problems may feel threatened and even guilty, so be prepared to be generous and supportive.

The emotional impact

Couples who are having problems conceiving may be having other difficulties too. And if they do go ahead with treatment for infertility they may find it very stressful – it can mean almost intolerable interference with their sex life and can even erode the love a couple feel for each other. The huge costs of treatment can also be a major source of stress and so it's vital for both partners to be fully committed to this course of action.

Being unable to have children can seem like a denial of basic human rights, and an infertile couple can experience feelings of injustice, disappointment, and grief. The unfulfilled desire for children is a major crisis in the lives of some couples and can make them feel bad about all aspects of life. One or both partners may become introspective and antisocial, and the relationship may break down under the strain.

The importance of counselling

With all the tensions that surround the treatment of infertility, couples need and deserve sound psychological support. If you do decide to start on a course of investigation and treatment, ask your doctor to refer you to a counsellor to help you cope with the stress. Don't feel you have to wait until you find yourselves well on into secondary referral; you need advice right from the start. Some procedures involve deep self-questioning, which strikes right at the heart of your relationship, and a couple will need a great deal of support. The treatment can also be lengthy and invasive, and there are many ethical issues surrounding assisted reproductive technologies, insemination, and the use of donors.

Psychological factors affecting fertility The way you feel can in itself affect your fertility by causing a hormone disturbance or impotence. So, without proper support, fertility treatment may make matters worse. On the other hand, doctors have plenty of anecdotal evidence that some couples suddenly conceive very soon after making the decision to have their infertility investigated. It's as if taking the decision to do something about the problem releases the psychological tensions that may have been stopping them getting pregnant.

Unexplained infertility

In the UK, 12 per cent of couples with fertility problems may have to face the fact that their infertility cannot be explained. In those couples it's tempting to consider radical treatments, but it's generally agreed that it's best for them to wait for up to three years, depending on the woman's age, to see if anything happens naturally. After this there are several treatments that can be successful, such as intrauterine insemination together with stimulation by clomiphene or follicle-stimulating hormone (FSH), GIFT (see p.49), or IVF (see pp.48–53). Drug treatments with bromocriptine are not effective. Investigations to find out whether there could be immunological factors involved may also be fruitful (see p.39).

Questions to ask

Even before you have professional counselling, it's a good idea to ask yourselves some searching questions, so that some of the issues are out in the open between you from the very beginning.

■ If you decided to have fertility treatment, would you tell friends and family, or would you try to keep it a complete secret?

■ If you intend to keep it a secret, can you be sure that the truth won't come out, perhaps destructively, at a time of crisis?

■ Could you cope with a multiple pregnancy?

■ What if one, some, or all of your babies died?

■ Having committed so much time and money to having a baby, how easy will you find it to let her go once she grows up?

■ How long would you be prepared to carry on with infertility treatment?

■ Would you consider using donor eggs or sperm?

■ Would you think about adoption?

Lifestyle changes

If you're to have the best possible chance of conceiving, you may both have to make some changes in your lifestyle.

■ Stop smoking – both of you.

■ Aim for a healthy lifestyle – eat a balanced diet and stay active.

■ Cut down on alcohol (women not more than two units per week, men not more than seven units per week). Women are advised not to drink alcohol at all when pregnant.

■ Overweight women can have ovulation problems, so losing weight helps. In one study, 12 out of 13 women who lost 6kg (13lb) or more began to ovulate and 11 out of 12 conceived. Keeping weight within the ideal range is also important for male fertility.

■ Don't use temperature charts to find ovulation days (fertile days) and don't confine lovemaking to fertile days; couples used to be advised to time intercourse for these days, but the stress involved can work against you.

■ Have penetrative sex two to three times a week.

■ Although very frequent sex can diminish the number of sperm in each ejaculate, don't abstain for longer than ten days or the sperm count will start to fall.

■ Women should take 400mcg folic-acid as supplements daily.

■ Stop taking recreational drugs. Many of them affect fertility.

Seeking advice

First of all, go to see your family doctor so you can talk about your worries and ask any questions. For many couples it's the woman who seeks advice first, but it's really important for you both to accept that whatever the reasons for your problems, you're both going to need investigation. So if at all possible, get things off to a good start and make the first visit a joint one.

If you're worried that your doctor won't have the time for the kind of detailed, relaxed conversation you need, ask for a longer appointment, perhaps at a time of day when things are less pressured. Or you could try going to the sexual health clinic in your local hospital or a family planning clinic. You don't need a referral from your doctor for either of these, and you should find a team of sympathetic experts to talk to.

What will happen first?

When you first see your doctor, ask how any treatment is likely to be managed. Each stage in the investigation and treatment of infertility should be fully explained to you in a way you can understand. You'll also be given lists of self-help organizations to get in touch with. Your family doctor may do the initial tests or may refer you to a specialist. Either way you'll be referred for all secondary tests and for further treatment to a dedicated specialist infertility clinic. You do have the right to insist that you're referred to such a unit.

Any infertility treatment is a stressful business, so it's important that the doctors caring for you are relaxed and friendly. The atmosphere of the clinic should be sympathetic so you feel that you'll be listened to properly. The clinic should also provide information on what will be involved, including the pros and cons of any alternative treatments.

Primary tests

The first tests can be initiated by your family doctor, but many doctors prefer to refer you. Your doctor will ask about your fertility history as a couple, including your ages, how long you've been trying to conceive, past illnesses or surgery, and any drugs you've been taking that might affect fertility (see column, opposite). The woman will also be asked about her menstrual cycle, how regular it is, how long her periods last, and whether they're painful. You'll both also be asked about your jobs in case either of

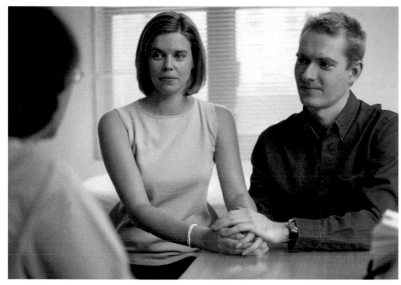

▲ **SEEING A COUNSELLOR** It's important to start any investigation of infertility with a thorough talk with your doctor, who'll be able to tell you about the treatment stages and refer you to a specialist fertility clinic where you can see a counsellor.

you could be exposed to dangers at work that may affect fertility. The doctor will also ask about any past sexually transmitted diseases, including chlamydia, and will look at past smear test results.

Primary tests for the woman:
- Smear test (if not done recently).
- Test for chlamydia (see p.44), which will be treated if found.
- Physical examination, including an internal examination.
- A simple blood test for progesterone levels in the second half of the cycle to confirm whether ovulation is taking place.

Primary tests for the man:
- Physical examination of the man's penis and testes.
- A semen sample, which will be sent for analysis at the fertility clinic where further investigations and secondary tests (see p.41) will be done.

Rapid referral for secondary tests
In some circumstances couples are referred as quickly as possible for secondary investigations at a specialist unit. These include:
- If either partner is over 35 years of age.
- If the woman has a history of amenorrhoea (absence of periods), or oligomenorrhoea (sparse or infrequent periods).
- Abnormal anatomy on internal examination of the woman or a varicocoele of the scrotum (see p.39) in the man.

Drugs that can affect fertility

Many medications can harm your fertility, affecting sperm, eggs, or sexual activity. Your doctor will want to know if you have been treated with, or have been using, any of the following drugs.

For men:
- sulphasalazine may lower sperm count
- nitrofurantoin may lower sperm count
- tetracyclines may lower sperm motility
- cimetidine may cause impotence
- ketoconazole may cause impotence and lower sex drive
- colchicine may lower fertilization power of sperm
- antidepressants may cause impotence
- propranolol may cause impotence
- chemotherapy can lower sperm count
- cannabis and alcohol may cause sperm abnormalities
- cocaine may lower libido as well as sperm motility and count.

For women:
- anti inflammatories (such as ibuprofen) may affect egg follicles
- chemotherapy can cause ovarian failure
- cannabis may stop ovulation and interrupt menstruation.

Workplace hazards

Working with harmful substances can be particularly dangerous for a man's fertility, as some of them can lower the sperm count.

At your first consultation, tell your doctor if you work with any of the following substances:

- pesticides

- X-rays

- solvents used in paint products

- heavy metals such as lead, mercury, or arsenic.

Male infertility

Problems with the sperm themselves are the most common cause of male infertility, although there are also anatomical problems that affect a man's ability to ejaculate. The study of male fertility is relatively new, compared to female fertility, but doctors now know much more about it and the role of sperm in particular.

Problems with sperm

Sperm are extremely vulnerable cells. They take seven weeks to form and can be affected by outside influences at any point in their development. Because of this, it's entirely possible for a man to give sperm samples on separate occasions that differ widely both in quality and quantity.

Testicular failure The cause of this is usually hard to establish, but it may be due to a chromosomal problem such as Klinefelter's syndrome (when a man has two or more X chromosomes rather than one), testes that did not descend properly after birth, a blow to the testes, such as a sports injury, or the man having suffered mumps as an adult.

Anatomical problems

Ejaculation problems	About one per cent of men find that they appear not to ejaculate at orgasm. This is because of retrograde ejaculation (a "dry run"), when the semen is ejaculated backwards into the bladder instead of forwards into the urethra.
Scrotum	A hydrocoele (a condition that occurs when there is an excess of normal lubricating fluid around the testis) or a varicocoele (which occurs when the veins of the scrotum and testes become enlarged, see opposite above) may be present. Both of these conditions raise the temperature of the testes, which in turn may inhibit sperm production.
Tubal blockage	Either or both of the vas deferens (the tubes that connect the testicles to the seminal vesicles where sperm are stored) may be obstructed. If this occurs it may be difficult or even impossible for the sperm to move out of the testis. A blockage of the vas deferens may exist from birth, or be the result of an infection, such as gonorrhoea.
Testicular failure	Sperm production may be non-existent, or may be inhibited. There is a very rare condition, testicular failure, in which the semen contains no sperm at all. Unfortunately, complete testicular failure, like complete ovarian failure, tends to be untreatable. This condition does not, however, always affect both testes.

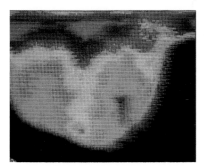

▲ **HEALTHY TESTES** This thermal photograph of normal testes shows how healthy testes (blue) are at a lower temperature than the body (orange, top of picture).

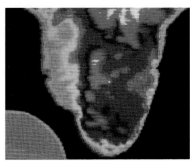

▲ **VARICOCOELE** The orange patches on the nearer testis are a varicocoele (enlarged veins); the orange colour indicates a raised temperature, which may affect normal sperm production.

The sperm count

Male fertility is checked by two sperm tests, which also look for any sperm abnormalities. Each millilitre of semen should contain at least 20 million sperm, most of which should be normal.

If there are fewer than 20 million sperm per millilitre or there's a high proportion of abnormal sperm, the semen is rated poor.

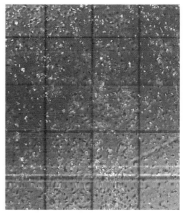

Good semen sample

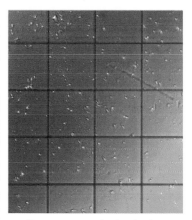

Poor semen sample, showing low sperm count

Low sperm counts By itself, a low sperm count does not mean infertility. Many men with low sperm counts father children, but conception tends to take longer. Unfortunately, when there are few sperm the majority tend to be abnormal or are not very active. Low sperm counts and sperm abnormalities may be caused by hormonal, anatomical, or immunological problems, or even environmental factors.

Immunological problems

Both men and women may produce antibodies to sperm, which can interfere with fertilization, but it's mainly a problem for men. This is because in men the antibodies are on the surface of sperm, in the semen, or in the blood: in women antibodies are found in the cervical mucus or in the blood. Antibodies are found in five to ten per cent of infertile couples, but two per cent of fertile men also have antibodies.

How antibodies affect fertility Most important are the antibodies that are attached to the sperm themselves: they can affect the way sperm move and their ability to penetrate a woman's cervical mucus and fertilize the egg. Antibodies can also affect the acrosome – the cap on the head of the sperm, which contains enzymes essential for egg penetration (see p.40).

How antibodies affect fertility treatments Antibodies on the surface of the sperm can interfere with in vitro fertilization (IVF) (p.50) and other kinds of assisted reproduction technology (ART) (see p.48). The antibodies can stop sperm moving and even destroy them. However, the presence of antibodies doesn't necessarily mean that a man can't conceive a child. Many specialists recommend that antibody testing is only carried out in couples with "unexplained infertility" (see p.35) and who've had all the other tests, because treatment is difficult and associated with serious side effects, so it's only justifiable as a research procedure.

Semen analysis

If you have to give a semen sample for analysis, follow instructions carefully to make sure that results are accurate and the test won't have to be repeated.

Taking the sample The man must not ejaculate for three days. He then produces a semen specimen by masturbating into a sterile plastic pot marked with name, date, and the time. The sample is protected from temperature extremes and delivered to the laboratory.

What's healthy? The laboratory would expect the following findings from a healthy semen sample.

Amount: 2–5ml (½–1tsp).

Numbers: more than 20 million sperm per millilitre.

Motility: more than one-half of the sperm wriggle.

Normality: more than one-third of the sperm are normal.

White blood cells: fewer than 1 million per ml of sperm.

▶ **COMPARING SPERM** If a sperm is to be able to fertilize an egg successfully, it needs to be properly formed. First, it must have a tail so that it can swim and reach the egg. Second, on the head of the sperm there must be a normal cap, called the acrosome, that contains enzymes that play an important part in egg penetration.

Male tests

When a couple have fertility problems it's usually the woman who wants to get advice early on, but there's no point in her doing this on her own. If a couple are having difficulty in conceiving it really doesn't make sense for the man to delay. A semen analysis should always be the first test to be done if fertility is to be investigated.

How men can be helped

Male infertility has nothing to do with virility. A man's sperm may be incapable of fertilizing an egg, yet he may be an excellent lover. In contrast, a man who is unable to make love to a woman may have perfectly viable, fertile sperm.

Studies suggest that sperm counts decreased during the 20th century because of environmental factors such as exposure to oestrogens in foodstuffs and chemicals used in the plastics industry that enter the food chain. At one time, much more was known about female infertility than

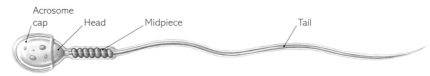

Acrosome cap · Head · Midpiece · Tail

▲ **NORMAL SPERM** Each sperm has a head that contains its genetic material, and a long tail for helping it move into the female reproductive tract so that fertilization can take place.

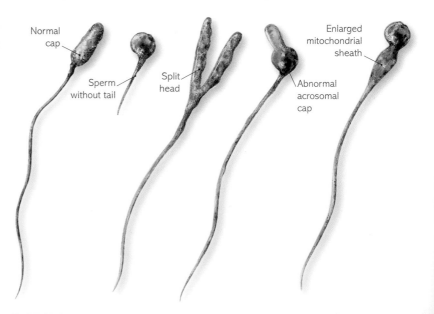

Normal cap · Enlarged mitochondrial sheath · Sperm without tail · Split head · Abnormal acrosomal cap

male, but fertility clinics now deal just as much with male problems and diseases. There's a greater chance than ever before that men who have low fertility or are infertile can be helped to achieve natural fatherhood.

Semen analysis

One of the first tests for a man is semen analysis. Sperm counts can vary according to circumstances, such as how often he has sexual intercourse and therefore two samples may be analyzed if the first shows problems.

The analysis checks the number of sperm in a sample, how well and how much they move, and their shape. Many specialists believe that even a relatively low sperm count may not affect a man's fertility. But if he has a low sperm count combined with many sperm that are malformed, move poorly, or both, or if there is a high white blood cell content, then it's likely that his fertility will be affected.

Low sperm counts There are several types of low sperm count. A semen analysis decides which of the following definitions apply to a particular sperm sample:

■ Azoospermia: there's no sperm in the semen, because the man cannot make sperm, he has a blockage affecting the sperm transportation, or he fails to ejaculate.
■ Oligospermia: fewer than 20 million sperm per millilitre of semen. A mild case is around 10–20 million, a moderate case is 5–10 million, and a severe case would be fewer than 5 million sperm per millilitre.
■ Aesthenospermia: sperm are unable to wriggle but count is normal.
■ Teratospermia: a high number of abnormal sperm. This is severe if the man has more than 70 per cent abnormal sperm, possibly caused by a chromosomal abnormality or by some kind of environmental damage.

Special tests

After routine semen analysis (see column, opposite), microscopic tests of sperm function would be done only at a specialist clinic as part of the secondary stage of investigation of a couple with infertility problems.

Special tests examine the ability of sperm to penetrate mucus so they can get through the cervix to the uterus, and from there to the tubes and egg.

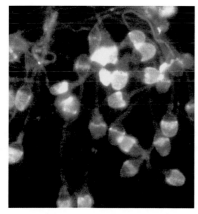

Normal sperm

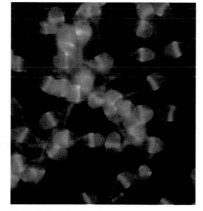

Defective sperm

◀ **NORMAL AND DEFECTIVE SPERM** The head of a normal sperm is surrounded by a cap, called the acrosome. This contains enzymes that enable the sperm to break through the outer membrane of the egg. If sperm don't have this acrosomal cap, they're incapable of fertilizing an egg. Sperm are tested by using chemicals that glow when they react with the acrosome. These pictures show defective sperm (left) and normal sperm (far left).

Polycystic ovary syndrome

Many women have benign ovarian cysts that don't affect fertility. But polycystic ovary syndrome (PCOS) interferes with ovulation and can therefore cause fertility problems.

PCOS is caused by FSH and LH not functioning properly, which is often linked to high levels of male hormones. The ovary becomes filled with "cysts" – actually immature follicles that fail to generate eggs. Sufferers have infrequent periods, a tendency to obesity, and excessive body hair.

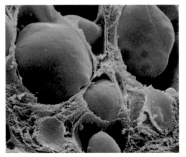

▲ DEVELOPING EGGS This hugely magnified picture shows part of a normal ovary, with eggs developing in their follicles.

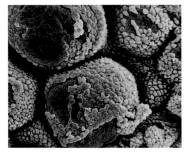

▲ POLYCYSTIC OVARY In PCOS, follicles develop into cysts so eggs fail to develop or remain immature and ovulation does not take place.

Female infertility

A huge amount of research has been done over the last few decades into the reasons for female infertility, and great advances have been made in the diagnosis and treatment of problems. The causes of female infertility tend to fall into four main areas and all of these types can now be treated with varying degrees of success.

Failure to ovulate

About one-third of female infertility is caused by failure to release an egg (ovulate). This is usually due to hormonal problems, but occasionally a woman's ovaries are damaged or, more rarely, have run out of eggs.

Hormonal problems In a woman with a normal ovarian cycle (see p.28) the hormones produced by the pituitary gland and the ovary are responsible for the healthy growth and maintenance of an egg. In many cases of infertility, too little of one or too much of the other hormone may be present. For example, at mid-cycle the hypothalamus should stimulate the pituitary gland to release massive amounts of luteinizing hormone (LH) and follicle-stimulating hormone (FSH) to bring about ovulation, but in 20 per cent of cases it fails to do so. Although there may be some LH and FSH, there's not enough for ovulation.

Alternatively, the pituitary gland may be damaged or malfunctioning, and either produce too little LH and FSH or none at all. Or, as a result of too much LH stimulation and not enough FSH, the ovaries may become polycystic (see column, left, for more information on this condition) and have difficulties producing mature eggs.

Problems caused by abnormal levels of hormones are often treated by fertility drugs. For 90 per cent of women whose infertility is caused by hormonal problems, modern drug therapy can bring about regular ovulation. Unfortunately, for reasons unknown, only about 65 per cent of these women will actually get pregnant.

Hormonal imbalance

Hormones may interfere with conception in other ways than influencing ovulation. For example, a fertilized egg needs progesterone in order to survive. If too little progesterone is produced or it's produced for too short a time, the egg may not survive. Known as inadequate luteal phase, this condition can be treated with drugs.

Hyperprolactinaemia In this quite common condition the pituitary gland produces too much of the hormone responsible for milk production. Often, there's no apparent reason why this happens. The condition can sometimes be caused by a small benign tumour developing on the pituitary gland, called a prolactinoma. This leads to low levels of LH and FSH, which causes infrequent or absent periods in women and lowered sperm production in men.

Fibroids and fertility

Fibroids are benign muscle tumours, anything from the size of a pea to a tennis ball, that form anywhere within the uterine wall. They don't necessarily affect fertility, but can make the uterus misshapen and may compress one or both of the Fallopian tubes.

Effects on fertility Fibroids very near to the surface of the uterine lining can interfere with the normal implantation of the embryo in the uterus. If they are near the junction of the uterus and the Fallopian tubes, they may stop the fertilized egg from reaching the uterus at all.

Fibroids are most common in women over the age of 35 and around 50 per cent of women develop fibroids by the time they are 45. There's often no cause for concern, but if fibroids do cause problems they can be removed in an operation called a myomectomy. This operation should not be undertaken lightly, however, as it carries a high risk of bleeding and may require a blood transfusion in as many as 50 per cent of cases.

Endometriosis

If you suffer from very painful periods (dysmenorrhoea), it's possible that you're suffering from endometriosis and this will need to be checked.

Endometriosis is a common condition in which cells from the endometrium (the lining of the uterus) spread to other sites in the ovaries, pelvis, and tubes. These respond to the cyclical changes of ovarian hormones and so they bleed internally when you're menstruating, causing severe abdominal and pelvic pain.

Endometriosis may affect fertilization, thus causing fertility problems. Ovarian cysts, known as endometriomas or "chocolate cysts", may also form and affect the woman's fertility.

Structural problems

Tubal damage	A previous ectopic pregnancy (see p.225), previous surgery, pelvic inflammation, endometriosis, or an infection, particularly chlamydia (see p.44), may cause blocked or damaged tubes that will prevent natural conception.
Problems with fertilization	In order to reach an egg and fertilize it, sperm must swim through the mucus in the cervix. If there is too little mucus, or if it's very thick, sperm cannot get through the cervical canal. If the mucus contains antibodies that attack the sperm directly, the sperm will never reach the egg so fertilization won't happen.
Damage to the ovaries	The ovaries may fail to produce mature eggs. Scarring, caused by surgery, infection, or as a side effect of radiation treatment, can damage the ovary. Alternatively, the supply of eggs may become exhausted earlier than normal. This can be due to the menopause or its premature onset, surgical damage, or radiation therapy.
Uterine conditions	The uterus may be congenitally abnormal in shape (although this does not necessarily cause infertility); contain scars, polyps, or fibroids; or be subject to adenomyosis (the inner lining of the uterus grows inside the middle layer, causing bleeding and cramps).

Chlamydia infection

Clamydia is the most common bacterial sexually transmitted infection, and it can cause fertility problems. Up to 70 per cent of women with it have no symptoms so they don't know they've been infected and aren't treated.

You'll be tested for chlamydia infection as part of your primary investigations because the condition can cause pelvic inflammatory disease (PID). One episode of PID has a ten per cent chance of causing blockage of the Fallopian tubes, with the risk rising to 50 per cent after three episodes.

The incidence of PID can be reduced by the following:

■ selective screening of high-risk women for cervical chlamydia infection, which can be done with a smear test

■ screening of all women aged 25 years or younger, and women who have had two or more partners in the last year, as they make up nearly 90 per cent of infections

■ any infertility test involving an instrument being inserted into the uterus can aggravate a cervical infection, so this shouldn't be done without first checking for chlamydia.

Testing for chlamydia infection includes a blood antibody test, cervical swabs for culture, and DNA tests on urine. Sexual partners must be told, assessed, and treated as chlamydia may play a part in male infertility too.

Female tests

One of the aims of the primary tests you'll have is to find out whether or not you are ovulating. If you are, the fertility clinic will start a range of more advanced tests to discover why you haven't been able to conceive. These tests will check the condition of your hormones, ovaries, uterus, and Fallopian tubes and look at how well they're functioning.

Hormone and ovulation tests

Measuring the levels of hormones in your blood during your menstrual cycle can give useful information. Generally levels are checked during the first three days of your cycle and again seven days before your period is due. The measurements show how your ovaries, brain, pituitary, and hypothalamus are interacting, and highlight any imbalance in your hormones that may be causing a problem with ovulation. Usually, your oestrogen, progesterone, and luteinizing hormone (LH) levels are measured and compared to normal ones. Other hormones that can affect a woman's ability to ovulate are follicle-stimulating hormone (FSH), testosterone, and prolactin, so blood levels of these will also be checked.

Ultrasound scanning With a simple scan your fertility specialist can check the development of your ovarian follicles and confirm that you're ovulating. Tracking of the follicle in this way is important if you're taking drugs to stimulate ovulation, as it can help avoid overstimulation, which can be dangerous. Your doctors will also want an accurate assessment of your follicular growth if they need to perform complex assisted conception procedures such as in vitro fertilization (IVF) (see pp.50–1).

Endometrial biopsy Under the influence of oestrogen and progesterone, the endometrium (lining of the uterus) changes through the menstrual cycle. There's a dramatic endometrial thickening and growth during the first half of the menstrual cycle before ovulation, because of the increased amount of oestrogen in the body. But if not enough oestrogen is made, the endometrium may not be sufficiently developed to allow the embryo to implant successfully. In a biopsy, a tiny sample of your endometrium is taken during the second half of the menstrual cycle. It's examined under a microscope when any changes that are caused by hormone levels will be visible.

Fallopian tube tests

The fallopian tubes are extremely delicate structures. Less than 4mm (⅛in) in diameter at their narrowest, they are easily damaged. Up to one-third of all of the women who attend an infertility clinic are found to have a problem with their Fallopian tubes. Once the primary tests have been completed, there are a number of tests that are carried out to check the Fallopian tubes. These tests are among the first investigations made when an infertile couple attend a specialist clinic.

Hysterosalpingogram Also known as HSG, this is an X-ray picture of the uterus and tubes, which can show up problems inside them. A special dye that can be monitored on an X-ray screen is slowly injected into the uterus and should pass into the Fallopian tubes. If it fails to do so, there may be some damage, distortion, or blockage in the tubes.

Laparoscopy This is one of the most useful tests for finding out whether a woman's tubes are damaged or blocked. The laparoscope (see below) is a slender telescope – only about the width of a fountain pen – that uses fibreoptics to look directly into your abdominal cavity. It gives a superb view of all the organs, allowing your surgeon to assess their health and giving information on adhesions, endometriosis, and ovarian disease. High-quality videos can also be taken through the laparoscope so that your doctors can refer to them later. Although you'll need to have a general anaesthetic, laparoscopy can usually be done as a day procedure.

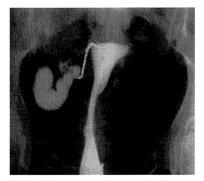

▲ **BLOCKED FALLOPIAN TUBES** This X-ray image, produced during a hysterosalpingogram (HSG), shows that the Fallopian tube on the right is blocked near the uterus. The dye hasn't been able to enter this tube.

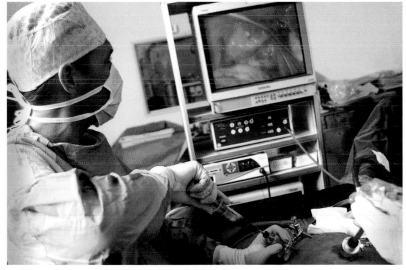

▲ **WHAT HAPPENS IN A LAPAROSCOPY** A thin tube is inserted into the patient's abdomen. An enlarged image from a tiny camera attached to the tip of the tube appears on the monitor, allowing the surgeon to assess the organs.

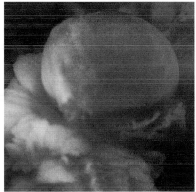

▲ **HEALTHY OVARY** Laparoscopy is useful for showing that organs are healthy as well as revealing any problems. This picture, taken through a laparoscope, shows a healthy ovary with a mature follicle that'll soon burst to release an egg. Eggs may be removed for use in IVF using laparoscopy (see p.50).

Treating PCOS

For some, weight loss is the solution to PCOS (polycystic ovary syndrome). If drug treatment is needed, its aim is to stimulate ovulation and produce a healthy egg.

Weight loss After losing weight, many women ovulate normally. UK guidelines state that no woman should start fertility treatment if her body mass index (BMI) is over 30. Being overweight increases the risk of problems in pregnancy.

Drug treatments

■ Clomiphene to induce ovulation

■ FSH injections in clomiphene-resistant women.

Treatments for female infertility

If a woman isn't ovulating, her ovaries can nearly always be encouraged to produce good-quality eggs by using fertility drugs. These drug treatments used to produce a large number of multiple pregnancies, but much more is now known about the correct dosage and treatment is very carefully controlled and monitored.

Drug treatments

Clomiphene This is the most common fertility drug, taken for five days at the beginning of each menstrual cycle. Clomiphene stimulates the release of follicle-stimulating hormone (FSH) by the pituitary gland. This acts on the ovaries and often triggers the ripening of a follicle and then ovulation, usually around five to ten days after the last tablet is taken. Clomiphene's advantages are that it's free from major side effects and has a low multiple pregnancy rate – only five to ten per cent. There's a possible link with ovarian cancer after 12 cycles, so if conception isn't achieved after about six cycles, you may be advised to try assisted reproduction technology (ART) instead (see pp.48–9). Increasingly, metformin, taken up to three times a day, is used as an alternative.

Clomiphene-resistant PCOS If you're suffering from polycystic ovary syndrome (PCOS) (see p.42), but you've failed to ovulate after several months' treatment with clomiphene, you could be given a course of FSH by injection. The success rates of this treatment are quite high. There's an ovulation rate of about 95 per cent per cycle and pregnancy rates of up to 25 per cent after three cycles.

Pulsatile GnRH "Hypothalamic" infertility with amenorrhoea is a rare cause of infertility resulting from the absence of a hormone called gonadotrophin releasing factor (GnRH), which is made in the part of the brain called the hypothalamus. The role played by GnRH in fertility is to force another part of the brain, the pituitary gland, to release FSH and LH, which in turn stimulate the ovary to ovulate. Women who are deficient in GnRH can be treated with hormone replacements. These are usually given in subcutaneous "pulses" to mimic normal secretions at 60, 90, and 120 minutes, in an increasing dose per pulse. Ovulation rates as high as

75 per cent and pregnancy rates up to 15 per cent per cycle can be achieved after GnRH replacement treatment.

Bromocriptine If a woman has high levels of the hormone prolactin in her blood, normal GnRH pulses may be suppressed, so she does not ovulate and cannot conceive. Bromocriptine (or related drugs such as cabergoline or quinagolide) is the best treatment for this condition – it suppresses prolactin production so the ovaries work properly again. After treatment with bromocriptine, ovulation rates can be as high as 75 per cent. If a woman does get pregnant, bromocriptine treatment should be stopped, but there are no known cases of miscarriage, prematurity, fetal abnormalities, or multiple pregnancies as a result of this drug.

Surgical procedures

Microsurgical techniques, involving laparoscopy (see p.45), have greatly improved doctors' ability to repair any damage to the Fallopian tubes. If you have clomiphene-resistant PCOS your doctors may suggest you have surgery such as ovarian drilling. In this operation, holes are drilled in the surface of your ovary with diathermy or laser to stimulate ovulation.

Tuboplasty (see below, right) Scarred and narrowed Fallopian tubes can be unblocked by an operation known as tuboplasty. A small balloon-tipped catheter is inserted into the blocked Fallopian tube. The balloon is then inflated to open the damaged tube and create a passage for fertilized or unfertilized eggs to pass through to reach the uterus. The balloon is then deflated and removed.

Fimbrioplasty Sometimes the frond-like ends of the Fallopian tube – known as the fimbriae (see p.28) – fuse together, blocking the opening of the tube and preventing eggs from entering from the ovary. Microsurgical techniques allow the blocked end of the tube to be peeled back and opened, giving free access for eggs once again.

Reversal of sterilization Reversal of female sterilization is an increasing part of the treatment of infertility. If the severed sections of the Fallopian tubes are rejoined, the woman has a good chance of achieving a normal pregnancy – rates are as high as 92 per cent – but this does depend on the expertise of the surgeons at your particular centre; some have a much lower success rate. Sterilization in which the tubes have been clamped with clips has the highest chance of being successfully reversed. However, IVF (see p.48) may be the treatment of choice for sterilized women, the pregnancy rate being about one in six.

Treating endometriosis

Female infertility caused by endometriosis can be treated quite successfully by surgery.

Laparoscopic surgery (see p.45) can be used to destroy all visible signs of endometriosis. This increases the chance of conceiving by almost 75 per cent in the first 36 weeks after treatment in women under the age of 40 with mild endometriosis.

Assisted reproduction technology (see p.48) may be an option for women who don't conceive after laparascopic surgery, whether or not they have tube problems, and for women with moderate to severe endometriosis.

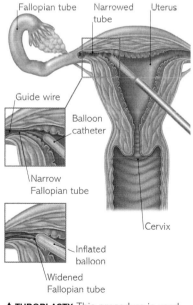

Fallopian tube   Narrowed tube   Uterus

Guide wire

Balloon catheter

Narrow Fallopian tube

Cervix

Inflated balloon

Widened Fallopian tube

▲ **TUBOPLASTY** This procedure is used to open up Fallopian tubes that have become scarred or blocked.

Medical risks of ART

ART gives many couples new hope and if all goes well can result in a healthy pregnancy and a bouncing baby. But it's important to remember that, even if you do conceive, the risks of the following are greater than usual:

■ high rate of multiple pregnancies (15 per cent)

■ high rate of ectopic pregnancies (4 per cent)

■ high rate of complications (15 per cent)

■ high rate of premature births (20 per cent)

■ high rate of Caesarean sections (15 per cent).

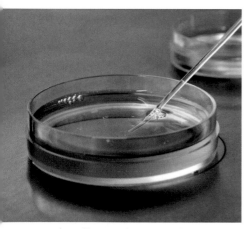

▲ **IVF** Harvested eggs are placed in liquid on a Petri dish and mixed with sperm. A fertilized egg(s) is then placed in the uterus for implantation.

ART
(assisted reproduction technology)

Assisted reproduction technology has helped many childless couples to become parents. Originally in vitro fertilization (IVF) was the only form, but now there are a number of techniques aimed at helping a couple conceive and give birth to a healthy child. The rewards are wonderful, but the emotional costs can be high, and any couple considering ART needs expert support.

What is ART?

ART describes a range of infertility treatments (see chart, oppposite). Through drugs, laboratory techniques, and even the use of sperm or egg donors, men and women can be helped to bring about sperm production, ovulation, fertilization, implantation, conception, and birth.

Why you may need ART

If you or your partner has problems with any stage in the chain of events leading to a healthy baby, you may need ART. Possible difficulties include failure to produce normal, active sperm, failure to ovulate, and failure of healthy sperm to penetrate and fertilize an egg.

Ethical considerations

The science of ART raises enormous ethical questions that affect the individual, the couple, the family, the community, and society. Most of us would say that if this technology helps a couple who are desperate for a child but have fertility problems, it is morally acceptable. But each situation can be complicated by experience, cultural background, the law, and religious teaching.

Remember, though, ethics is not an exact science. There is no absolute moral right and wrong. To impose a moral imperative unwillingly on another person is nothing less than tyranny and flies in the face of enhancing the moral dignity of a couple and their children.

Discussing alternatives Each member of a couple has a unique perspective and interest. In addition, there are the interests of the potential child to consider. I don't feel that doctors have the right to question a couple who opt for treatment for infertility. To my mind, the only option is to offer the couple expert counselling so they can discuss alternatives like adoption and the use of donor sperm or eggs.

It's important for specialists to understand that an infertile couple are in a vulnerable position and need impeccable investigation and therapy.

Contentious issues Most people agree that there is no moral problem with ART using the sperm and eggs of partners, the only objection being from the Roman Catholic Church. The use of donor eggs, sperm, or even embryos, however, is highly sensitive. Opponents say it violates marriage vows and blurs a child's genetic makeup, but evidence points to a reassuring track record for such children. In the UK the children now have the right to learn the names of donors when they reach 18, if they choose.

Cryopreservation (freezing of donor sperm or pre-embryos) This is another area of concern. Despite religious opposition, cryopreservation has proved to be very useful in improving pregnancy rates while avoiding multiple pregnancies. It's worth remembering that most moral arguments against it object only to the fact that some pre-embryos will not survive. In principle, cryopreservation preserves individual human life.

Moments of strain

Undergoing any form of ART is stressful for any couple. The biggest strains happen at key moments in the process.

■ **During ovarian stimulation** anxiety about techniques and the hormonal effects can lead to fear and tension, which constrains sexual needs.

■ **During laboratory investigation** couples fear that embryos might get mixed up or damaged.

■ **After embryo transfer** there may be worry about implantation problems or other complications.

49

ART: What the initials mean

IVF	In vitro fertilization (see p.50). Fertilization takes place outside the body, in a glass dish (in vitro means "in glass"), and the fertilized embryo or embryos are placed into the uterus. Helpful for: a woman with damaged Fallopian tubes, or who has severe endometriosis; cases of immune problems; unexplained infertility; and older women who have deteriorating egg production.		underneath the zona pellucida (the outer layer of the egg). This helps men with low sperm counts.
		MIST	Micro-insemination sperm transfer. See SUZI above.
		ICSI	Intra-cytoplasmic sperm injection. An amazing technique in which a single sperm is selected, specially treated, and injected directly into the egg itself (see p.52). When fertilization has taken place by IVF, the embryo is transferred in the usual way.
GIFT	Gamete intra-Fallopian transfer. Sperm and egg are mixed outside the body and immediately transferred into the Fallopian tube so that fertilization can happen "naturally". GIFT is cheaper than IVF, but can only be used for women with healthy Fallopian tubes.		
		MESA	Micro-epididymal sperm aspiration. The surgical extraction of sperm from the epididymis is needed for men who have no sperm in their ejaculate, because of a blocked vas deferens. It precedes ICSI.
ZIFT	Zygote intra-Fallopian transfer. Like GIFT, except a very young embryo is transferred to the Fallopian tube following IVF.		
		TESE	Testicular sperm extraction. This is like MESA, except the sperm are collected from the testes for ICSI.
SUZI	Sub-zonal insemination. A type of IVF in which sperm are carefully selected and injected		

The typical pattern of an IVF treatment

Several difficult and complex steps have to be got through so that you can have your baby: harvesting your eggs; fertilization of the eggs by healthy sperm; implantation of at least one embryo into your uterus; pregnancy to term; and delivery of a healthy baby.

Ensuring a good egg supply

So that you have the best chance of a successful pregnancy through in vitro fertilization (IVF) treatment, more than one egg will be collected and fertilized prior to implantation. Normally a woman only sheds one egg during each ovarian cycle, but with IVF a few days after the end of your period your ovaries will be stimulated with drug treatment such as gonadotrophin releasing factor (GnRH) analogues followed by follicle-stimulating hormone (FSH), so that your ovaries produce a number of eggs simultaneously.

Over the next week or so, you'll need to go to the fertility clinic every day so that the development of your eggs can be carefully monitored with

IVF procedure

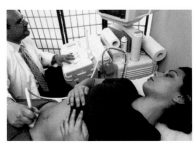

▲ULTRASOUND SCAN A scan helps to determine when a woman's eggs are mature enough for collection for IVF.

▶ EGG COLLECTION Here under general anaesthetic, a gynaecologist uses ultrasound to guide a thin, hollow probe through the vagina toward the ripened eggs. The eggs are then drawn into the probe using gentle suction. The probe is then withdrawn.

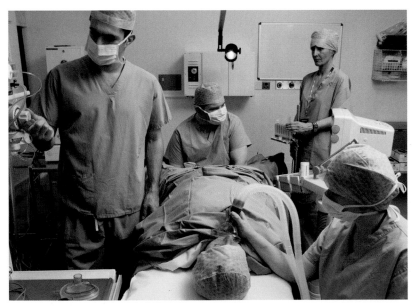

ultrasound scans. As the eggs mature, the follicles containing them swell and produce increasing amounts of oestrogen. A series of blood tests will detect this increase in oestrogen and the growth of follicles can be precisely measured and tracked by a daily scan.

Collecting the eggs

When ovulation is imminent, your mature eggs will be collected at your clinic under ultrasonic guidance. Then they're ready for fertilization by your partner's (or donated) sperm.

The egg-retrieval procedure may be carried out under light or even a local anaesthetic, instead of a general anaesthetic. You'll need to spend only a few hours at the fertility clinic for this.

Confirming conception

The harvested eggs are mixed with semen, and 18 hours later they're inspected under a microscope to find out if any have been fertilized. It's uncommon for all the eggs to be fertilized and develop into embryos, but two or three usually do. The fertilized eggs are incubated for 48 hours or more, when they will have divided into about two to four cells. Provided they show no signs of abnormality, a maximum of two embryos are transferred (see p.53) to your uterus. Because of the risks of a multiple pregnancy, however, you may be advised to have only one embryo transferred and you'll need to discuss this with your specialist.

Retrieving and returning eggs

Once her partner's sperm have been tested for viability, the woman is given fertility drugs to stimulate her ovaries.

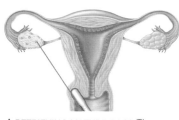

▲ **RETRIEVING MATURE EGGS** The woman is then carefully monitored using ultrasound until her eggs are mature, when they will be collected from her ovaries and transferred to a Petri dish for fertilization.

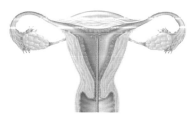

▲ **RETURNING FERTILIZED EGGS** Once the eggs and sperm have been mixed outside the body, a successfully fertilized egg is injected through the cervix into the uterus for implantation.

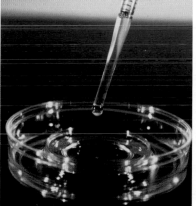

▲**FERTILIZATION** The eggs are transferred to a petri dish, where droplets of sperm are added. If fertilization is successful, the embryos are incubated for 48 hours and then transferred into the woman's uterus.

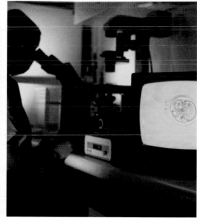

▲**EMBRYO CHECK** Here a specialist is checking an IVF embryo (visible on the screen). Doctors need to make sure that the embryo is healthy before it is introduced into the mother's body.

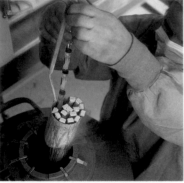

▲ **FROZEN SPERM** Sperm frozen in liquid nitrogen can be used during ICSI (Intra-cytoplasmic sperm injection) procedures. This works particularly well for men with a low sperm count or for sperm with poor movement, as the sperm can be stored and then injected directly into the prepared egg.

Advanced ART

Micromanipulation, an extraordinary technique in which not only eggs but individual sperm can be manipulated by the embryologist, makes it possible for a man with a very low sperm count and virtually no active sperm to fertilize his partner's egg. Living proof of the success of this advanced technology are the many thousands of babies conceived by ART who are now alive and well.

Micromanipulation

Intra-cytoplasmic sperm injection (ICSI) (see p.49) is one technique that uses micromanipulation. A prepared egg is placed under a microscope and injected with an individual sperm. Sperm may be collected by masturbation or from a testis using surgical techniques such as MESA or TESE (see p.49). Once fertilized, the embryo is incubated and implanted when it's reached two to four cells in size. ICSI may be offered to couples who don't conceive by other methods. The first ICSI pregnancy was in 1988. However, there's some controversy about this technique. For example, there's concern that an egg could be fertilized with a sub-standard sperm, possibly resulting in a damaged or unhealthy child. But although the pregnancy rate with ICSI is not quite as high as with IVF, the babies born so far have been normal, with no chromosomal abnormalities.

Embryo transfer

All forms of IVF (see p.49) involve taking an embryo, usually between two and three days old, from the incubating dish in the laboratory and placing it inside a woman's body. Sadly, two out of three embryo transfers fail to

▼ **TIMETABLE FOR IVF** Below is a timeline showing the steps in IVF through drug treatment to embryo transfer.

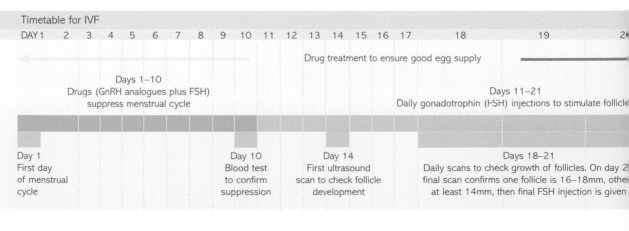

Timetable for IVF

| DAY 1 | 2 | 3 | 4 | 5 | 6 | 7 | 8 | 9 | 10 | 11 | 12 | 13 | 14 | 15 | 16 | 17 | 18 | 19 | 2 |

Drug treatment to ensure good egg supply

Days 1–10
Drugs (GnRH analogues plus FSH) suppress menstrual cycle

Days 11–21
Daily gonadotrophin (FSH) injections to stimulate follicle

Day 1
First day of menstrual cycle

Day 10
Blood test to confirm suppression

Day 14
First ultrasound scan to check follicle development

Days 18–21
Daily scans to check growth of follicles. On day 2 final scan confirms one follicle is 16–18mm, othe at least 14mm, then final FSH injection is given

implant. Successful implantation depends on the age of the mother, how receptive her uterus is, and the quality of the embryo. One of the problems with this treatment is that doctors still don't know when is the best time to transfer an embryo. Studies suggest that delaying the transfer of an embryo to the uterus can increase the chances of implantation. But in one study, there was no difference between embryos placed 44 hours after insemination and those that were placed after 68 hours.

Pregnancy rates do increase with the numbers of embryos that are placed, but so does the risk of multiple pregnancies. Twin or triplet pregnancies have a far greater risk of complications, such as miscarriage, prematurity, and possible abnormality, so parents are increasingly advised to have only one embryo transferred.

Cryopreserved embryos It's possible to thaw cryopreserved (frozen) embryos (see p.49) or eggs from liquid nitrogen (-273°C/-523°F) and transfer them. The embryo is thawed slowly, at a rate of 8°C (17°F) per minute. Not all embryos survive this process in a good enough state to implant. Placement in the womb is done at a point in the menstrual cycle 100 hours after the LH (luteinizing hormone) peak – determined by serial blood tests. Pregnancy rates vary from one in six to one in four.

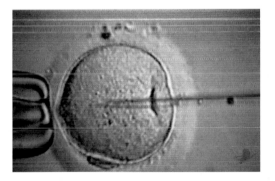

◀ **ICSI (INTRA-CYTOPLASMIC SPERM INJECTION)** In this procedure, an egg is placed under a microscope and then injected with an individual sperm. If the egg is fertilized, it is placed inside the woman's uterus ready for implantation, a process known as "embryo transfer" (see opposite).

Many doctors feel that ART has gone as far as it can – the pregnancy rate has reached 22 per cent, the same as the natural chance to conceive. But, there is still much to learn and to do:

■ superovulation of the ovaries – increasing the number of eggs a woman produces – will probably be achieved

■ further studies will be made on embryos before transfer

■ more research on implantation of the embryo in the uterus

■ more research on male infertility, perhaps as the result of refinement of ICSI (see left) or the invention of some other method of sperm treatment

■ more investigation into cryopreservation techniques to improve egg freezing methods and the low pregnancy rate with freeze-thawed embryos

■ research into in vitro maturation of eggs.

The stages of fertilization

21	22	23	24	25	26	27	28	29	30	31	32	33	34	35
	Day 22 Sperm collected; eggs collected – 6–8 eggs fertilized by ICSI and put in incubator	Day 23 Eggs checked for initial fertilization	Day 24 Eggs checked for first cell division	Day 25 Two 2- or 4-cell embryos transferred to womb				Days 26–35 Daily progesterone dose to support embryo						
	IVF			Embryo transfer									Day 35 Blood test and scan to confirm pregnancy	

Questions to ask yourselves

If you're thinking of using donors, or a surrogate mother, you'll need to have some specialized counselling to help you through what can be a difficult process.

Using donors can cause tension and disagreement between partners and it's important to try to be sympathetic to each other's reactions. Sometimes one partner may feel that a donor is being used because of poor sexual performance, or procreative failure, and this can cause emotions of guilt or even feelings of subconscious accusation or blame. You also need to think about how you would feel towards a child conceived this way. Ask yourselves these questions:

■ if you were to have a child using donor sperm, or eggs, or both, would the fact that the child wasn't "yours" prevent you from loving her as your own?

■ would you feel jealous if a donor conceived a child with your partner when you couldn't?

■ would you tell your child about how she was conceived, or would you try to keep it a secret?

■ if your child was conceived using donor eggs, or sperm, or both, how would you cope if she wanted to trace her genetic history in later life? And would you be willing to help her?

Using donors

Many childless people have been helped to become parents by using sperm, eggs, and even embryos given by other people. Surrogacy is also a form of donation – a woman donates her uterus to bear another couple's biological child. Emotional costs can be high, and all the issues need to be talked about openly. Clinics provide counselling for couples thinking of using donors.

Donor insemination

The use of donor sperm can be an option in the following situations: when the male partner is sterile or has a very low sperm count that doesn't respond to treatment; when either partner carries a hereditary abnormality; or when a mature, stable, single woman wants a child but not a partner.

Donor insemination (DI) can seem an ideal solution for people in these situations, but there are a number of points that need careful thought. First, the feelings of your partner – some men feel inadequate or even jealous of donors who impregnate their partners. These feelings can affect your life together, and your child once she is born. In addition, some women are repelled by the way they are going to conceive or by the fact that a different man's sperm is used at each visit.

Most couples feel hesitant about this method of conception and it's very stressful, so good counselling is important. You can insist that there's no mention of DI in your maternity records, and yours and your partner's names can be given on the birth certificate. In the past donors were anonymous, but since 2005, children conceived in this way have the right to find out their parent's identity when they reach 18 if they so wish. This applies only to children born after the new ruling came into force and the changes are explained to all potential donors. As before, donors have no legal or financial responsibility and cannot be forced to meet a child.

Egg donation

If a woman is unable to produce an egg herself, donor eggs may be used during IVF treatment. Egg donation does have the advantage that both of you are involved: your partner fertilizes the egg, and you will carry and give birth to the baby. However, it's more complicated than sperm donation – hormonal drugs have to be taken and the eggs collected by surgical techniques (see p.50) – so donor eggs are hard to come by. The main sources are relatives, unrelated donors (who, like sperm donors, no longer have the right to anonymity), and IVF patients who may donate extra eggs produced during their treatment.

There can be problems with egg donation. For example, eggs donated by IVF mothers have an increased risk of chromosomal disorders because IVF patients tend to be older than average, but donations are not accepted from women over 35. When relatives or friends donate eggs there can be tensions later.

If you're not producing eggs, you probably won't be menstruating, and this means that the lining of your uterus (endometrium) will be thin and incapable of nourishing a developing embryo. You'll need to be given drugs to stimulate it to thicken so that the embryo can implant.

Embryo donation

A couple who have been through IVF treatment may sometimes wish to donate unused frozen embryos to a childless woman. The embryo is implanted and the woman gives birth to the "adopted" child. Feelings run high on this and many sensitive issues have been raised. For example, how would the donor parents feel if their own child, or children, die? And what are the chances of the siblings meeting and perhaps having children together?

Selecting semen and embryos

Semen Fresh semen is frozen and stored before being used for donor insemination. After collection, the semen is put into a sterile vial and frozen by immersing it in liquid nitrogen. It's then stored while the clinic tests the donor to make sure that he's free of infections, such as hepatitis B or HIV, that could be passed on via his semen. Once it's been checked that the donor was free of infection when he made his donation, the semen is tested for harmful microorganisms, such as bacteria; if these tests prove negative, semen can then be used for insemination.

Up to 50 per cent of sperm in the semen are unlikely to survive the freezing and thawing. This fall in sperm numbers is partly offset by the fact that it's the healthiest, most robust sperm that will survive the process. Donor insemination is carried out under exactly the same conditions as artificial insemination with sperm from a partner (see p.49) – that is, by IVF, ICSI, or in natural cycles.

Embryos Storage of frozen embryos (see p.53) prevents embryo wastage if several embryos have been fertilized – no more than two are placed in any cycle because of the risk of multiple pregnancy – or they could be donated to help another infertile couple.

Surrogate mothers

A surrogate mother is a woman who bears a child on behalf of another. Surrogacy is physically straightforward but fraught with possible moral, legal, and emotional difficulties.

Full surrogacy This is the simplest form of surrogacy: a surrogate mother conceives and carries the child of an infertile woman's partner. Insemination may be indirect (the surrogate is artificially inseminated with the man's sperm) or direct (the man has sexual intercourse with the surrogate).

Partial surrogacy In this arrangement an egg from the woman who is unable to conceive is fertilized with her partner's sperm and then implanted into the surrogate mother's uterus.

Surrogacy problems When the child is born she's handed over to the couple who commissioned her. They then legally adopt the child and the surrogate mother has little or no further involvement. Sometimes, however, the surrogate can find it very hard to part with the child, especially if she is the genetic mother.

There can also be problems if the child is born with abnormalities or if the surrogate wants to keep up a close relationship with the child and is not allowed to do so. There's also the possibility that the commissioning parents may find it hard to accept the child fully and lovingly as their own.

Miriam's casebook

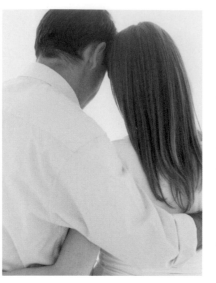

Infertility

Peter, 29, and Jane, 27, have been trying for a baby for three years without success. Peter had non-specific urethritis (NSU) three years ago and was treated at a genito-urinary (GU) clinic. The problem hasn't come back. Peter also had mumps when he was 12. Jane wants some medical advice about what she and Peter should do next, but Peter isn't keen to see their doctor. In the end, Jane visits their doctor on her own.

Sharing responsibilities

For whatever reason, many men find it difficult to talk about the possibility of being infertile. Infertility is not linked with virility and it's helpful if men can separate these two things in their minds. If a man is found to have less than perfect fertility, there's now a lot that can be done to help him and his partner conceive successfully. In half of all infertile couples the infertile partner is found to be the man, but as I explained to Jane, the investigation of their fertility is best undertaken as a couple.

Primary tests

Jane's doctor said more or less the same, and after about a week of soul-searching, Peter agreed to go along with Jane. The doctor took Peter's past attack of NSU (non-specific urethritis) very seriously – any sexually transmitted disease can interfere with fertility. The mumps virus, which may cause inflammation of the testes and damage future sperm production, can also result in problems. Peter had mumps at the age of 12, when his testes were extremely vulnerable. At the end of the first visit, the doctor asked Peter to go to the fertility clinic for semen analysis. He explained that both Jane and he would need primary tests. Jane's would be in

the form of a smear test, a test for chlamydia, an internal examination, and blood tests to confirm that she was ovulating. Peter would have a physical examination of his penis and testes as well as semen analyses.

As the doctor explained, it made sense to start by checking the form and health of Peter's sperm, but Peter hated the idea of going to the fertility clinic and having to supply semen samples. He found the process cold, clinical, and inhuman. He felt torn. He wanted to do what was necessary, to please Jane if nothing else, but he felt isolated and persecuted. His morale fell lower and lower at the thought of finding out that their difficulties with conceiving lay with him.

Getting advice

Jane did her best to reassure Peter and show her love for him, but he went deeper and deeper into his shell, refused to talk about the problem, and became very uncommunicative. Jane felt increasingly estranged from Peter. He felt unloved, and they stopped having sex altogether. Jane, feeling desperate, suggested that they should get some counselling. Peter cut short the conversation by leaving the room. All seemed lost when the results of the semen analysis came back. Peter's sperm count was low – 5–10 million – and fewer than 30 per cent of his sperm were active.

At this point I insisted that both Peter and Jane give serious thought to seeing a counsellor if only to outline the possibilities open to them through fertility treatment. It was a great struggle, but Peter finally swallowed his pride and made an appointment to see a fertility counsellor with Jane so that they could be prepared for what was to come.

Secondary tests

The counsellor explained that, although a low sperm count with low motility is, of course, a blow, Peter does have some sperm, and some are mobile. This means that even if Peter's sperm fail the egg penetration test, they could use an advanced form of ART called ICSI (see p.49) in which an individual sperm would be injected into one of Jane's eggs and could lead to a successful pregnancy and a healthy baby.

Starting IVF

An IVF treatment programme (see p.50) won't be straightforward for either of them. Jane will have to be heavily involved too, even though her fertility is normal. To increase the chances of having several eggs on which to perform ICSI with Peter's sperm, Jane will have to undergo drug treatments and serial tests to make sure her ovaries produce several eggs at the same time rather than the usual single egg. This part of the treatment will take around three weeks and both Peter and Jane would be well advised to prepare for the effect of the fertility hormones on Jane, which may make her moody, irritable, and even weepy and tearful. She'll have to make daily visits to the fertility clinic for ultrasound scans during the third week, which will mean she'll have to make special arrangements at work and will need Peter to help her out and support her.

In many ways, the greatest impact of Peter's infertility will fall on Jane. Even though Jane is desperate to have a baby, it's easy for resentment to build, especially if the initial treatments aren't successful and she has to undergo several IVF treatment programmes. Peter's involvement is

When you don't conceive as quickly as you thought you might, do seek advice and professional support.

■ Be open-minded about the possible causes of infertility, take professional advice on your specific situation, and share the responsibility as a couple for finding out more.

■ Keep talking with each other about your thoughts and feelings, and support each other every step of the way.

■ Try not to feel embarrassed or self-conscious about talking with your doctor or other healthcare professionals about your fertility issues. The more open you are, the sooner you will get to the root cause.

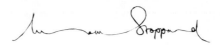

comparatively slight – he will have to provide two specimens of semen for each treatment programme, and that in itself could cause estrangement from Jane. If he's not careful it'll be all too easy for Peter to feel shame and guilt and to resent Jane for putting him in this position. It could all backfire, so it's really important for Peter and Jane to share their thoughts with each other.

Seeking support

No couple should face such a painful situation without psychological support and I think Peter is beginning to accept that. Their fertility clinic has a team of counsellors and Peter and Jane have made an appointment. Once they've had all the different steps of the fertility programme explained to their satisfaction and all their questions have been answered (I suggest that they sit down and make a list together), I strongly advise them to keep on talking about their feelings to each other and to their counsellor, every step of the way. If and when they succeed in conceiving, it'll all be worthwhile.

You and your developing baby

There's nothing as exciting as the month-by-month development of your baby. And the more you understand about how he grows, the better you'll be able to build a relationship with your baby even before he's born.

Your pregnancy is divided into three periods, or trimesters, according to the way your baby grows and develops. The first trimester starts at the date of conception and represents the first 12 weeks of your baby's life. The second trimester ends at 26 weeks, and the third with the birth of your baby.

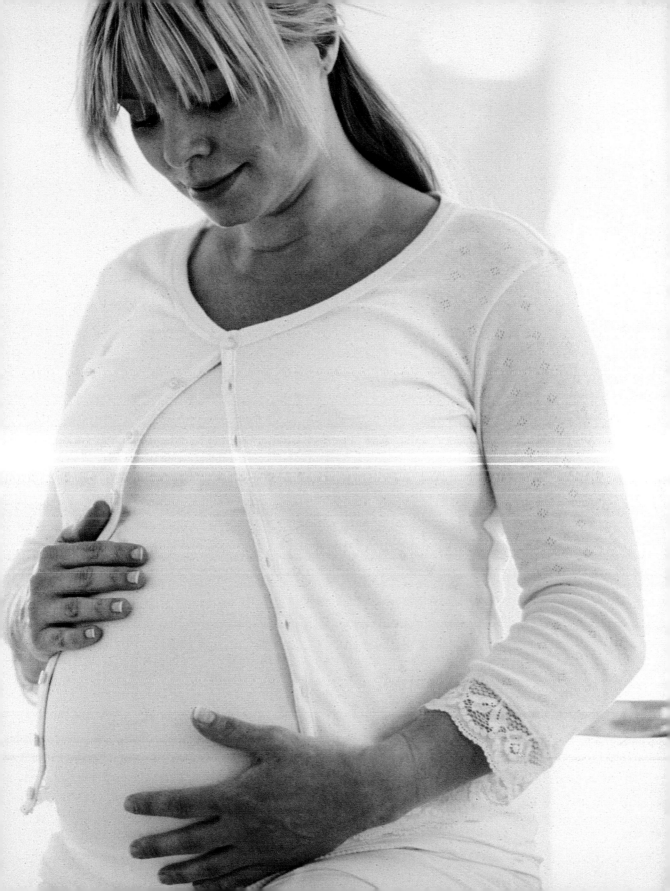

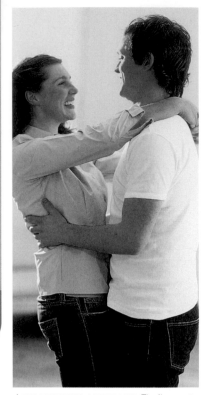

▲ **DISCOVERING A NEW LIFE** Finding out that you're pregnant can be one of the most special moments of your life.

Pregnant!

Many women "know" when they've conceived. This intuitive feeling is probably due to the early outpouring of female hormones. First of all, you'll have high levels of progesterone (which you don't experience unless you're pregnant). Then fetal tissues start to produce human chorionic gonadotrophin (hCG) as soon as the embryo is implanted in the uterus, about a week after fertilization.

Suspecting that you're pregnant

A few classic signs can make you suspect that you're pregnant before you do a test to make sure.

Missed period You may miss a period within two weeks after conceiving your baby. Although pregnancy is the most common reason for a missed period, it's not the only one, so don't take this as an absolute sign of pregnancy. There are other things, such as jet lag, severe illness, surgery, shock, bereavement, or great stress, that can cause you to miss a period. Periods don't always stop in pregnancy, though. Some women have light periods up to the sixth month, or even all the way through.

Wanting to urinate more often As soon as your progesterone levels rise and the embryo starts to produce hCG, blood supply to your pelvic area increases, which leads to pelvic congestion. This affects the bladder, which becomes irritable and tries to expel even the smallest quantity of urine. This is why most women feel like they want to pass urine more often than usual. This can happen as early as one week after conception.

Tiredness The very high levels of progesterone in your body have a sedative effect and this is one of the reasons for tiredness when you're first pregnant. Early in your pregnancy your metabolism speeds up to support your developing baby and your vital organs, which are having to do so much more work than usual. This can make you feel so tired that there's nothing you can do but sleep. And if that's how you feel, you must rest – for your sake and your baby's.

Morning sickness Although it's most common in the morning, sickness can come on at any time of day. It's more likely if you don't eat often enough and your blood sugar is allowed to drop.

Odd tastes Your saliva often reflects the chemical content of your blood, and as hormone levels rise, the taste in your mouth can change – many women describe it as metallic. You may also notice that certain foods taste different from usual, and that you stop liking some tastes that you usually enjoy (coffee is a common example).

Some women begin to crave certain foods – and occasionally want to eat strange things such as coal. There's no real scientific explanation for this. It may be the body's way of trying to make up for deficiencies in certain minerals and trace elements, but it's best to control cravings for inedible substances.

Smell You may notice that your sense of smell becomes more acute when you're pregnant, and everyday odours such as cooking smells make you nauseous. Perfume may also affect you this way, and the way your own perfume smells on you may also change, because your skin's chemistry alters.

Breast changes Right at the start of pregnancy, you may feel changes in your breasts. They may become quite lumpy and sore to the touch; your nipple area may feel very tender and sensitive, and your nipples will also deepen in colour. The veins in your breasts may start to look larger and more obvious too.

Confirming that you're pregnant

Once you suspect that you might be pregnant you'll want to confirm it as soon as possible. There are a number of tests you can have that can be done at different intervals following conception. Some are more accurate than others. At one time women had internal examinations, but now that most women have an ultrasound scan at around 12 weeks (see p.180) these are rarely needed.

Urine tests The pregnancy hormone human chorionic gonadotrophin (hCG) can be detected in your urine. Urine tests can be done at home, in hospital, at your doctor's surgery, at family planning clinics, or at a chemist. These tests are more than 99 per cent reliable. They can be carried out as early as two weeks after conception, although you'll get the most reliable result if you wait a little longer (see also p.62).

Blood test This test is carried out by your doctor, usually only when there's a problem such as bleeding or pain, or after a cycle of assisted reproduction. The test accurately detects the hCG in the blood as early as two weeks after conception – about the time your next period is due.

Telling the world

You'll want your partner, and possibly close family, to know the news as soon as you find out.

Doctor Your doctor may confirm your pregnancy, so will know immediately. If not, it's important to get in touch with your doctor as soon as you can to talk about birth options and antenatal care.

Employer You may want to talk to your employer before you go to your antenatal clinic (see p.174) for your first visit, probably when you're about three months pregnant. You don't have to tell your employer this early though.

Friends and acquaintances Many women put off telling people they're pregnant until the end of the first trimester. This is understandable, but it's probably fine to spread the news once your pregnancy's confirmed, although miscarriages can happen up to 14 weeks (or unusually, beyond).

Is your test result right?

There are a number of things that can affect the accuracy of pregnancy tests.

■ If urine is incorrectly collected or stored there can be errors.

■ If the test is performed too early, the concentration of hCG will be too low to detect. It's important to know when your period was due. If your periods are usually irregular or infrequent this can make it harder to confirm pregnancy.

■ If you've taken fertility drugs containing hCG these can change the results. Contraceptive pills, antibiotics, and painkillers shouldn't have any effect.

■ If the equipment used for a urine test is too hot, the result may be false. Urine must be room temperature at the time of the test.

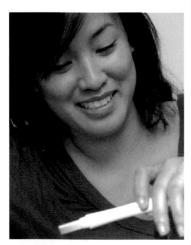

▲ TAKE CARE Follow the kit's instructions very carefully and don't use the test if it's been damaged in any way or is past its use-by date.

Home testing

You'll probably prefer to find out whether or not you're pregnant in the privacy of your own home. There's a range of pregnancy testing kits available from chemists. They're all simple to use and give immediate results that are more than 99 per cent accurate.

How the tests work Urine tests check for the presence of hCG, the hormone that's made by the developing embryo. Two of the main types, the ring and the colour tests, involve mixing a chemical solution with a sample of your urine. The chemicals react according to the amount of hCG in your urine. The reaction is shown by a colour change in the tube or window strip, or coagulation is prevented, causing a dark ring to appear in the tube. A third test can be done by simply placing the absorbent part of the test strip in contact with the urine.

Although signs of hCG may be detected in urine as early as two weeks after conceiving, most kits advise using the test between one and four days after the first day of your missed period. If you do perform the test early, repeat it two weeks later when the hCG is more concentrated and the result will be more reliable. Most kits provide two tests.

Taking the test Use a sample from the first urine you pass in the morning because it will contain a higher concentration of hCG. Don't drink anything before the test as this will dilute the sample. Make sure you collect your sample in a clean, soap-free container. If you can't do the test immediately, store your urine sample in the refrigerator, but don't keep it for more than 12 hours. Always follow instructions exactly.

Unexpected result Sometimes you may have a positive first test but a negative second test, followed by your period starting a few days later. Don't worry. Half of all conceptions don't become established pregnancies, as the fertilized egg fails to implant in the lining of the uterus and there's a natural termination. Your first test may have been positive because it was done before the fertilized egg was lost. To avoid this error do the test around the time of your first missed period. If there's a weak but positive result, repeat the test a few days later with a fresh sample.

When will your baby be born?

You'll want to know the estimated date. There are usually about 266 days or 38 weeks between conception and birth. This is the same as 40 weeks from the start of your last menstrual period (LMP) because ovulation, and therefore conception, is normally two weeks after the start of your period (see chart, right). You can work out the approximate date of your baby's arrival by calculating from the first day of your last period. The estimated date of your baby's delivery (EDD) is therefore at 280 days (40 weeks) from the first day of your last period. How accurate this date is depends on whether you have a regular 28-day cycle. If your menstrual cycle is shorter or longer, your delivery date may be earlier or later.

Medical staff use the EDD when monitoring your baby's development and checking the expected rate of growth. Sometimes too much emphasis is put on this date, leading to unnecessary intervention, and doctors may want to induce labour if they believe your baby is overdue. However, risks to you and your baby don't rise much until after 42 weeks, and most doctors are prepared to let a pregnancy continue, without inducing, if tests show the baby is not at risk (see p.260).

How the EDD chart works
Find the first day of your last period on the chart by looking for the month in bold type on the left-hand side, and look along the line until you find the actual date of your LMP. Then look at the figure below it. This is your baby's estimated date of delivery (EDD).

Your baby's arrival

Don't be anxious if your baby doesn't show signs of arriving on the day you'd expected. About 85 per cent of babies born from normal pregnancies are delivered within a week before or after the date predicted.

The EDD is used to give you an approximate idea of when to expect your baby to be born. It's best to be flexible and not to see this as the exact day you'll go into labour and deliver your baby. A healthy pregnancy may last for anything from 37 to 42 weeks.

Your estimated date of delivery

January Oct/Nov	1 8	2 9	3 10	4 11	5 12	6 13	7 14	8 15	9 16	10 17	11 18	12 19	13 20	14 21	15 22	16 23	17 24	18 25	19 26	20 27	21 28	22 29	23 30	24 31	25 1	26 2	27 3	28 4	29 5	30 6	31 7
February Nov/Dec	1 8	2 9	3 10	4 11	5 12	6 13	7 14	8 15	9 16	10 17	11 18	12 19	13 21	14 22	15 23	16 24	17 25	18 26	19 27	20 28	21 29	22 30	23 1	24 2	25 3	26 4	27 5	28			
March Dec/Jan	1 6	2 7	3 8	4 9	5 10	6 11	7 12	8 13	9 14	10 15	11 16	12 17	13 18	14 19	15 21	16 22	17 23	18 24	19 25	20 26	21 27	22 28	23 29	24 30	25 31	26 1	27 2	28 3	29 4	30 5	31
April Jan/Feb	1 6	2 7	3 8	4 9	5 10	6 11	7 12	8 13	9 14	10 15	11 16	12 17	13 18	14 19	15 21	16 22	17 23	18 24	19 25	20 26	21 27	22 28	23 29	24 30	25 31	26 1	27 2	28 3	29 4	30	
May Feb/Mar	1 5	2 6	3 7	4 8	5 9	6 10	7 11	8 12	9 13	10 14	11 15	12 16	13 17	14 18	15 19	16 21	17 22	18 23	19 24	20 25	21 26	22 27	23 28	24 1	25 2	26 3	27 4	28 5	29 6	30 7	31
June Mar/Apr	1 8	2 9	3 10	4 11	5 12	6 13	7 14	8 15	9 16	10 17	11 18	12 19	13 21	14 22	15 23	16 24	17 25	18 26	19 27	20 28	21 29	22 30	23 31	24 1	25 2	26 3	27 4	28 5	29 6	30	
July Apr/May	1 7	2 8	3 9	4 10	5 11	6 12	7 13	8 14	9 15	10 16	11 17	12 18	13 19	14 21	15 22	16 23	17 24	18 25	19 26	20 27	21 28	22 29	23 30	24 1	25 2	26 3	27 4	28 5	29 6	30 7	31
August May/June	1 8	2 9	3 10	4 11	5 12	6 13	7 14	8 15	9 16	10 17	11 18	12 19	13 21	14 22	15 23	16 24	17 25	18 26	19 27	20 28	21 29	22 30	23 31	24 1	25 2	26 3	27 4	28 5	29 6	30 7	31
September June/July	1 8	2 9	3 10	4 11	5 12	6 13	7 14	8 15	9 16	10 17	11 18	12 19	13 21	14 22	15 23	16 24	17 25	18 26	19 27	20 28	21 29	22 30	23 1	24 2	25 3	26 4	27 5	28 6	29 7	30	
October July/Aug	1 8	2 9	3 10	4 11	5 12	6 13	7 14	8 15	9 16	10 17	11 18	12 19	13 21	14 22	15 23	16 24	17 25	18 26	19 27	20 28	21 29	22 30	23 31	24 1	25 2	26 3	27 4	28 5	29 6	30 7	31
November Aug/Sep	1 8	2 9	3 10	4 11	5 12	6 13	7 14	8 15	9 16	10 17	11 18	12 19	13 21	14 22	15 23	16 24	17 25	18 26	19 27	20 28	21 29	22 30	23 31	24 1	25 2	26 3	27 4	28 5	29 6	30	
December Sep/Oct	1 8	2 9	3 10	4 11	5 12	6 13	7 14	8 15	9 16	10 17	11 18	12 19	13 21	14 22	15 23	16 24	17 25	18 26	19 27	20 28	21 29	22 30	23 31	24 1	25 2	26 3	27 4	28 5	29 6	30 7	31

Paternity leave

To qualify for paternity leave, an employee must: have or expect to have responsibility for the child's upbringing; be the biological father of the child or the mother's husband or partner (including same-sex partners); have worked continuously for their employer for 26 weeks ending with the 15th week before the baby is due.

Employees can choose to take either one week's or two consecutive weeks' paternity leave (not odd days). They can choose to start their leave: from the date of the child's birth; from a chosen number of days or weeks after the date of the child's birth (whether earlier or later than expected); or from a chosen date later than the first day of the week in which the baby is expected to be born. Leave can start on any day of the week on or following the child's birth but must be completed within 56 days of the actual birth of the child. If the child is born early, leave must be completed within the period from the actual date of birth up to 56 days after the first day of the expected week of birth.

During paternity leave, most employees are entitled to Statutory Paternity Pay (SPP), but some companies offer more generous packages, so ask your employer about this. Employees are entitled to return to the same job after paternity leave and can't be dismissed for taking it.

Your rights

A pregnant woman has certain rights and benefits depending on her circumstances. There are two state benefits available. These are Statutory Maternity Pay (SMP) and Maternity Allowance. Some employers offer more generous maternity packages than those provided by law. Any Citizens' Advice Bureau or Social Security office can help you work out what you're entitled to.

Who qualifies for Statutory Maternity Pay?

Provided you have been on a fixed-term contract, or employed full-time or part-time for more than six months, you will be entitled to up to 39 weeks of statutory maternity pay (SMP). In order to qualify for SMP, you need to have been employed by the same company for a minimum of 26 weeks by the time you reach the 15th week before your expected delivery date – in other words, around the 26th week of your pregnancy. Your SMP will be 90 per cent of your average weekly pay for the first six weeks, followed by the basic SMP or 90 per cent of your earnings (whichever is lower) for the remaining 33 weeks. SMP is paid to you regardless of whether you decide to return to work. The rules are explained in leaflets that you can get from your local Social Security Office, Citizen's Advice Bureau, or antenatal clinic. You can also get free prescriptions and dental treatment while you are pregnant and for 12 months after the birth, and you may be entitled to free milk and vitamins for yourself and any children under five if you're on a low income.

Who qualifies for Maternity Allowance?

If you are self-employed, have changed your job, or have at times been unemployed during your pregnancy, Maternity Allowance is for you, on condition that you have been employed or self-employed for a minimum of 26 weeks during the 66 weeks ending with the week before your expected delivery date.

The weekly Maternity Allowance that you receive depends on what your average earnings have been. You are entitled to the standard rate for 39 weeks, or 90 per cent of your earnings, whichever is lower. You can start to claim Maternity Allowance from the 11th week before your baby is due, until the day after your baby's birth. Your local Social Security office or Job Centre can provide all the details and give you a claim form to fill in if you are eligible.

Maternity benefits

WHEN	WHAT TO DO	WHY
As soon as you know you're pregnant	1 Ask your doctor or midwife for form FW8. 2 Tell your dentist if you need treatment. 3 Check leaflets MV11, H11, and G11, and tell the Social Security office if you're getting supplementary benefit. 4 Tell your employer, especially if your job is dangerous, as your employer must find you an alternative job or suspend you on full pay.	1 Apply for free prescriptions. 2 Apply for free dental treatment. 3 Check your right to free glasses, free milk and vitamins, help with hospital fares. 4 No loss of pay for keeping antenatal appointments; protection against unfair dismissal.
As soon as you can	If you're unemployed or sick, check leaflet N117A and ask your Social Security office about the Maternity Allowance claim.	This can affect the amount of Maternity Allowance you may get.
20 weeks	Ask at your antenatal clinic for forms BM4 and Mat B1. Apply BM4, and give Mat B1 to your employer.	You can apply from now for Statutory Maternity Pay or Maternity Allowance.
15 weeks before expected week of childbirth	Tell your employer in writing: the date you want to stop work; the week the baby is due; and whether you intend to return to your job.	To protect your right to maternity pay, and return to work.
29 weeks	If getting supplementary benefit, claim single payments for maternity clothes and baby's needs.	Statutory Maternity Pay or Maternity Allowance are paid from now.
As soon after the birth as you can	1 If you've had more than one baby, fill in BM4X. 2 If your baby was late, fill in form BM9. 3 Register your baby's birth as there are time limits, see below. 4 Send off CH2 or CH11A if you're a single parent. 5 Check low income benefits and find out about child tax credit.	1 Extra maternity grant for each baby. 2 To claim extra maternity allowance. 3 To get the birth certificate. 4 To get child and one-parent benefit. 5 To see if you qualify for supplementary benefits, free prescriptions, dental treatment, spectacles, milk, vitamins, hospital fares, or help with rent and council tax.
3 weeks after birth	Register your baby (if you live in Scotland).	Latest date.
6 weeks after birth	Register your baby (the rest of the the UK).	Latest date.
3 months after the birth	If you haven't already, apply for Maternity Allowance for single or multiple births.	You may lose out on a Maternity Allowance if not claimed by now.
28 days before returning to work	Write to your employer stating the date when you wish to return to work.	To help them plan for your return.

Your weight gain

In the first three months you'll probably put on about 1–2kg (2–4lb), if you haven't had too much problem with nausea.

Your baby will weigh only 48g (1¾oz). The rest of the weight is made up of your baby's support system (the placenta and amniotic fluid), your enlarged uterus and breasts, and the extra amount of blood in your body. Your own fat stores will make up about the same weight gain as your baby.

First trimester

When you're pregnant the three trimesters are your major milestones. The trimesters aren't three periods of exactly three months each – they're of different lengths, defined by the way a baby grows and develops. The first trimester starts with the presumed date of conception.

In the first trimester, your body adjusts to being pregnant. At first you won't look any different, and you might not feel different either, but the activities of your hormones will soon start to affect you in various ways. You might experience lots of mood swings, you may want to make love more or less often, and you may find that your appetite changes and you start feeling like simpler, blander food than usual.

Physical changes

Your pregnant body is having to work very hard to accommodate the developing embryo and the placenta. When you're pregnant your body's metabolic rate increases and is between ten and 25 per cent higher than normal. This means that all the body's functions are stepped up. Your cardiac output rises steeply, almost to the maximum level that will be kept up throughout the rest of your pregnancy. Your heart rate rises too, and will go on doing so until the middle of the second trimester. Your breathing becomes more rapid as you now need to send more oxygen to your baby and breathe out more carbon dioxide.

Because of the action of increased levels of oestrogen and progesterone in your body, your breasts quickly become larger and heavier. They're usually tender to the touch from very early on, too. There's an increase in fatty deposits in your breasts and new milk ducts grow. The areola around the nipple becomes darker and develops little nodules called Montgomery's tubercles. Underneath your skin, a network of bluish lines will appear as the blood supply to your breasts increases.

Your uterus becomes larger even in early pregnancy, but you won't feel it through the abdominal wall until the end of the first trimester, when it begins to rise above your pelvic brim. While the uterus is still low in your pelvis, it'll start to press upon your bladder as it gets bigger, so you'll

◄ **EARLY CHANGES** At this stage you may not look pregnant, but your uterus will already be enlarged and your breasts may feel tender and heavier.

almost certainly find that you need to urinate more often. The muscle fibres of your uterus begin to thicken until it becomes very solid indeed. Even so, you probably won't notice your waistline changing until the end of this first trimester.

Taking care of yourself

When you're pregnant you'll need extra carbohydrates and protein to supply your growing baby and the placenta, as well as your uterus and breasts, so it's vital to eat healthily right from the start. You'll need extra fluids, too, so try to drink at least eight glasses of liquid a day. Avoid drugs, caffeine, junk food, alcohol, and smoking throughout the whole of your pregnancy. Make sure, too, that you get plenty of rest.

Clothes You'll feel much happier in comfortable clothes. While you won't need to buy any maternity clothes just yet, there's nothing worse than wearing something that's tight and uncomfortable, even if it's only for a few days, so try to keep one step ahead of your increasing size. You'll almost certainly find that you need to wear a larger bra from early on, and it's best if this is a properly fitted maternity bra (see What to wear, p.162).

Your antenatal care

Your doctor may confirm that you're pregnant, or you may make an appointment with the antenatal clinic as soon as you've had a positive test result. If this is the case, you may not be seen until your next trimester. At the first visit to the clinic, your midwife will ask you about your own and your family's medical histories. You'll also be given a thorough physical examination, including urine and blood tests.

Making plans

Your doctor will talk to you about choices for childbirth in your area – what hospitals you could go to and what arrangements could be made for a home birth. Some doctors' surgeries offer antenatal care, whether complete or shared with your hospital. Now is the time to start thinking about the type of delivery you want and where you're most likely to get it. Books like this one can help you decide what sort of birth you would prefer to have as well as give you in-depth information on everything to do with pregnancy, birth, and baby care.

Some women feel like buying their unborn baby a little gift, such as a teddy bear, as soon as they know they're pregnant, but many feel that doing anything more than this is to tempt fate. You might like to start keeping a daily journal of your health and feelings during the first trimester, so that you'll have a complete record of your pregnancy.

Your pregnancy

Finding out that you're pregnant is very exciting – especially if it's the first time. Here are some of the early physical signs that you will be aware of.

■ Your breasts will grow larger, heavier, and feel more sensitive.

■ You'll notice more pigmentation on your nipples, and any moles and freckles will get bigger.

■ You may feel very tired.

■ You'll probably have some feelings of nausea, especially first thing in the morning.

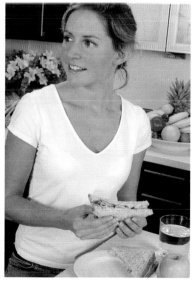

▲ **YOUR APPETITE** It's important to eat well throughout your pregnancy, but in the early weeks you may feel like eating some unusual foods or go off foods that you normally enjoy. You may notice a metallic taste in your mouth.

Your weight gain

In the second trimester, you'll probably put on about 6kg (13lb) in weight.

Of this, only about 1kg (2lb) will be your baby. The rest of the weight is made up of your baby's support system (such as the placenta and amniotic fluid), your enlarged uterus and breasts, and the extra blood and fluid in your body. Your fat stores will be about the same amount of weight as your growing baby.

Second trimester

By this time your pregnancy will be well established and many of the little problems you may have had during early pregnancy will have disappeared. If you're over 35 years old or have a family history of congenital abnormalities, for example, you'll be offered screening, which may include amniocentesis.

Physical changes

Your nipples may begin to make colostrum – your baby's first food – and leak slightly from time to time. Your waistline gradually starts to disappear and you'll now "look" pregnant. You may notice you have more pigmentation on your areolae and on freckles and moles (see p.158). Your gums may become slightly spongy, probably because of the action of pregnancy hormones. There's no reason why you should have more dental decay during pregnancy, though, and there's no truth in the saying "a tooth lost for every child".

Digestion The hormone that helps your cervix stretch to allow your baby to be born also affects other muscles in your body. All the muscles of your intestinal tract will be relaxed and this can cause many of the minor discomforts during your pregnancy.

You may suffer heartburn because the sphincter, or muscular ring, at the top of the stomach is more relaxed than usual. This allows the acid contents of your stomach to come back into your gullet, causing discomfort. Your gastric secretions are also reduced, so food remains for longer in the stomach.

Because your intestinal muscles are relaxed you'll also have fewer bowel movements and although this does allow your food to be absorbed more completely, it can also lead to constipation in pregnancy.

Your increasing size You'll notice your shape changing, but many women are told they look small-for-dates during the second trimester. If this happens to you, don't worry. How big you'll look at this time depends

◀ **GETTING BIGGER** Once your uterus has grown above your pelvis, you'll notice your waistline will begin to disappear.

on many different things, including your particular height and build; whether this is your first pregnancy or not, because uterine muscle tends to get stretched after the first child; and the size of your baby. If your doctor's happy with the way your pregnancy is going, then you can be too.

Taking care of yourself

During this trimester you'll gain the most weight of your pregnancy (about 6kg/13lb) and it's vital to keep on eating well (see p.128). You may find your posture changes as the muscles of your abdominal wall become more and more stretched to make room for your growing uterus. As your uterus gets bigger, your centre of gravity changes because you're carrying more weight in front. Try not to start leaning backwards or you may get backache (see Check your posture, p.160).

Backache You may have some backache because the increased blood flow to the whole of your pelvis causes some softening and relaxation of the ligaments of the sacrum, which attach your pelvic bones to your spine at the back. Also, the ligaments and the cartilage at the front of your pelvis loosen and the mobility of these joints is slightly increased.

To help prevent backache, sit with a straight back and try not to slouch. You'll find it best to sit on a hard chair or the floor. Always bend with a straight back. Don't lift anything heavy if you can help it (see also p.160). If you do need to lift anything from the floor, bend from your knees and lift from a crouching position.

Your antenatal care

You'll have regular urine and blood pressure checks. If necessary you'll have tests for chromosomal defects. From this time, too, your doctors or midwives will want to measure that your baby is growing enough. They will feel your abdomen to check the size and shape of your uterus and the height of the fundus (see p.178), and they'll listen for your baby's heartbeat.

During the fifth month you'll probably have an ultrasound scan (about weeks 18–22), and you'll have the special thrill of seeing your baby for the first time. You'll be able to hear your baby's incredibly fast heartbeat, too (see column, p.178), and you may see your baby moving.

Preparing for your baby

Towards the end of this second trimester, you'll probably be feeling well and full of energy so it's a good time to start shopping for some of the equipment you'll need. It's a good idea to do at least some of these things now rather than to wait until the third trimester. By then you'll rapidly be getting bigger and you might not feel like going shopping.

Your pregnancy

You'll start to feel more comfortable with being pregnant now. You'll love the feeling of your baby moving inside you and you'll be energetic and full of life.

■ You'll feel like making love again – or more often – some women have their first orgasm or multiple orgasms at this time.

■ Your abdomen will become rounded and you'll "look" pregnant.

■ Your pigmentation will increase and you may notice a darker line developing down the centre of your abdomen (see p.158).

■ You might suffer from indigestion and rib pain.

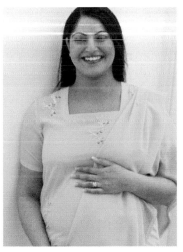

▲**HORMONAL EFFECTS** As the placenta takes over the production of pregnancy hormones, your hormone levels should begin to balance out. You'll feel calmer and more positive than you did in the first trimester. You'll look better, too, with shiny hair and clear, glowing skin.

Your weight gain

During the final months you'll probably put on about 5kg (10lb) in weight.

Of this, about 3–4kg (6–9lb) will be your baby. The rest is made up of your baby's support system (the placenta and amniotic fluid), your enlarged uterus and breasts, and the extra blood in your body. Your own fat stores will usually account for about the same weight gain as your baby.

Third trimester

At this time you might start to feel anxious about labour and wish you could have your baby now. Don't worry – this doesn't mean there's anything wrong. Your feelings of urgency are caused by metabolic changes in your brain. Subtle shifts happen in each trimester, bringing about the tiredness of the first, the elation and energy of the second, and now the anxiety of the third.

Physical changes

You're rapidly getting bigger now and you're bound to feel tired. You may not be sleeping as well as usual at night and you'll need to rest more and take naps during the day (see opposite). As your ligaments stretch and give way, you might start to find walking around uncomfortable. Once your baby has settled into your pelvis, you'll find you won't feel so breathless because there's less pressure on your diaphragm.

Breathing Because your diaphragm can't move as much when your baby grows bigger, you breathe more deeply when you're pregnant. You take in more air with each breath, which allows for better mixing of gases and the more efficient consumption of oxygen. This lifts your ventilation rate from the normal 7 litres (12pt) of air per minute to 10 litres (17½ pt) per minute, an increase of more than 40 per cent. However, your oxygen requirements are only 20 per cent more. This leads to overbreathing, which means that you breathe out more carbon dioxide per breath than is normally the case. The low level of CO_2 in the blood causes a shortness of breath, which you may find bothersome during this trimester. Relief from this should come when your baby engages in your pelvis and there's less pressure on your diaphragm.

Possible problems Some women suffer from hypertension (high blood pressure – see p.178) in later pregnancy. Major warning signs of this are swollen and puffy hands, wrists, ankles, feet, and face. Your doctor or midwife will check for these at your antenatal visits. Pre-eclampsia (see p.224) may interfere with the functioning of your

◀ **THE LAST WEEKS** You'll be much bigger now and you may find it harder to move around and get comfortable. You'll really be aware of your baby's presence.

placenta and prevent it carrying nutrients to your baby efficiently. If you do develop pre-eclampsia you may have to go into hospital.

Caring for yourself

As the third trimester goes on, the extra weight you're carrying may cause more backache and make you feel tired all the time. You'll probably find it difficult to sleep in the last weeks, because it's hard to get comfortable in bed. Don't take sleeping pills – they'll make your baby sleepy too. Take your time with everything and make sure you get enough rest. Take catnaps during the day and be sure to give yourself some quiet times when you can relax. If you don't feel like making love or it's difficult because of your increasing size, you may find that massage helps you relax. Eat lots of fresh fruit and vegetables and drink at least eight glasses of fluid per day as you'll probably pass urine more often. You may be constipated at times.

Your antenatal care

You'll go for checkups more often during this trimester. Your doctors may suggest you have a number of different tests to assess your baby's health and wellbeing, such as ultrasound or fetal heart rate monitoring. At each stage you should be told what's being done and why. Unlike the special tests in the first and second trimester – chorionic villus sampling, amniocentesis, and cordocentesis (see pp.184–87) – none of the tests at this time are invasive of your uterus. You'll have regular urine and blood pressure tests, and your feet and hands will be checked for possible swelling, although such swelling may be normal if there aren't any other symptoms. From your 36th week up to the start of labour, you'll go to the antenatal clinic more often than you did in the earlier months.

Preparing for your baby

By the time you're nearing the end of your third trimester, you'll need to have clothing and equipment ready. You never know – your baby might arrive early. You may find yourself thinking more and more about the labour and some women find that they worry obsessively. Try not to be too anxious. No one can predict what will happen during your labour, as every woman's experience is unique, but most births go without a hitch.

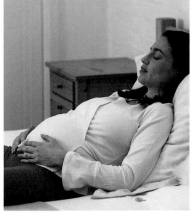

▲ **TAKE A BREAK** If you often find yourself short of breath in the later stages of pregnancy, it'll help to sit in a semi-propped-up position whenever you can. Try not to overdo things.

Your pregnancy

In this trimester, practical matters such as going to childbirth classes and getting your baby's clothes and room ready will vie with daydreaming and fantasizing about the new arrival.

■ You'll probably get tired easily, although you may find it hard to rest.

■ You'll notice Braxton Hicks contractions (see p.270) more and more.

■ You'll have visited the hospital where you're going to give birth and met the staff. If you're planning a home birth you'll need to get everything ready.

■ You might worry about whether you can tell when you're in labour or not. Even for an experienced midwife or doctor, it can be difficult to know when labour has really started. Don't be afraid to ring your midwife or hospital delivery ward for advice if you're in any doubt.

Mother

At the end of the first month, you probably won't be sure that you're pregnant, although you may have your suspicions.

Symptoms You'll notice few, if any, symptoms, although you may feel slightly premenstrual and pass urine more often than usual. Your breasts may feel sore and heavy and your nipples may tingle. You may even feel sick.

Ovulation cycle Once the embryo has implanted on the lining of your uterus, your normal cycle stops. The corpus luteum (see p.28) in the ovary continues to make progesterone, which prevents you having periods and keeps the pregnancy healthy and viable.

Cervix The hormone progesterone makes your cervical mucus thicker, forming a plug. This stays in place until the end of your pregnancy, when it comes out (the show).

Uterus The wall of your uterus softens so that the embryo can become firmly embedded. Your uterus starts to get bigger almost from the moment of implantation.

First six weeks

Your fertilized egg becomes a ball of cells (known as a blastocyst), which floats into your uterus and implants itself in the lining. The basis for your baby's future development is now laid down.

Your baby's progress

Once it has implanted, the embryo begins to make chemicals that have two functions. First, they signal to your body that the embryo has arrived and this triggers changes in your body: your ovulation cycle stops; the mucus in your cervix thickens; your uterine wall softens; and your breasts begin to grow. Second, your immune system is suppressed so that the embryo is not treated as foreign and rejected, but is allowed to grow. Also, an outer layer of the ball of cells becomes a protective cocoon around the embryo. This cocoon will create the beginnings of the placenta and the support system in which the embryo will grow: the amniotic sac (the watery balloon in which it will float) and the chorion (a safety cushion around the amniotic sac). The yolk sac (which will make blood cells until the liver takes over) forms from the inner layer. The chorion grows finger-like projections, the chorionic villi, with which the cocoon burrows into your uterine lining.

Your baby at six weeks of pregnancy

The beginnings of the spinal cord appear

The embryo has gill-like structures that will later become the jaw, neck, and part of the face

The rudimentary heart of the embryo bulges out

Baby's vital statistics By the end of the sixth week of life, the embryo will be about 4mm (⅛in) long. It will weigh less than a gram (0.03oz)

The cells specialize Throughout these early weeks, the embryo's cells become more specialized. There are now three layers of them. Each layer will create different organs of your baby's body. The innermost layer makes a primitive tube that later develops into the lungs, liver, thyroid gland, pancreas, urinary tract, and bladder. The middle layer will become the skeleton, muscles (including the heart muscle), testes or ovaries, kidneys, spleen, blood vessels, blood cells, and the deepest layer of skin, the dermis. The outer layer will provide the epidermis, sweat glands, nipples (and breasts, if your baby is a girl), hair, nails, tooth enamel, and the lenses of the eyes.

The embryo's support system

The villi, finger-like projections, of the growing placenta intermingle with the mother's blood vessels in the uterine wall in such a way that they eventually become surrounded by "lakes" of blood. The mother's blood flows in and around these spaces and, because it is divided by only a cell or two from fetal blood, exchange of nutrients and waste between fetus and mother can take place in these blood spaces. The placenta is a hormone factory pumping out hormones, such as human chorionic gonadotrophin (hCG), that support a healthy pregnancy. Until the sixth week, the embryo's blood cells are supplied by the yolk sac. After the end of the third week, the blood circulation is pumped by the baby's own heart. Until week eight the baby is known as an embryo, after which it is called a fetus, Latin for "young one".

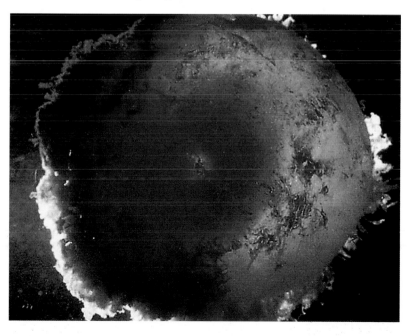

Baby

Probably even before you know you're pregnant, the embryo reaches a critical stage in development so it's vital to plan for pregnancy.

Spinal cord During the second week of life, a dark mark appears on the embryo's back. This marks the position of the spinal cord.

Heart By the end of the third week, the embryo has a heart that's now beginning to beat.

Sensitivity In the third week, the embryo enters a sensitive phase of development when all the major organs are forming. Embryos are generally robust but can be harmed by drugs, alcohol, smoking, infections, and so on.

◀ **THE DEVELOPING EMBRYO**
Surrounding layers of chorion and amnion protect the embryo, and blocks of tissue that will become the vertebrae can be seen to have started forming. Between these grow bunches of nerves.

Mother

1
2
3
4
5
6
7
8
9
10
11
12
13
14
15
16
17
18
19
20
21
22
23
24
25
26
27
28
29
30
31
32
33
34
35
36
37
38
39
40

Some women find that morning sickness is one of the first signs of pregnancy. Other changes happen that may not be as noticeable.

Metabolic changes Very early in your pregnancy your metabolic rate begins to increase. As a result you need to take in more protein and calories.

Circulatory changes Your total blood volume begins to rise. About 25 per cent of this is being used by the placental system.

Genitals The blood supply to your vagina and vulva increases quite rapidly and they both become a purplish colour. Your vaginal walls become softened and relaxed, and an increasing amount of a watery substance is made so you'll have more discharge while you're pregnant.

Breasts Your breasts may start to swell or feel tender and heavier than usual. The skin around your areola starts to become softer and lighter; this area is known as the secondary areola.

Tiredness You are likely to get tired more easily than usual.

Up to ten weeks

This is a time of very rapid and crucial development – your baby quadruples in size. The embryo is lying in the centre of a large placental cocoon and is still very tiny. As the embryo develops, its cells are constantly changing to make new structures.

Your baby's progress

Inside the tube that will eventually become your baby's brain and spinal cord, the cells multiply at an amazing rate, then move away to the areas where they will become active. The nerve cells that will form the brain travel along pathways that are being laid down by glial (glue) cells. These cells allow the nerve cells to move towards each other, connect, and become active. Your baby's head is growing rapidly in order to make room for the enlarging brain, and the body is becoming less curved. A neck begins to develop and the primeval tail disappears.

The skin now starts to develop into its two layers, and the sweat glands and sebaceous (oil-producing) glands begin to form. Hair then starts to grow from the hair follicles so that the skin becomes downy.

Your baby at ten weeks of pregnancy

The face begins to develop and eyes and nose appear

Fingers and toes are forming

The heart beats and can now be seen on ultrasound

The tail is reabsorbed

The body begins to straighten up

Baby's vital statistics By the end of this month your baby's crown to rump length will be 2.5cm (1in). Your baby will weigh about 3g ($\frac{1}{10}$oz)

All the major organs develop. The heart achieves its final form and beats strongly. The stomach, liver, spleen, appendix, and intestine develop. The intestine becomes so long it forms a loop, the circulatory system is established, and most muscles begin to take on their final form.

Facial features   Under the skin on the baby's face, a primitive bone structure develops and these bones are now fusing together. One of these goes down between the eyes and ends on either side of the nostrils, thus forming the nose and the middle of the upper lip. Two others appear under the eyes, forming the cheeks and sides of the upper lip. Two more grow under the mouth, fusing to form the lower lip and chin. There's already some pigment in the eyes, which are covered and very far apart. The inside and outside parts of the ears begin to form and the taste buds start developing. The tooth buds of all non-permanent teeth are in place.

Arms and legs   The baby's embryonic limbs continue to develop. Wrists and fingers appear on the arm buds, which become longer and project forwards. The arms become bent at the elbow. Touch-pads form on the fingertips. Leg buds sprout, then develop three distinct sections – thigh, calf, and foot. Toes start to appear. At this stage, your baby's arms and hands grow faster than her legs and feet. This trend will continue after your baby's been born – she'll be able to grasp objects long before she starts walking.

Baby

Nutrients pass from you into the placenta and the umbilical cord to feed your baby, who needs more and more nourishment to support the rapid growth.

Heart rate The baby's heart beats 140–150 times per minute, which is about twice the rate of yours.

Body shape The baby's head is still very large in comparison to the body and is bent forwards on the chest. The body begins to straighten and get longer.

Internal organs All organs are now in place and most major structures will have been formed.

Reflexes Your baby can respond to touch, although you won't be able to feel any movements yet.

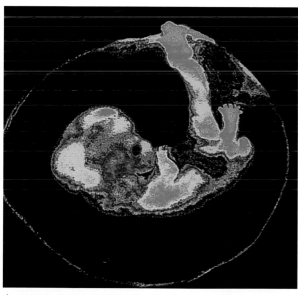

▲ **COLOUR-ENHANCED SCAN** The developing umbilical cord and placenta can be clearly seen in the top right-hand corner of this ultrasound scan.

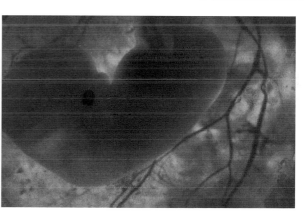

▲ **EXTERNAL FEATURES** At this stage the embryo's eyes already have some pigment and there are visible signs of nostrils, lips, and ears. The rudimentary ears now divide into inner and outer sections, the eyelids form, and the tip of the nose can be seen. The embryo's muscles are starting to build and by the seventh week of life, the first embryonic movement can be detected using ultrasound. This picture shows the embryo at about six weeks after conception.

Mother

1
2
3
4
5
6
7
8
9
10
11
12
13
14
15
16
17
18
19
20
21
22
23
24
25
26
27
28
29
30
31
32
33
34
35
36
37
38
39
40

You'll probably start to feel better during this month, particularly if you've been suffering badly with nausea and vomiting.

Weight You'll probably begin to put on weight as your baby and his support system grow rapidly.

Hormones Your hormones begin to settle down and you'll be much less up and down emotionally.

Fundal height Your developing baby is causing the fundus (see External examination, p.178) of your uterus to rise through the pelvic brim where it can be felt. You'll probably have an ultrasound scan at this time to confirm dates.

Outlook If you've been anxious about your pregnancy, you'll probably feel more relaxed now as the risk of miscarriage is less than three per cent.

Circulatory system Your cardiac output has reached almost the maximum level that will be kept up throughout the rest of your pregnancy. To lower blood pressure, the arteries and veins in your extremities relax, so your hands and feet are nearly always warm.

Up to 14 weeks

By 14 weeks after your last period, all of your baby's major organs have formed and his intestines are sealed in his abdominal cavity. He's starting to grow and mature.

Your baby's progress

By the 11th week of pregnancy, your baby is recognizable as a human being, and he's now called a fetus (offspring) rather than an embryo. His head is very large compared to the rest of his body – by 14 weeks it's about one-third of his whole length. His eyes are completely formed, although his eyelids are still developing and remain closed. His face, too, is completely formed. His trunk has straightened out and the first bone tissue and ribs appear. He has nails on his fingers and toes and he may have some hair. The external genital organs are now growing and doctors may be able to tell your baby's sex by ultrasound. His heart is beating between 110 and 160 times per minute and his circulatory system is continuing to develop. He swallows amniotic fluid and excretes it as urine. His sucking reflex is getting established – he purses his lips, turns his head, and wrinkles his forehead. The muscles he'll use after he's born for

Your baby at 14 weeks of pregnancy

His external ears move up from the neck (where they were gill-like growths) to their places on the side of his head

His eyes move round to the front of his face but are still wide apart

His head and neck extend and grow

Fine hair covers his whole body

External sex organs are different now

Baby's vital statistics By the end of this month his crown to rump length will be 9cm (3½in), and he'll weigh 48g (1¾oz)

breathing and swallowing are also being exercised. In fact, by the end of this month your baby will begin to move around vigorously, but you probably won't be able to feel his movements until the fourth month.

Blood-cell production While your baby will go on relying on the placenta for his nourishment, oxygen, and the clearance of waste until he is born, he has to have a system of blood-cell formation that will eventually support life outside the womb. Towards the end of this month, the yolk sac becomes superfluous as its task of producing blood cells is taken over by your baby's developing bone marrow, liver, and spleen.

His support system

The placenta is developing very quickly, making sure that there's a rich network of blood vessels to provide your baby with vital nourishment. Now the layers thicken and grow until the chorion and membranes cover the entire inner surface area of the uterus. The umbilical cord is now completely mature and is made up of three intertwined blood vessels wrapped in a fatty sheath. The large vein carries nutrients and oxygen-rich blood to your baby, while the two, smaller, arteries carry waste products and oxygen-poor blood from your baby back to the placenta. The umbilical cord is coiled like a spring because the sheath is longer than the blood vessels. This allows your baby plenty of room to move around without the risk of damaging his lifeline.

Baby

Your baby is fully formed; now he needs to mature. He's very active at this stage, although you won't feel him yet.

Bones In the form of flexible cartilage, the bones in his body are rapidly growing.

Movements He jerks his body, bends his arms and legs, and has hiccups.

Jaws These already show 32 permanent tooth buds.

Amniotic sac He floats comfortably in a warm bath of amniotic fluid. At 37.5°C (99.5°F), the temperature of the amniotic fluid is higher than your own body temperature. He has plenty of room to move.

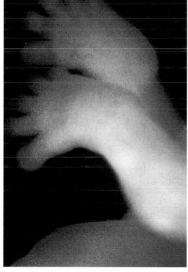

▲ **FEET AND HANDS** Your baby's fingers and toes are growing rapidly and becoming fully formed.

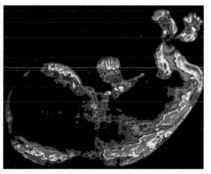

▲ **12-WEEK-OLD FETUS** Your baby's features are more clearly defined. He now has a definite chin, a large forehead, and a button nose. His eyelids are forming across his fully formed eyes, and he's beginning to respond to what happens outside the womb – if his mother's abdomen is poked, he'll try to wriggle away. An ultrasound scan would show that he's moving, but you won't feel his movements for at least another month.

Mother

1
2
3
4
5
6
7
8
9
10
11
12
13
14
15
16
17
18
19
20
21
22
23
24
25
26
27
28
29
30
31
32
33
34
35
36
37
38
39
40

You're showing many signs that pregnancy is advancing well, although you may not have gained much weight. You'll probably have extra energy.

Nipples They're darkening in colour as your skin becomes more deeply pigmented. They may tingle, feel sore, and the surface veins are becoming prominent.

Heart This is working twice as hard as before, putting out enough blood (6 litres/10½pt per minute) to keep up the increasing needs of your vital organs. Your uterus and skin need twice as much blood as usual and your kidneys 25 per cent more.

Abdomen You may develop a dark line, called the linea nigra, down the centre of your abdomen. Your uterus has been forced out of the pelvic cavity into your abdomen by your growing baby and can be felt on examination.

Quickening
Towards the end of this month you'll probably feel your baby moving – a bubbling, fluttering sensation like butterflies, little fishes, or wind!

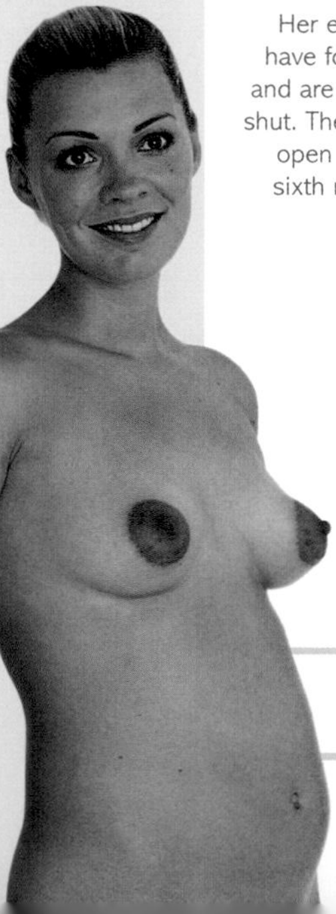

Up to 18 weeks

The second trimester starts from the fourteenth week of pregnancy. Your baby is steadily growing and if you have a scan now it'll be possible to tell your baby's sex. If your doctors think it necessary, they may suggest you have various tests around this time to rule out any abnormalities. The length of your baby's thighbone will be measured, as well as the diameter of her head. The head measurement will be used to confirm the EDD.

Your baby's progress

She's looking more human now, with legs longer than her arms and the parts of her legs in proportion. Her skeleton continues to produce more bone and those parts with sufficient calcium can be seen on X-ray. She now has the same number of nerve cells as an adult. The nerves from her brain begin to be coated in a layer of myelin (protective fat). This is an important step in their maturation because it helps the passage of messages to and from the brain. Connections between nerves and

Your baby at 18 weeks of pregnancy

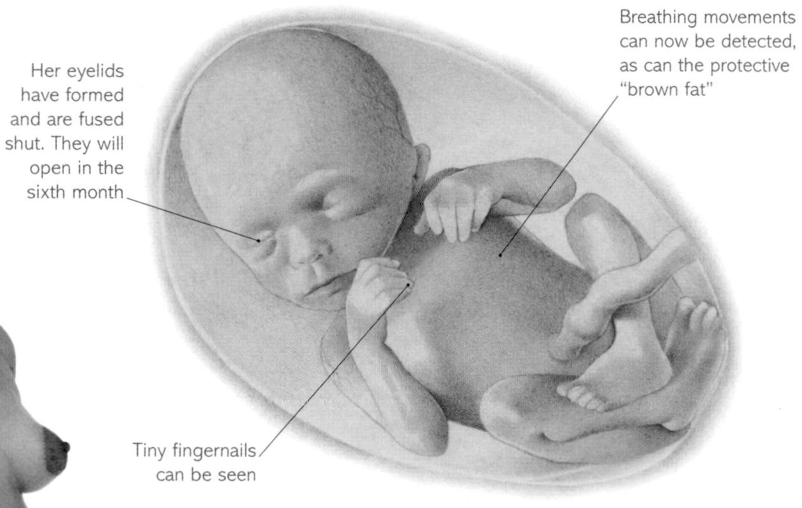

Her eyelids have formed and are fused shut. They will open in the sixth month

Breathing movements can now be detected, as can the protective "brown fat"

Tiny fingernails can be seen

Baby's vital statistics By the end of this month her crown to rump length will be 13.5cm (5½in), and she'll weigh 180g (6oz)

muscles are set up so that your baby's well-formed limbs can move around their joints when the muscles are stimulated to contract and relax. Her movements aren't yet under the control of her brain, though. Nor do you notice them yet because she's not big enough to activate nerve endings on your uterine wall. Second-time mothers tend to feel their baby's movements sooner (see p.194).

Your baby's external genital organs are taking on a more distinctive look. A girl's vaginal plate, the beginnings of her vagina, is developing, and a boy's testes are well on their way to descending into the scrotum.

Her support system

The placenta is making the increasing amounts of hormones (chorionic gonadotrophin, oestrogen, and progesterone) that are needed throughout pregnancy. It's also making an assortment of other hormones that keep your uterus healthy and play an essential part in the growth of your breasts in preparation for breastfeeding your baby. The placenta forms a barrier against general infection, although not viruses such as rubella (German measles) and AIDS, and poisons such as alcohol and nicotine.

The placenta is firmly attached to the uterine wall (usually the upper part). By the end of week 16, the placenta has grown to about 1cm (⅓in) in thickness and is 7–8cm (3½in) across. It continues to grow until term, when it will weigh about 500g (1lb), and measure 3cm (1¼in) thick and 20–25cm (8–10in) across.

Baby

Your baby's skin is transparent and her blood vessels can be seen clearly. Her bones, which are beginning to harden throughout her body, can also be seen.

Taste buds They've begun to develop on her tongue.

Ears As the tiny bones inside her ears harden, she begins to hear sounds – your voice, your heart, and your digestion rumbling.

Lungs They are developing and she "breathes" the amniotic fluid. She'll continue to receive oxygen via the placenta until she's born.

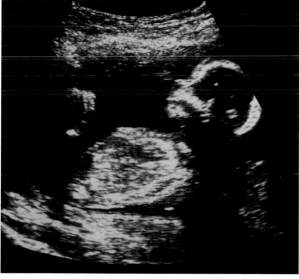

▲ULTRASOUND SCAN At this time, you'll clearly see smaller features, such as your baby's nose, clearly on a scan. Her head is still large compared to her body.

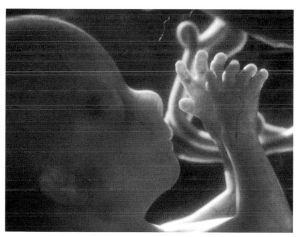

▲HEAD AND FACE Her face is looking more human and she's starting to frown and squint. Eyebrows and eyelashes start to grow, and the hair on her head is coloured by pigment cells. Her eyes look straight ahead although they're still widely spaced. The retinas of her eyes are sensitive to light, although they're still covered by her eyelids, and she's aware of bright light outside of her mother's body.

Mother

Around this time, well into your second trimester, you'll probably notice that your energy and sense of fun have come back and any nausea should have disappeared.

Movements If you didn't feel your baby move earlier, you'll certainly notice him now.

Abdomen Your waistline has disappeared and you may notice stretchmarks.

Skin Dilated blood vessels may cause tiny red marks (spider naevi) to appear on your face, arms, and shoulders. These should fade after the birth.

Minor complaints Your gums may become spongy, probably because of hormonal influences. You may have constipation, heartburn, and bladder infections.

Metabolic changes Your thyroid gland becomes more active and you may perspire more heavily than usual. You may feel short of breath when you exercise.

Up to 22 weeks

By this time your baby has grown enough to have developed a nervous system and muscles that allow him to move around inside your womb, and he may be very active. Because he's still so small, he can swim up and down and be in any position at any time.

Your baby's progress

Up until about 19 weeks after your last period, your baby grows very rapidly. Now this growth rate slows down, apart from his weight gain, and he matures in other ways. He begins to build up his defence systems.

A sheath begins to form around the nerves in his spinal cord to protect them from possible damage. He also has his own primitive immune system, which will help to defend him from some infections. To make body heat and keep up his temperature, your baby needs some specialized fatty tissue. This is provided by a substance called "brown fat", which began to form during the fourth month. Now, deposits of brown fat begin to build up in areas of his body such as his neck, chest, and crotch. This will continue until term. One of the reasons that babies born prematurely are

Your baby at 22 weeks of pregnancy

His eyes and eyelids are now well developed

His ears have developed

Fine hair (lanugo) covers his body

Baby's vital statistics By the end of this month his crown to rump length will be about 17.5cm (7in) and he'll weigh about 450g (1lb)

so vulnerable is that they haven't had time to build up enough of this brown fat, and so they cannot keep themselves warm.

His skin will continue to grow, although it'll be red and wrinkled because there's so little fat underneath it. His body begins to get plumper from now on. The sebaceous glands (oil-producing glands in the skin) become active and make a waxy, greasy substance called vernix. This protects his skin during its long immersion in the amniotic fluid.

Your baby's body is also covered with fine hair called lanugo. Nobody's quite sure why babies have this hair, but it may help to regulate the body temperature, or it may help hold the protective vernix in place.

His movements As his nerve fibres become connected and his muscles continue to develop and grow stronger, his movements become more purposeful and coordinated. He embarks on his own athletics programme – stretching, grasping, turning – to build up his muscles, improve his motor ability, and strengthen his bones.

Sex organs A boy's scrotum is solid at this stage. A girl's vagina starts to become hollow and her ovaries contain about seven million eggs, which will be reduced to about two million at birth. By puberty, she'll have between 200,000 and 500,000 eggs and she'll release only 400–500 of these during her adult life – around one per month until menopause. Nipples and underlying mammary glands develop in both sexes.

Although he's well developed, your baby cannot yet survive outside your womb. His lungs and digestive system aren't fully formed, nor can he keep up his own body heat properly.

Vernix Skin glands make this waxy coating to keep his skin supple.

Taste He's now able to tell sweet from bitter.

Touch His skin is now sensitive to touch and he'll move in response to any pressure that's put on your abdomen.

Teeth Hidden in his gums, many of his "baby" teeth have already been formed.

Heartbeat This can now be heard by less sensitive stethoscopes.

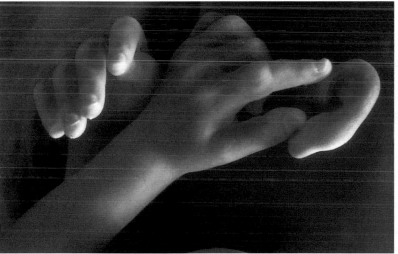

▲ **HIS HEARING** Your baby can hear the sounds of your blood flowing through your blood vessels, your heart beating, and your stomach rumbling. He can hear sounds from outside the uterus and will respond to sound, rhythm, and melody from now on. Sing and talk to your unborn child. After birth, he'll probably be soothed by the same songs, and he'll feel safe and secure when he hears his parents' voices.

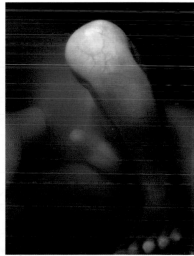

▲ **YOUR BABY'S GENITALIA** Your baby's sex was determined at conception. This ultrasound scan shows a direct view of the external genitals, revealing that this 17-week-old fetus is male.

Mother

Your baby's movements are well established now and you'll feel some every day. When she hiccups, for example, you'll feel a sudden jerk.

Weight You'll be putting on weight at the rate of about 500g (1lb) per week. Don't worry if you are told you look "small for dates". Your size will depend on many things such as your build, how tall you are, the way you move, and the amount of amniotic fluid inside. It's the size of your growing baby that counts and that can be checked by ultrasound scanning.

Aches and pains As your baby grows, and your uterus along with her, they push upwards against your ribcage. It'll rise by about 5cm (2in) and your lower ribs will spread outwards. This can give you rib pain and, because your baby is now beginning to press upon your stomach, you may also start to have bouts of indigestion and heartburn (see p.208). As your uterine muscle stretches, you may get stitch-like pains down the sides of your abdomen.

Up to 26 weeks

Your baby is growing taller and stronger, and her movements are becoming more complex. She's also showing signs of sensitivity, awareness, and intelligence. A baby born after 24 weeks of pregnancy is legally viable and could survive with specialized intensive care in a neonatal unit.

Your baby's progress

She's still red and skinny, but she'll soon start to put on weight. Her skin may look very wrinkled, but this is because she doesn't yet have much fat to plump it out. Her body is growing faster than her head and by the end of this month her proportions are about the same as those of a newborn. Her arms and legs have their normal amount of muscle, her legs and body are in proportion, and her bone centres are beginning to harden. Lines start to appear on the palms of her hands.

The brain cells she'll use for conscious thought now start to mature, and she begins to be able to remember and learn. (In one experiment, babies in the womb were trained to kick in response to a particular

Your baby at 26 weeks of pregnancy

Her skin has lost the translucent look it had before and has become opaque and reddish-looking. It's still wrinkled because she hasn't yet built up enough fat deposits

Her body is still thin, but more in proportion to her head

Baby's vital statistics By the end of this month her crown to rump length will be 25cm (10in) and she will weigh just under 1kg (2lb)

vibration.) The genitals of a boy and girl look completely different by this time; if your baby is a boy, testosterone-producing cells in the testes increase in number.

Her hearing Your baby can hear sound frequencies that you can't hear. She'll move more in response to high frequencies than to low ones. She'll also move her body in rhythm with your speech. If she hears a piece of music often, she may realize it's familiar to her when she grows up – even if she can't remember ever hearing it. Some musicians have said that they "knew" unseen pieces of music, and later found out that their mothers played these to them while they were in the womb.

She'll also learn to recognize her father's voice from this month onwards. A baby whose father talks to her while she's in the womb can pick out her father's voice in a roomful of people immediately after she is born. She'll respond to it emotionally – for example, if she's upset, she'll stop crying when she hears her father talking and calm down.

Her breathing Inside her lungs, more and more air sacs are forming. They'll continue to increase in number until she's about eight years old. Around them, the blood vessels that will help her to absorb oxygen and expel carbon dioxide are multiplying. Her nostrils have opened, too, and she's beginning to make breathing movements with her muscles, so that her system has plenty of breathing practice before she's born.

Baby

She continues to grow slowly and steadily. If she's born prematurely, she'd have a slim chance of survival now.

Lungs The bronchi (the main tubes leading from her windpipe to her lungs) are growing, although they aren't yet mature.

Brain The patterns of her brainwaves are now like those of a full-term newborn child. The source of these brainwaves is thought to be the cortex, the highly evolved part of the brain. She's now developed patterns of sleeping and waking.

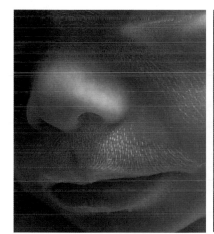

▲ **YOUR BABY'S FACE** The features of this six month old fetus are already very like those of a newborn baby. Lanugo, the downy hair on a baby's skin, forms patterns because of the oblique way in which the hair roots are positioned in the skin.

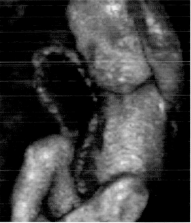

▲ **ULTRASOUND** This coloured 3-D ultrasound scan shows a 26-week-old fetus in the womb. The umbilical cord can be clearly seen. At this stage, the baby will be moving around a good deal and may respond to sounds such as drum beats by jumping up and down.

Mother

1
2
3
4
5
6
7
8
9
10
11
12
13
14
15
16
17
18
19
20
21
22
23
24
25
26
27
28
29
30
31
32
33
34
35
36
37
38
39
40

This ends your second trimester. You may start to feel tired and, knowing that your baby just needs to mature, you may begin to think more about his birth.

Colostrum Your breasts will probably have made this sweet, watery fluid, which is less rich than breast milk and easier to digest. It will provide your baby with his first few meals before your milk comes through (see also p.326).

Urination Your growing baby will now be pressing against your bladder and you'll feel like passing urine more often.

Sleeping problems You'll find it hard to get comfortable if you're big. Lying on your side with one knee to your chest and the other stretched out will probably be the most comfortable position.

Low back pain You may get some backache because of an alteration of your centre of gravity caused by the enlarged uterus plus the slight loosening of the pelvic joints. Wearing low-heeled shoes and sitting with a straight back on a hard chair or the floor will help. Don't lift heavy objects if you can help it.

Up to 30 weeks

Your baby's now so big that when a doctor or midwife examines you she can check his position and the way he's lying. This is the last month he can turn a somersault.

Your baby's progress

Great changes take place in your baby's nervous system this month. His brain grows larger (to fit inside the skull, it has to fold over and wrinkle up until it looks like a walnut), and his brain cells and nerve circuits are all fully linked and active.

Also, a protective fatty sheath begins to form around his nerve fibres, just as a similar sheath formed earlier around his spinal cord. This fatty sheath keeps on developing until early adulthood. Thanks to this, nerve impulses can travel faster and your baby is now able to cope with more complex types of learning and movement.

Your baby starts getting ready for birth. (If he were to be born prematurely at this stage, he'd have an excellent chance of survival. Even though he might have some breathing problems and difficulty in keeping himself warm, modern special care facilities would help him thrive.) He's beginning to gain some fat underneath his skin, which starts to smooth out, lose its wrinkles, and look more rounded. His coat of hairy lanugo

Your baby at 30 weeks of pregnancy

His hands are now fully formed and his fingernails are growing

His eyelids are open and he can now see and focus

Fat builds up under his skin

Baby's vital statistics By the end of this month his crown to rump length will be 28cm (11in), and he'll weigh about 1.5kg (3lb)

may reduce to just a patch on his back and shoulders. The membranes that sealed and protected his eyes while they were growing will have fulfilled their function by the beginning of this month. His eyes are now fully formed and his eyelids have separated, allowing his eyes to open. He continues to develop the swallowing and sucking skills that he'll need as soon as he's born.

His breathing Your baby has developed his mature breathing rhythm, and the air sacs in his lungs are starting to get ready for the first breath he'll take in the world outside your uterus. The air sacs line themselves with a coating of special cells and a fluid (surfactant) that will prevent them from collapsing.

His movements He'll find he has less room to move about in and may move around less. He'll wriggle uncomfortably if you're in a position that doesn't suit him (see p.194).

Orientation During his weeks of "gymnastics practice", your baby has done more than increase his muscle tone – he's developed the ability to position himself in space. He'll probably continue to lie with his head upwards during this month, although if he's maturing fast he may turn upside down and settle into place ready for delivery (engage) rather earlier than usual. This is more common in first babies. Babies can continue turning up to 36 weeks.

Baby

Your baby continues to gain weight and to mature. His kicking keeps him in touch with you.

Temperature He now begins to control his own body temperature.

Fat White fat begins to build up under his skin.

Red blood cells His bone marrow has now completely taken over responsibility for the making of red blood cells.

Urine He passes urine into the amniotic fluid at the rate of about 500ml (1pt) every day.

Genitals The testes of boy babies descend first into the groin and then into the scrotum. Premature boy babies will usually have undescended testicles.

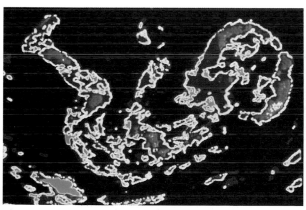

▲ **YOUR BABY GROWS** His body is growing plumper as fat builds up under his skin. His eyebrows and eyelashes are fully developed, and the hair on his scalp is growing longer. His eyelids have opened, and he begins to practise seeing and focusing – the limitations of his field of vision (20–25cm/ 8–10in) at birth is thought to be related to how far he's able to see while in the womb. As the ultrasound above shows, he now has the proportions of a newborn baby.

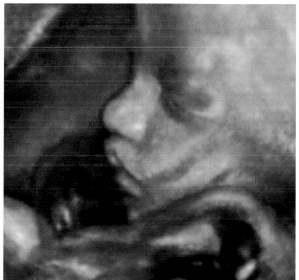

▲ **HIS FACE** The baby's maturing profile can be seen clearly in the 3-D ultrasound scan above.

Mother

You'll probably be having antenatal checks more often now. Your carers will monitor your blood pressure and urine and check your baby's position.

Contractions Your uterus hardens and contracts as a sort of practice for labour. These are known as Braxton Hicks contractions. They will last only about 30 seconds and some women are not even aware of them.

Pelvis Your pelvis has now expanded and may ache, especially at the back.

Blood Some women may have a low haemoglobin level at this stage of pregnancy.

Abdomen Your baby's getting bigger so that your uterus is pushed hard against your lower ribs, and your ribcage may become quite sore. Your abdomen is so stretched that your navel sticks out and the increased pigmentation of the linea nigra can make it look very prominent.

Up to 34 weeks

Thirty-four weeks after your last period, your baby is perfectly formed. All her proportions are exactly as you'd expect them to be at birth. She still has some maturing to do, though, and some more weight to gain before she's ready to be born.

Your baby's progress

Her organs are now almost fully mature, except for her lungs. These aren't yet completely developed, although they're making increasing quantities of surfactant, the fluid that will stop them collapsing once she begins to breathe air. She makes strong movements that can be felt on the surface of your abdomen. Almost all babies born at this time survive.

Her eyes, skin, nails, and hair Her irises now contract in response to bright light, and also to allow her to focus, although she won't need this skill until after she's born. Her skin is now pink rather than red, because of the deposits of white fat underneath it. Fat deposits build up under her

Your baby at 34 weeks of pregnancy

Fingernails reach tips of her fingers

There may be a lot of hair on her head

Her face is now smooth, with most of the wrinkles gone

Your baby is putting on weight; about eight per cent of her weight is fat

Baby's vital statistics By the end of this month her crown to rump length will be about 32cm (12in), and she'll weigh about 2.5kg (5lb)

skin to provide energy and regulate her body temperature after she's born. The protective vernix that covers her skin is now very thick. Her fingernails now reach the ends of her fingers but her toenails are not yet fully grown. She may have quite a lot of hair on her head.

Her position Some babies take up the head-downwards position about now, but there's still plenty of time – most don't engage until after 36 weeks. She may remain in the breech (bottom-down) position (see p.307) until birth, although most babies do turn on their own.

Her support system

From this month the placenta layers may start to thin. To make oestrogen, the placenta converts a testosterone-like hormone that's made by your baby's adrenal glands. By this month these glands are as big as those of an adolescent, and every day they produce ten times as much hormone as an adult's adrenal glands. They'll shrink rapidly after birth.

The amniotic sac, or bag of waters, contains a large amount of fluid, most of which is the baby's urine – she can produce as much as 500ml (1pt) of urine every day. Excess vernix, nutrients, and products necessary for the maturing of her lungs are also in the amniotic sac. The umbilical cord is large, strong, and tough. A firm, gelatinous substance surrounds the blood vessels and this prevents kinks or knots forming in the cord that could affect your baby's blood supply.

Baby

Your baby's main activity now is to settle into a head-down position and adjust to her lack of space in the uterus.

Eyes She can now focus and blink.

Weight gain She'll have gained at least 1kg (2lb) since last month. Most of this is increased muscle tissue and fat.

Lungs Your baby's lungs are still developing so that she can adjust to breathing outside the uterus. If she were to be born at this stage, she'd almost certainly have breathing difficulties, although she would have an excellent chance of survival.

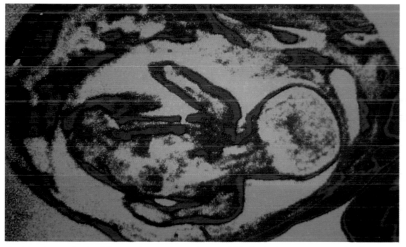

▲ **YOUR BABY'S SIZE** It's now becoming rather a tight fit in the uterus, especially if your baby's large. Because of this she may start to move less, although you should still be able to feel her moving (see pp.194 and 195). Her body, like that of the baby in the scan above, will now start to become tightly curled as her elbow and knee space is restricted. Quite a few babies are bottom-down (breech) at the start of this month (see column, p.259), but most will have tipped head-down by term.

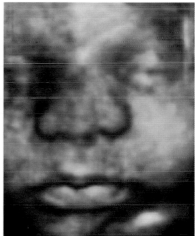

▲ **HER HEAD AND FACE** This coloured 3-D ultrasound scan shows the well-developed features of a 32-week-old fetus. Her irises can now dilate and contract. She can also close her eyelids and has begun to blink.

Mother

1
2
3
4
5
6
7
8
9
10
11
12
13
14
15
16
17
18
19
20
21
22
23
24
25
26
27
28
29
30
31
32
33
34
35
36
37
38
39
40

When you see your doctor or midwife at this stage, they'll be checking that all is going well.

Engagement In most first-time mothers, the baby's head drops down into the pelvis at about 36 weeks. In subsequent pregnancies it's normal for your baby's head not to engage until later, sometimes not until labour has started.

Posture You may tend to make up for extra weight at the front by leaning backwards. Your centre of gravity has altered, so you may bump into things or drop them.

Sleeping and resting It may be more and more difficult for you to get a good night's sleep as your large abdomen makes it hard to get comfortable. Put your feet up and rest as much as you can.

Nesting instinct You want to do things like clean the cooker! Try to resist it – you'll need all your energy for giving birth.

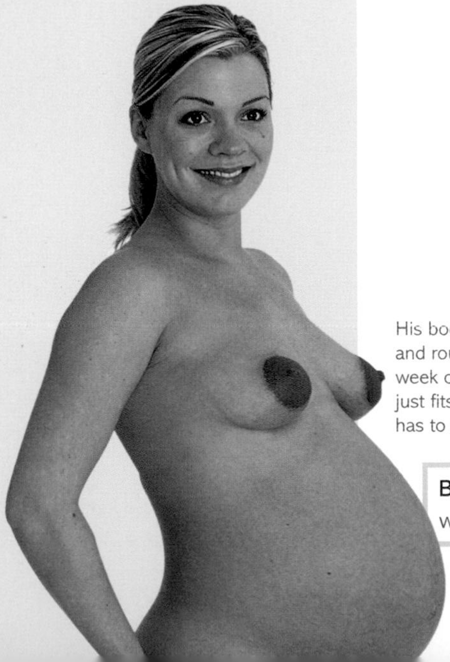

Up to 40 weeks

Most women have their fertile time about 14 days after the first day of their menstrual period. Because of this doctors set an artificial, but convenient, timescale of 40 weeks, calculated from the date of your last menstrual period (see p.63). A baby actually reaches "full term", meaning he's fully developed, after about 38 weeks.

Your baby's progress

During this month your baby will usually shed most of the fine hair (lanugo) from his body. There may be some small patches left in odd places and perhaps some in his body creases.

His skin is smooth and soft, and there is still some vernix left on it (mostly on his back), which will help his passage down the birth canal. He'll be almost chubby before birth. His fingernails are long and may have scratched his face – they'll need trimming after birth. His eyes are

Your baby at 40 weeks of pregnancy

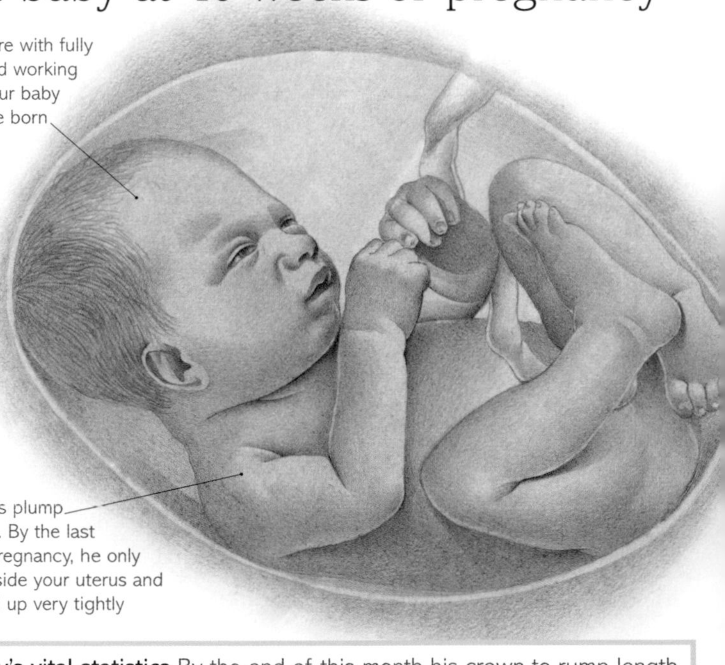

Fully mature with fully formed and working organs, your baby waits to be born

His body is plump and round. By the last week of pregnancy, he only just fits inside your uterus and has to curl up very tightly

Baby's vital statistics By the end of this month his crown to rump length will be about 35–37cm (14–15in), and he'll weigh 3–4kg (6½–9lb)

blue, although they may change in the weeks after birth. When he's awake his eyes are open. In these last weeks, your baby produces increasing amounts of a hormone called cortisone from his adrenal glands. This helps his lungs to mature and prepare for his first breath.

Meconium Your baby's intestine is filled with a dark green, almost black, substance called meconium. This is a mixture of the secretions from his alimentary glands together with the lanugo that's been shed from his body, pigment, and cells from the wall of his bowel. It'll be the first bowel motion he'll pass after birth, but he may pass it during delivery.

Immune system His own system is still immature, so to make up for this he receives antibodies from you via the placenta. These protect him against anything that you have antibodies for, such as flu, mumps, and German measles. After he's born, he'll keep on getting antibodies from you via your breast milk.

His support system

The placenta now weighs 500g (1lb), measures 20–25cm (8–10in) in diameter, and is 3cm (just over 1in) thick, thus creating a wide area for the exchange of nourishment and waste products between yourself and your baby. There's now more than 1 litre (2pt) of water in the amniotic sac.

The hormones made by the placenta are stimulating your breasts to swell and fill with milk. These hormones also cause swelling in your baby's breasts, whether it is a boy or a girl. This will go down after birth.

Your baby prepares to be born; his lungs mature and the last of his brown fat is laid down.

Reproductive organs The testes of most boy babies will have descended by now. In a girl baby, the ovaries are still above the pelvic brim and don't reach their final position until after birth.

Movements Although your baby's movements will be much less strong than they were earlier, you should still be able to feel him kick.

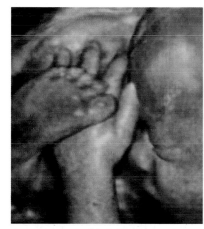

▲ **A TIGHT FIT** In this 3-D ultrasound scan of a full-term fetus, the head and a foot and hand are clearly visible. At this stage it's a tight fit in the uterus and the baby has to lie curled up.

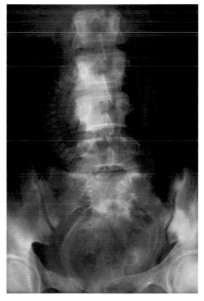

◀ **PREPARED FOR BIRTH** As your baby gets heavier and matures, he'll tip head-down in your uterus. In this colour-enhanced X-ray of a baby ready for birth, the baby's head can be seen settled deeply into the mother's pelvis.

Preparing for fatherhood

Most men have strong nurturing instincts and most, given half a chance, make excellent fathers. No one feels confident about parenthood and the prospect of becoming a father can be daunting. A little thought and preparation in advance can go a long way to boosting morale and to giving a man a sense of fulfilment.

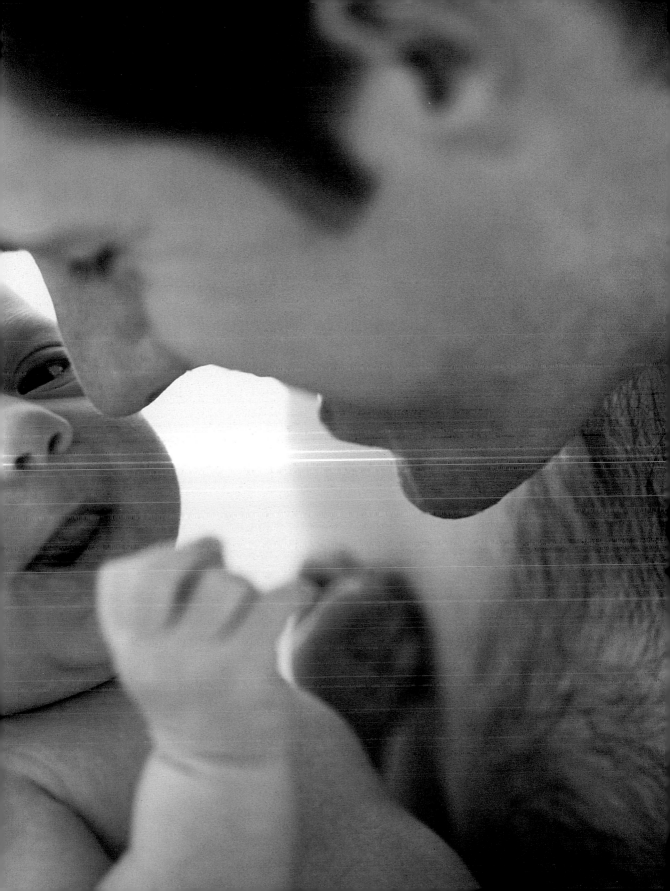

21st-century dads

Today, most men take it for granted that they share tasks that used to be seen more as a mother's responsibility. Dads are just as capable as mums of bathing the baby, doing the weekly shop, and taking children to and from school.

■ More and more men are becoming stay-at-home dads and the main carers of their children while mums go out to work.

■ Many fathers are fitting family matters, like the school run, helping in the classroom, or taking their child to the doctor, into their working day.

■ Most fathers love to share the bedtime bath and story routine, especially if they've been away from their children all day.

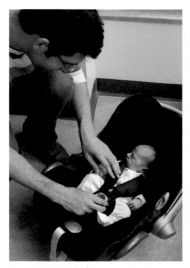

▲ SHARING Most men want to be an involved father from the moment their child's born. Men are just as capable of the nurturing role as women.

Becoming a dad

This chapter is for dads. Fathers often take a back seat in books like this and I'd like to correct that bias. Your baby doesn't have any notion about the difference between mothers and fathers. She just wants to be loved and cared for. Men can do these things just as well as women and caring for your baby helps build your relationship with her for the future.

Making room for fathers

With a little planning and a generous heart, both of you can enjoy sharing all the aspects of caring for your baby. After all, baby care means loving your baby, encouraging your baby, teaching your baby, watching your baby grow and develop, and establishing bonds with your baby that will probably be the strongest you ever make with anyone. Being a parent is perhaps the most important job any of us do. Who in their right mind doesn't want to be a part of all that?

No one has trouble defining a mother's role. Mothers care for children: they feed, comfort, dress, and bathe; they encourage, teach, carry, undress, put to bed, and maybe sing to sleep. We all know this because it's what our mothers did for us when we were children. Defining a father's role is more difficult and many men are struggling to come to terms with what it means to be a modern father. Really what's needed is for fathers to be much more involved with the day-to-day business of child care – for them to be more like mothers.

Your baby doesn't mind Babies and young children are happy to be cared for by their father or mother. What your baby needs is comfort, warmth, and security from her parents. Although she'll soon learn to tell her mother and father apart, she's not going to make value judgments based on what mothers and fathers ought to do. Apart from breastfeeding, there's nothing a woman can do for a baby that can't be done by a man.

The need for parenting Babies don't need mothering and fathering, they need parenting. They need the most important adults in their lives to be models of what parents do for their children. When this happens, the next generation of fathers won't be at a loss to know what a father's role should be. A child will only start to look to one parent rather than the other for her needs if this is what she learns she should do from her

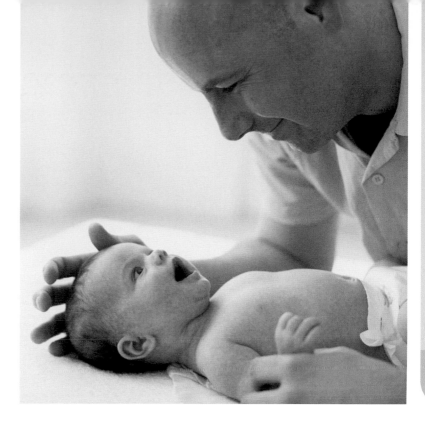

▶ **A CARING DAD** Caring for your baby helps build your relationship and that's a powerful argument for parenting being equal and shared.

experiences. If you, as a father, never change her nappy, hold her when she cries, or play and laugh with her, of course she'll relate more to the parent who does do all those things.

Your feelings about having a family

However much you long for a family, the decision to go ahead and have a child needs the same reasoned, clear-eyed evaluation you'd give to any other major change in your life, such as buying a house or a new car. It helps to be open with one another about your feelings and to put into words some of the thoughts and questions that may be lurking in the back of your mind. Even if you think you both really want a baby because you love each other and it seems like the natural thing to do, it's still a good idea to talk about all the issues involved. Have you thought about how a baby will affect your way of life? Does having a child seem the right thing for you as a couple, or are you just reacting to pressure from others, such as the potential grandparents? Do you both have the same desire for a baby?

A different kind of parenting

A father used to be a protector, out at work all day and with little direct involvement in the care of children. Now, fathers and mothers are equal partners at home. Both may be working, full or part time, and sharing the financial responsibilities and the juggling of caring for home and family. Some couples may decide they don't want to use any form of child care and so one of them takes a career break to stay at home. In an increasing number of couples it's the father who opts to be the carer while his wife earns the money. One reason why such families are often strong and successful units is because they make their plans carefully and take account of both partners' talents. But whatever practical arrangements you make, providing a stable, loving, and open environment in which to bring up children is what matters the most.

Bonding with your baby-to-be

It's never too early to start bonding with your baby. Babies can hear sounds outside the womb by five or six months. If you talk to your baby, he'll get to know your voice even before he's born – in fact, he'll be able to hear your low-pitched voice more clearly than his mother's. To help you bond with your baby:

■ gently massage your partner's tummy and feel your baby move

■ talk and coo softly to your baby, and kiss and nuzzle him through your partner's skin

■ listen to your baby's heartbeat – a cardboard tube, such as the inner tube of a toilet roll, can make a good amplifier

■ go to ultrasound scans with your partner and watch your baby develop (see p.180)

■ read as much about pregnancy and birth as you can so you can talk things over together

■ talk over names for your baby together – this gives your unborn baby a personality and you can start relating to him

■ check the dates of antenatal classes and talks on childbirth and plan ahead so you can go too

■ if you really want to know how your partner feels, find out about the Empathy Belly – a device that you can wear, which mimics many of the physical changes of pregnancy.

The expectant father

The moment you find out that you're going to be a father is one of the most exciting of your life and you'll probably feel just as emotional about the news as your partner does. Talk to your partner about the pregnancy and get involved in plans for the birth. Allow your unborn baby to become as big a part of your life as you can. After all, this great event is something that's happening to both of you, not just to your partner.

Understanding your feelings

For the first couple of months your partner will look much the same as usual and you may find the fact that you're expecting a baby hard to take in. Don't worry if your feelings about the pregnancy aren't the same as hers at first; your experiences are very different. A couple doesn't suddenly become one person with one set of feelings just because they're having a baby together. Later on, when you see your partner's body beginning to change and you've seen your baby on an unltrasound scan and felt his first movements, the idea of having a child of your own will become more real.

You may find at this time that your feelings of joy and excitement are mixed with fears and worries about how your life will be affected and whether you'll be able to cope financially. There's no doubt that having a child can be an extra financial burden, especially if one of you is going to give up your job to care for your baby, but don't rush into making life-changing decisions. You may find that having time to spend with your child becomes much more important to you than making more money or offering material possessions.

Getting involved

When you're an expectant father you're likely to feel not quite in control of things. You may feel something of an outsider and well-meaning female friends and relatives may assume you're not really involved and seem to push you out of what they see as their territory. Medical professionals, such as obstetricians and midwives, will understandably direct their conversations to your partner more than to you.

Take the initiative Don't just step back and allow your female relatives and friends to become more involved than you. Talk to your friends and colleagues: some may tease you at first but you'll probably find other fathers will be keen to share their experiences with you. Try to find out as much as you can about the pregnancy so that you can understand what's happening in your partner's body. Go with her to the scans so that you can see your baby developing, talk about the fact you're going to be a father, and ask as many questions as you want.

Plan for the birth together

Talk to your partner about the type of birth that she wants (see p.106) and how best you can be involved. Plan to talk to your employer about taking time off for antenatal appointments and classes as well as for the birth and afterwards, so that you can spend some time at home with your partner after your baby is born.

The birth plan Go through the birth plan together (see p.122), but don't impose your views. If she feels strongly about certain aspects, such as trying for a drug-free labour (see p.282), respect her feelings but make sure you both know the pros and cons. Some men worry they'll feel squeamish at the birth but few are. Witnessing the birth of your child is probably one of the most moving things that will ever happen to you, and holding your baby in the first few seconds after the birth not only helps bond the two of you, but is a tremendous emotional experience.

It's your baby too

There's no need to hold back any of your feelings or thoughts. Feel free to:

■ express your concerns

■ talk frankly to your partner about sex so it doesn't become an issue

■ be involved in all arrangements and plans for the birth

■ go to antenatal classes

■ go to antenatal appointments to hear your baby's heartbeat and see him move on the ultrasound

■ visit the hospital and meet the doctors and midwives

■ be present at the birth.

How you can help

WHAT TO DO	HOW IT CAN HELP YOU
Talk to your partner	The best way to understand how your partner is feeling and what's going on in her body is to talk to her. Ask her what it feels like when your baby moves; go over your plans for the birth together; find out if she's got particular discomforts. It'll also help her to share her experiences with you.
Go to antenatal classes	If you go to antenatal classes (especially father-only sessions) you'll have a chance to learn about what will happen at the birth and talk through your own worries. This will help you to work out the best way to support your partner and to be more involved in making decisions about the birth.
Talk to other fathers	Get to know the other expectant fathers at antenatal classes – they'll probably be feeling much the same as you and be glad to have someone to talk to. Talk to friends and colleagues who have babies; find out what their experience was like and ask their advice.
Read about pregnancy	Read pregnancy and parenting books and any leaflets you're given. The more you understand about what's going on during the pregnancy, the more familiar it will become and you'll appreciate more how your partner is feeling. You'll also be able to give your partner support if she's worried or anxious about anything.
Ask questions	Go to antenatal appointments with your partner so that you can meet the professionals and be present at the examinations. If you're a first-time parent, there'll be things you don't understand and need to know more about. If you ask questions of professionals they're more likely to involve you.

Coping with the unexpected

A labour that doesn't go to plan can be scary for both of you. It helps to be prepared in advance and accept that unexpected interventions may be necessary.

■ Well before your baby is due, talk to your partner about any special situations that could come up. Make sure you know her views and preferences. Bear in mind, though, that she may change her mind when it comes to the point.

■ Unless it's an absolute emergency, talk through any interventions suggested and ask questions if anything isn't clear. But remember that the final decision is hers.

■ If your medical attendants suggest something you know your partner wants to avoid, try to buy time. For instance, if labour has slowed, suggest a change of position before starting measures to accelerate labour.

■ If the medical team decides the labour needs monitoring with high-tech equipment, try not to be distracted by it. Concentrate on your partner, not the machines.

■ If the medical team does have to intervene, it's not your partner's fault. These things happen.

■ Whatever happens, talk about it afterwards with your partner, but also with friends and, if necessary, health professionals. You'll have a lot of feelings to work through.

Dads at the birth

When the due date is near, make sure your partner can always get in touch with you easily. Your support during the labour and birth will be a huge comfort to her and you have a practical role too. Trust your intuition and judgment as to what's needed and ask for feedback.

During labour

Your partner will need you with her once labour starts. You may feel that the medical staff have everything under control and there's not a lot you can do, but there is and it's important for you to be there and to be loving and intimate with your partner. Whatever you're feeling like yourself, try to be slow and gentle, quiet and reassuring. Don't try to do too much and get in the way of the medical staff or become an irritation to your partner; always give her space when she wants it. Be positive and don't criticize her; she needs plenty of praise, encouragement, and sympathy to keep her going.

Practical help There are lots of things you can do to help your partner cope with the discomfort and the pain of giving birth. Get her a warm hot-water bottle if she's got backache, refresh her with sprays of water or a cool flannel if she's too hot, and give her sips of water if her mouth is dry. If she wants to go without pain relief, encourage her while it seems reasonable, but if she asks for it, don't put her off. She's the one who's in pain. You'll certainly have talked about it beforehand and she may at that time have been quite adamant that she didn't want pain relief. But if she changes her mind in labour don't argue with her; nobody can possibly know how they're going to feel when giving birth until it actually happens.

Seeking explanations Talk to the midwife or doctor if you don't understand what's happening, or if you're worried. They're there to help both of you, and they have your partner's and your baby's best interests at heart. At the same time, don't let the hospital staff and their machines become the focus of your attention. Your job is to support your partner.

Your partner's moods Keep your sense of humour; if your partner shouts – or swears – at you, or seems to get angry or overwrought, take it in your stride. It's her way of coping with a very stressful situation and quite often happens, particularly at the transition phase of the first stage of labour (see p.273). Treat it as a positive step towards the birth – it's a sign that the second stage of labour isn't far off.

Second stage and birth

Helping your partner and watching your baby being born is an overwhelming experience for all fathers. The second stage is hard work for mothers, but there are ways you can really help your partner during this stage, so that you can feel as involved in your baby's birth as possible.

Practical help If you've been going to antenatal classes together, you'll already have worked out together the positions that your partner thinks will be best for her when giving birth. Help her to get into the position she feels is right, and support her there. This may not be the one she thought of using, nor even be among the ones you've practised. That doesn't matter; just support her in whatever position she feels comfortable in at the time. Keep encouraging her all the time throughout the second stage, and keep in physical contact so she knows you're with her all the way.

The moment of birth If you can see your baby's head as it crowns, describe it to your partner or hold a mirror for her so she can see the head too – this will be a huge encouragement to her. Don't get in the midwife's way, though, as she'll need to be able to monitor your baby's progress second by second. Once your baby is fully out, let your partner know what sex it is, even if you'd been told this during the pregnancy. It's a good idea to say that you have a son or a daughter, not just "it's a boy", or "it's a girl"; the words "son" and "daughter" express family feelings. If the midwife agrees, clamp and cut your baby's cord yourself. It's a fantastic moment – the moment your baby really becomes an individual being.

Sharing feelings When your baby is born, share the first minutes of your child's life with your partner. You'll probably be very emotional and if you feel like weeping, don't hold back. By all means photograph or film your partner and baby, but don't do this instead of helping them if they need you. They're more important than anything else.

Meeting your baby

This is the moment you've waited nine months for, the moment when you can take your baby in your arms together for the first time. Everything you've just gone through will feel worthwhile. Your midwife will probably lay the baby on your partner's tummy or give him to one of you to hold while the cord is clamped and cut; take your shirt off so your baby can feel and smell your skin. Hold him close to your face and let him look up into yours. Share this moment and savour it; this is a meeting that will change both your lives forever. You'll never forget this experience – the moment when you claim your new status as parents.

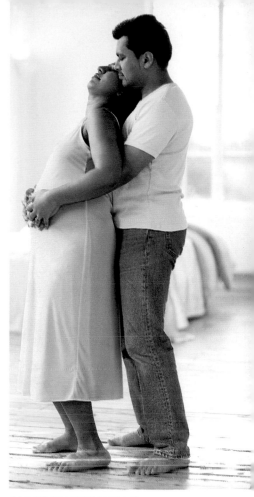

▲ **POSITIONS FOR LABOUR** Support your partner in whatever position she finds most comfortable for giving birth. Many women like to stand or squat and being held by their partner provides warmth and loving reassurance.

▼ **HELPING AFTER A CAESAREAN** If your partner has had a Caesarean delivery, she'll need plenty of rest so she can heal and recover. She'll need your help with lifting and carrying in the first weeks after the birth.

After the birth

You may feel as emotionally exhausted as your partner after the birth, but don't forget how physically exhausting labour and birth is for a woman. Because your partner is so tired she may not appear to experience quite the same emotions as you.

Your partner's reactions You'll probably feel a wave of euphoria once your baby's born, but, particularly if labour has been long and arduous, your partner may be just too tired to enjoy this same "buzz" immediately. Just hold her close and let her know how proud you are of her and of your new son or daughter. Stay with them both for as long as possible after the birth, and help get them settled into the postnatal ward.

Valuing your role Be ready to congratulate your partner on her achievement, and let her know how much you appreciate her. But although all your thoughts will be with her, don't belittle your own contribution and the support you've been able to give. You may think you haven't really been much help – this is a common feeling for fathers who've seen their partners struggling through labour. Most mothers, though, say just how important it was to have the emotional support and encouragement from their partner throughout the labour and birth.

Saying hello Take the chance to hold your baby while your partner is being stitched, or checked. Let her look into your eyes and hold her close, just 20–25cm (8–10in) from your face. She'll be able to see you and smell you, and she'll learn to recognize you from the very beginning (see p.316). Remember, too, that sight is not her only way of experiencing this new world, and that the sense of touch is very important to babies. Take your shirt off and hold her against your skin or gently stroke her – both are strong ways of bonding with your new baby.

Caesarean deliveries

Even if your partner has chosen in advance to have a Caesarean delivery (see p.308) she'll still be anxious, because it's quite a major operation. But if she has to have an emergency Caesarean after labour has started, she may feel distressed, bewildered, and helpless. There's much you can do to smooth the way for her. If she's finding it difficult to talk to the doctors, make sure you find out exactly why they want her to have a Caesarean. Although she has to give her permission for the operation, she may still not be quite clear afterwards what the reasons were, so it's important for you to help her understand them.

Caesarean under regional anaesthesia Unless your partner particularly wants a general anaesthetic or the operation is too urgent, ask if it can be done under spinal anaesthesia. This means you can share the experience and meet your new baby together. You don't have to watch what's going on; you'll both be shielded by the surgical drapes. But if you find the operation distressing or you feel faint – and many people do, even nurses – leave the room quickly. Don't hang on, the medical staff have enough to do without caring for you.

Caesarean under general anaesthetic If the Caesarean is done under general anaesthetic, your partner may not regain consciousness for an hour or more, and you'll probably be given your baby to hold for much of this time. Do cherish this very special time with your baby: father–child bonding can often be at its best following a Caesarean section birth, because the early time you have together is so precious.

Sudden birth – the father's role

Occasionally labour comes on with such speed that a mother is overwhelmed by the desire to push before her partner can get professional help, let alone take her to the hospital! Although the second stage can take a couple of hours, it may not, and babies have been known to be born after a couple of pushes. If it looks as if this is about to happen, there's no need to worry – most emergency births are perfectly straightforward.

What to do first Don't leave your partner alone for more than a minute or two; she needs to know that you are right by her. Help her get into a comfortable position, then telephone the doctor or midwife. If you can't get hold of them, call the emergency services and ask for an ambulance. Wash your hands well and get a heap of clean towels ready. Fold one and put it to one side for the baby. If you've got time, find some old sheets or plastic sheeting to cover the floor and furniture.

During the birth Watch for the top of your baby's head appearing at the vaginal opening. When you see it, ask your partner to stop pushing if she can and just pant. This will give her vagina a chance to stretch fully without tearing. Feel around your baby's neck to find if the cord is looped round it. If it is, hook your finger under the cord and draw it over her head. Hold your baby firmly as she emerges – she'll be slippery – and give her straight to her mother to hold. Wrap her immediately in a spare towel so she doesn't get cold. Don't touch the cord. If the placenta is delivered before medical help arrives, put it in a dish or plastic bowl so that it can be checked by the midwife or doctor.

Home alone

When you go home after the birth, leaving your partner in hospital, you may feel lonely and possibly a bit "flat". Don't worry, there's plenty that you can get on with.

■ Get on the phone and tell friends and relatives the good news.

■ Take the chance to catch up on sleep. You've had an exhausting time, too, during the labour and you'll be better able to support your partner when she comes home if you've had some rest.

■ Fit a baby seat in your car, if you haven't already got round to doing this.

■ Catch up with the washing and cleaning at home and stock up on food, so everything is ready and welcoming when your partner and your new baby come home.

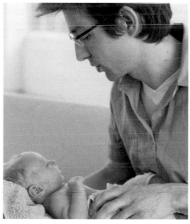

▲ **CARING FOR YOUR BABY** If your baby has been born at home it's easy for you to get involved right away. Tasks such as bathing her and changing her nappies give you time to bond with her.

What a new dad needs

As a new father, you may feel that your relationship with your partner is one-way traffic at this time, with you giving all the support. It's reasonable to expect something back and your partner should try to:

■ recognize your difficulties. It'll help both of you if she can accept that this is a confusing and emotional time for you too

■ give you some of her time. Caring for your baby will be time-consuming but it's good for you as a couple and as new parents if she can try to devote some time to your relationship

■ allow you to make mistakes. If your partner gave birth in hospital, she'll have had more time to get used to your baby. She'll need to let you get used to handling and caring for your baby, too – and not criticize if you fumble at first

■ be open about when to resume sex. You may feel like it before she does, but be understanding. Accept that it's probably better to be content with loving, non-penetrative sex until after she's had her six-week postnatal visit and she's had a chance to discuss contraception with her doctor.

▶ **SPENDING TIME TOGETHER** Time spent with your new baby and your partner is irreplaceable. Even if you have to go back to work soon after the birth, try to spend as much time together as you can, especially in the early days.

Getting to know your new baby

The first few weeks with your new baby are such an important time. You'll need to get to know her and start feeling comfortable in your new role. Your contribution is vital so spend as much time as you can with your baby.

The first few days

After the birth, you may be feeling an intense joy and elation that you want to share, while your partner seems a bit distant as her body recovers from labour and she tries to get breastfeeding started. Don't worry – there's plenty you can do that will involve you with both mother and baby.

Take the initiative Don't wait to be asked to share your baby's care. Take the chance to learn how to do all the practical things your baby needs while your partner's still in hospital. It will help you bond with your baby, and allow your partner to get some rest.

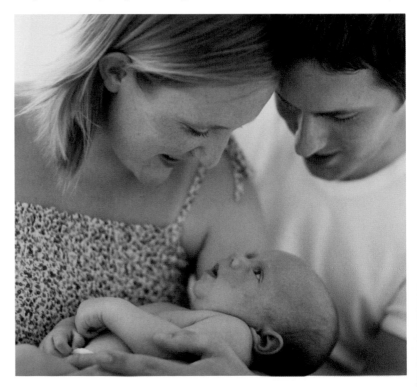

Get to know your baby Use these early days to establish a close relationship. Even if your partner is in hospital, change your baby's nappies and get used to handling her. Talk to her, hold her close so that she can focus on your face, or simply hold her if she's asleep. Bring her to your partner when she needs to be fed, and try to be there to help when she has her first bath.

Be ready for your partner's mood swings Some time during the first week your partner may get the "baby blues". They can happen as a reaction to the sudden withdrawal of the pregnancy hormones and to all her new responsibilities. These "baby blues" are temporary and shouldn't last more than a week to ten days. Your partner may try to hide her feelings so as not to worry you or because she fears you won't take her seriously. Don't belittle her or make light of her state of mind – she has a lot to cope with. If her baby blues last more than two weeks, speak to your doctor to head off postnatal depression (see p.361).

The new relationship

Concentrate on building your relationship with your baby from the start and spend as much time as possible with her. Don't isolate yourself or just see yourself as the breadwinner – most fathers are entitled to some paternity leave nowadays so take full advantage of this. Being an equal partner in your baby's care will be enormously rewarding to you and will help your family as a whole.

Give your baby love Babies need as much love and cuddles as they can get, and there's no difference between a mother's love and a father's love, except, of course, when your baby is hungry and needs breastfeeding. At all other times, she'll be just as happy with your closeness and attention. Being close and loving with your baby will mean that she learns to feel secure and content with both of you. This will help her settle and also take some pressure off your partner.

Support your partner Your partner will be very tired in the early weeks after the hard work of the labour and birth, and from the physical and emotional responsibility of breastfeeding. Give her as much time and space as you can for coping with the feeding and reassure her constantly that she's doing a great job. Your support can make all the difference. If you've gone back to work and your partner's at home with the baby, phone home during the day and do as much as you can for your partner and your baby in the evenings and at weekends. Perhaps you could develop your own special routine with your baby.

What a new mum needs

As a new father, you may be tempted to concentrate only on the day-to-day business of looking after the baby. Remember that your partner has strong emotional needs too. Try to:

■ recognize her vulnerability. A new mother feels very exposed, both physically and emotionally, in the days after the birth

■ appreciate the depth of her feelings. Try to accept the strength of your partner's overwhelming involvement in your baby. Even if this seems to exclude everyone else, don't see it as a rejection of yourself

■ protect her privacy. One of your most important roles is to make sure your partner isn't exhausted by visitors. Help her get enough time and space to get used to breastfeeding and to recover from the labour and birth.

Sleep routines

Understanding the way your baby's sleep patterns work will help you to tune into her needs, particularly at night.

Your baby's sleep needs She'll spend 50–80 per cent of the time in light sleep, when she wakes very easily. Her sleep cycle – light, deep, light – is shorter than an adult's, and she's vulnerable to waking each time she passes from one sleep state to another. Your baby isn't waking to spite you. She's programmed to wake up for all kinds of reasons – when she's wet, hot, cold, unwell – because her survival depends on it.

Having a sleep routine Your baby has to be deeply asleep before she'll settle so try a soothing sleep routine – gentle rocking, quiet songs, and talking softly. When she first falls asleep, lay her down and gently pat her shoulder at about 60 beats a minute for a few minutes. She's deeply asleep when her eyelids don't twitch and her limbs feel limp.

Time together If you're back at work and you find your baby's usually asleep by the time you get home, ask your partner if she can nap more in the afternoon so that she's awake when you arrive. This might not work so don't blame your partner. Instead, try getting up earlier to spend time with your baby before work.

Night duty

WHAT TO DO	HOW IT CAN HELP
Prepare yourselves for broken nights	Many babies continue to wake once or twice during the night well beyond 12 months. If you're both prepared for this, you'll find it easier to cope.
Share the burden	Take turns to get up when your baby wakes. You may both be back at work or one of you may be staying at home while the other goes out to work, but remember that looking after a baby is also a full-time job.
Adjust your sleep pattern	Broken nights are not necessarily sleepless nights. By adjusting to a new sleep pattern, you'll find that you're able to wake, attend to your baby, and then go back to sleep immediately.
Keep your baby close	Have your baby's cot by the side of your bed so you don't have to disturb yourselves too much when she wakes for a feed. Put her back in her cot when you're ready to go back to sleep.
Stay together	Sleeping apart so only one of you is disturbed may seem a tempting solution, but it could undermine your relationship with each other and with your baby. Keep this as a last resort – if one of you is ill or particularly tired.
Avoid sleep deprivation	Long-term sleep deprivation can affect your health. It's better for you both to lose some sleep than for one of you to take all the burden and become completely exhausted.

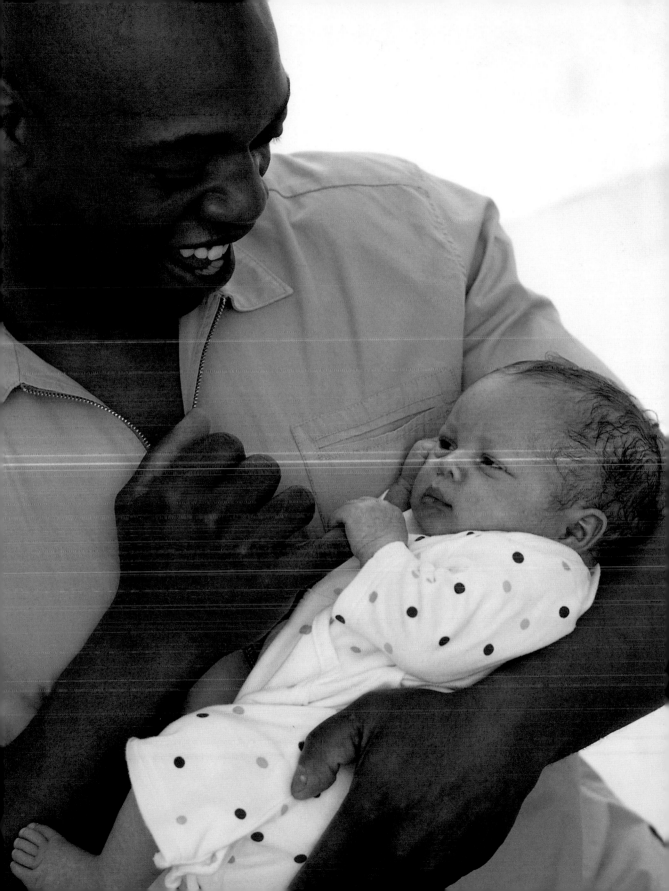

The birth of your choice

There are so many choices to make about the way you'll give birth to your child and it's important to know all the options. In theory, there's no reason why you shouldn't have exactly the kind of birth you want, but it's up to you and your partner to make sure you're able to take an assertive, informed part in the way your labour and delivery will be handled.

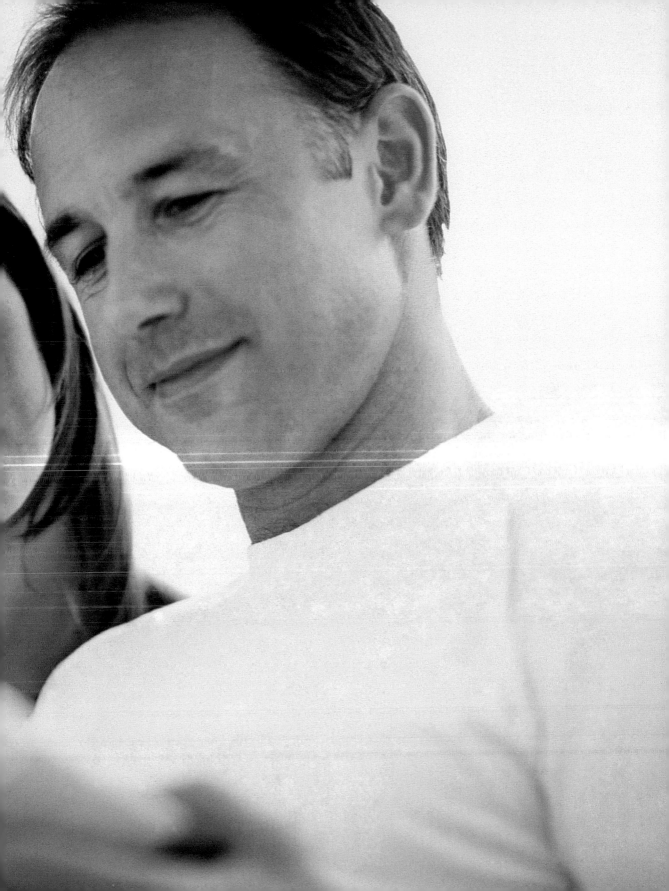

Active birth

Whether you opt to have your baby in hospital or at home, you'll be encouraged to have an active birth, in which your partner or other assistant, such as a birth coach, is also involved.

An active birth means that you're not lying down in bed for the labour and delivery. Mothers are encouraged to move around, supported by their partners, and get actively involved in the process of childbirth in whatever positions feel most comfortable.

Most childbirth classes include guidance on preparing yourself for an active birth and there's no doubt that movements and positions that help aim contractions downwards, pushing the baby towards the floor, make labour more efficient. Squatting, kneeling, sitting, or standing can all help to reduce pain and make labour easier, shorter, and more comfortable. A mother who's free to move around as she wishes may be less likely to need an episiotomy, forceps, or a Caesarean section.

The choices for childbirth

Women today want to be in control of their health, including the birth of their children, and the medical profession has generally responded enthusiastically to changing desires and needs. The "choices" for childbirth have never been greater, nor our wishes more paramount. Most of us want to have our children more naturally, and this option is available, at home and in hospital.

The modern natural birth

Most women would like childbirth to be as natural as possible: they want the process of birth and delivery to be familiar so they don't feel nervous or afraid; they like to have a calm, friendly atmosphere, in which they're allowed to take up the positions that are most comfortable for them and there's no undue pressure to take pain-relieving drugs; and they prefer to avoid any unnecessary medical intervention. Female bodies are well designed for giving birth; the soft tissues of the birth passage open so that a baby is gently squeezed out. Breathing and relaxation techniques can make birth even easier to manage, and most women now have plenty of chances to learn these techniques.

Most of the natural childbirth philosophies include some form of psychological re-learning to help you reduce your expectation of pain and raise your pain threshold. Learning special breathing techniques is usually central to the philosophy. There are slight variations in the different types, but all teach you intense concentration on breathing patterns and the ability to relax your body at will. The best way to experience a totally natural birth is in a dedicated centre or at home, but most general hospitals now accept that women want to give birth in the position they find most comfortable.

The modern managed birth

Normal pregnancies and uncomplicated births are almost entirely managed by teams of midwives and, although they may take place in hospital, the trend is towards less medical intervention. In a managed birth, labour is actively controlled for the safety of both mother and baby. A highly controlled birth in hospital is essential for some women who may have complications during pregnancy, labour, and birth – if you're expecting twins, for example.

In a hospital setting all the modern obstetric procedures are available, whether your birth is complicated or not. Epidural anaesthesia is literally on tap and electronic fetal monitoring may be necessary. Consequently, medical intervention is more common in hospital: there are more inductions and Caesareans, and the use of forceps or ventouse is more common. Although these practices are of course helpful in the percentage of births in which intervention is needed, it's now recognized that the routine use of them isn't justified (see Issues to think about, p.109). However, most women find a hospital setting makes childbirth the event they expect it to be, and they feel more secure there. Amenities such as birthing pools are now available in most hospitals.

Home birth

In many European countries healthy women may choose to have their baby at home if their pregnancy has been straightforward. In the United Kingdom, some doctors encourage women to have a home birth, even with a first baby, but in the United States it's more difficult. Arranging a home birth in the UK can still be tricky, and you do need to be very sure it's the best option for you. Always keep an open mind about transferring to hospital if things aren't going well.

Some doctors may feel that a home birth isn't as safe as a hospital birth. But there's always some risk attached to giving birth, and statistics have proved that in some circumstances a hospital birth can actually be less safe than a planned home birth (see p.114). Unplanned out-of-hospital births can be extremely dangerous, though, whether it's a teenager trying to conceal an unwanted pregnancy or a couple who don't manage to get to the hospital in time, so their baby is born on the way.

Birthing pools

More and more women like to spend at least some of their labour in water.

Birthing pools are more often used for easing pain during labour, rather than for the birth itself. There can be some danger if the baby is delivered under water and the head isn't lifted out right away.

Most hospitals now have birthing pools available, or you may be able to hire a portable pool (see Useful addresses, p.370). Water births must always be supervised by a qualified attendant.

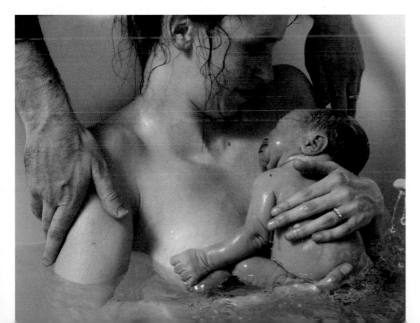

◀ **YOUR BIRTH ASSISTANT** Every woman going into labour should have someone other than medical and nursing professionals to help and encourage her. Research shows that good emotional and physical support from a trusted helper, such as your partner or a close relative or friend, can reduce a labouring woman's need for pain-relieving drugs.

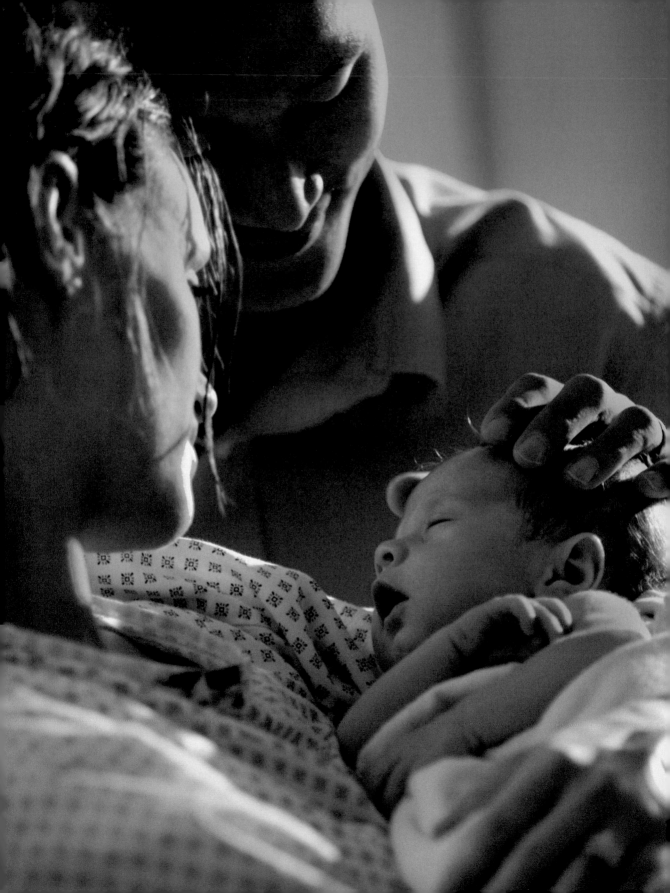

Issues to think about

There's more detailed information on the following subjects in other parts of this book, but this might be a good time to start thinking about certain issues. If you're aware of the arguments against some of these medical practices, you'll be more confident about questioning them, if you need to, with your medical and midwifery attendants. Generally they should be happy to go along with your wishes, but occasionally you may be told that to continue with a particular option will put your baby and you at serious risk – for instance, if your baby is showing signs of distress and you're still determined to continue with a totally natural childbirth. In this situation it's good to have an alternative birth plan ready (see column, p.123) and to be prepared to change it if need be.

This doesn't happen very often, though, so don't give in to medical intervention you're not happy about until you feel you've had proper answers to your questions. There can sometimes be intervention because midwives and doctors want to get a baby out quickly. An episiotomy, for instance, may be made necessary when you're encouraged to deliver your baby's head before the skin and muscles in your perineum have been given a chance to stretch. Given time, very few women need an episiotomy – as Michel Odent has proved (see p.113).

Nothing by mouth There's no medical or scientific rationale for starving a woman during labour. In fact, quite the opposite. Sometimes a labouring woman has a sudden need for energy and wants sugar. Other women don't feel like eating anything but they certainly need fluids; labour is hard work and uses up lots of energy, which causes sweating, and a woman must replace the fluids that she's lost through her skin. That said, if there's a high risk of a woman having an emergency Caesarean section, it's safer to give an anaesthetic on an empty stomach.

Moving rooms In most hospitals you should be able to labour and deliver your baby in the same room, without having to move. Depending on the unit, you may need to be moved to an operating theatre if you have to have an emergency Caesarean section. Otherwise, you should have peaceful surroundings, in a room equipped with good lighting, oxygen, and a suction apparatus to clear out the baby's air passages.

Induction Starting labour artificially is not a new idea, but it only became an easy procedure in the second half of the 20th century. However, labour should only be induced for medical reasons such as pre-eclampsia, high blood pressure, or post-maturity, when induction can save the lives of mothers and babies.

The case for home birth

A planned home birth can be one of the safest ways to have your baby.

A British all-party report concluded that although 94 per cent of all births take place in hospitals, they're no safer, and may be less safe, than home births.

In Australia, a study of 3,400 home births reported a lower perinatal mortality rate, and less need for Caesareans, forceps, and suturing for an episiotomy or a tear, than in women delivering in hospitals. The mothers taking part in the study were not all "low risk": the figures included 15 multiple births, breech deliveries, women who had previous Caesareans, and women with previous stillbirths. The group was older than the national average. Fewer than ten per cent had to transfer to hospital.

Episiotomy

An episiotomy is an incision that helps deliver a baby's head, but it isn't always needed.

If you've already had an epidural, you probably won't need any further anaesthetic before an episiotomy. If you haven't, you'll need a local anaesthetic in your perineum to numb the nerve supply, known as a pudendal block.

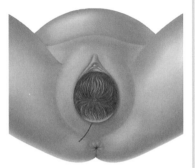

▲ **THE MEDIO-LATERAL CUT** This episiotomy cut is angled down and away from the vagina and the perineum into the muscle.

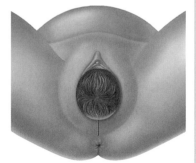

▲ **THE MID-LINE CUT** This cut is made straight down into the perineum, between the vagina and anus.

Amniotomy This means that the membranes (the bag of waters) surrounding the baby are artificially ruptured. This procedure is often referred to as artificial rupture of the membranes (ARM). It's not routine and is generally only done early in labour if the baby's heart rate is abnormal. Amniotomy is done for three reasons. The first is so that electronic fetal monitoring equipment can be set in place; the second is to check if the amniotic fluid contains meconium (this is the baby's first bowel movement and its presence may indicate fetal distress); the third reason is that once the bag of waters has been removed, the baby's head can then press hard on the mother's cervix, so helping along the dilatation of the cervix and completion of the first stage of labour.

Fetal monitoring For this, a heart-rate sensor is strapped to the mother's abdomen. A low-risk mother is monitored only intermittently through her labour, although some units prefer to monitor for about 20 minutes on admission so there's a permanent record of the baby's heart rate in case of problems later on. A mother with a high risk of problems is generally advised to have continuous monitoring. Fetal monitoring should not mean a woman has to keep still. Although movement is limited, you can sit on the bed and may be able to stand. Obviously having a "window" into the uterus during labour is of great value, but machines can go wrong, and they need trained staff to use them correctly. If machines are not working properly, or interpreted incorrectly, this can lead to unnecessary intervention. Also, using a machine to monitor the baby may switch attention from the mother to the machine, which can be very upsetting for a labouring woman.

Forceps These tong-shaped instruments (like large sugar tongs) are used to ease the baby's head out of the birth canal. Forceps have saved the lives of many babies and their mothers, and can reduce the need for a Caesarean section for a baby that's stuck up in the pelvis. The use of forceps does mean that an episiotomy is likely but not inevitable. Ventouse extraction (see pp.306 and 307), in which a cup is attached to the baby's head by suction, is increasingly being used instead of forceps but still does not always avoid the need for episiotomy (see below).

Episiotomy This is a surgical cut to enlarge the vaginal outlet at delivery, and is the most commonly performed operation in the West. Episiotomies are used in order to avoid tears, which have ragged edges and are difficult to stitch together. Also, they can take longer to heal. But you can avoid tears if you stop pushing while your baby's head is being born, and allow your uterus to ease out the head gradually rather than suddenly. If your baby's head is delivered suddenly, you are likely to tear so an episiotomy will be done if the perineum is under stress.

If an episiotomy is done too early, before your perineum has thinned out, muscle, skin, and blood vessels are damaged and there may be heavy bleeding. Tissues are crushed by the scissors as they are cut and this can lead to bruising, swelling, slow healing, and a perineum that is stitched too tightly. This tightness can be very uncomfortable during the postnatal period, and may even leave a painful scar, which can prevent you making love for months afterwards. If you want to avoid an episiotomy, it's a good idea to make it clear in your notes and birth plan that you don't want it to be done unless entirely necessary. If you do have to have an episiotomy, you have the right to have a local anaesthetic in the perineum before it's done, so insist on that.

Breech birth   Research shows that normal vaginal delivery is riskier than a Caesarean for a breech birth. Most breech babies are delivered by Caesarean section, but usually with epidural anaesthesia. Relatively few midwives have experience of breech deliveries so a breech baby will generally be delivered by a doctor.

Time   What hospitals judge to be the normal length for labour differs from place to place. For example, the "right" length for the second stage can be two hours or 30 minutes, or somewhere in between, depending on the obstetrician or midwife. In fact, the length of labour varies from woman to woman, and from birth to birth, and it's the marrying of what's normal for you with the hospital's policy that may cause problems. In most cases, if the first stage is thought to have gone on too long, the membranes are ruptured (if this hasn't been done already), or an oxytocin drip is set up to increase the rate and strength of contractions. If the second stage is taking a long time, your midwife may suggest an episiotomy or forceps delivery. Many midwives, though, say it's usually obvious when labour is going well, but is just taking some time, rather than being slow because something's wrong.

Being together   It's rare for babies to be separated from their mothers after the birth unless they need special care or the mother asks for her baby to be taken away for a while. But your partner won't be able to stay with you in the hospital, as there just aren't the facilities in most places, and this can be difficult for him after all the excitement and emotion of the birth. Before you go into hospital, ask how long your partner can stay with you after the birth. Many women say that they were too excited to sleep afterwards, and wished that they had someone to talk to.

When you need an episiotomy

There are times when an episiotomy is needed to make sure that your baby can be delivered safely.

■ If the birth is imminent and your perineum hasn't had time to stretch slowly.

■ If your baby's head is too large for your vaginal opening.

■ When you aren't able to control your pushing and you can't stop when you need to and then push gradually and smoothly.

■ When your baby is in distress.

■ If you need a forceps delivery (see p.306). With forceps, an episiotomy is likely but not obligatory.

■ If your baby is in a breech position and there's a complication during delivery.

The Bradley method

This birth preparation technique was developed by Dr Robert Bradley. It's also known as husband-coached childbirth, and the involvement of a woman's partner is a key feature.

The Bradley method teaches women to accept the pain of labour, and to go with the flow under the guidance of her husband or partner, friend, or counsellor. The coach attends the antenatal classes with the mother, helps her with her exercise and breathing routine, and comforts, coaxes, and coaches her through labour and delivery.

The danger of this is that most women need to be distracted from the pain, to focus outside of themselves, so that they can cope. Going into the pain can be totally overwhelming.

Also, each labour is completely individual and may be very unlike what you've practised, and a woman often reacts to giving birth in a different way than she'd imagined. Some birth partners can become so enthusiastic about the coaching that they lose sight of the woman and her needs.

Childbirth philosophers

The teaching and ideas of a number of people have changed women's attitudes to antenatal and postnatal care and led to alterations in the atmosphere and procedures surrounding childbirth in the Western world. Most of these theories seek to help a woman to follow her body's lead, in a loving and intimate environment.

Dr Grantley Dick-Read

Dr Dick-Read was the first obstetrician to realize that fear of giving birth was a main cause of pain in labour. He introduced the idea of natural childbirth, not only to the medical world but also to mothers. He recognized the need for proper education of mothers through antenatal classes and careful teaching, and also for emotional support, in the hope of eliminating fear and tension. His teaching was so basic that it's now taken for granted by all centres, and there's no method of childbirth that doesn't rely on his teaching, including breathing exercises, breathing control, and complete relaxation. Dick-Read's watchword for mothers was preparation – not only with information, but also by seeking help, reassurance, and sympathy.

Frederick Leboyer

Leboyer was influenced by the psychiatrists Reich, Rank, and Janov, who shared the belief that later problems in life stem from the trauma of birth. His concerns are less with the mother and more to do with the baby's experience of labour and delivery, and how this affects that baby once grown up. The Leboyer method works best viewed as an attempt to help people understand what a newborn baby sees, hears, and feels.

In his book *Birth Without Violence*, Leboyer suggests that the birthing room should have soft lighting, and there should be as little noise and movement as possible to lessen birth's trauma. Leboyer also believes that immediate skin-to-skin contact is essential to calm the baby, and that she should be laid on her mother's stomach as soon as she's born. He also says that the newborn should then be bathed in warm water as this is the closest she can get to the nurturing environment of the uterus.

Not all of this fits in with the physiology of what actually happens at birth. A baby needs to feel air on her face to stimulate her lungs to breathe for the first time: placing her in warm liquid may not be sufficiently stimulating for her to continue breathing. Many professionals say that there is no proof that Leboyer's theories work. However, it's only right that every baby be welcomed into the world with reverence, so even if you don't agree with all of Leboyer's ideas, it's still interesting to read about his suggestions for a gentler birth.

Dr Michel Odent

When he worked as a general surgeon, Dr Odent was extremely shocked when he first saw women pushing their babies uphill against the forces of gravity because their feet were held in stirrups. He realized that this meant stronger contractions were needed, which were more painful, and labour was much slower and more exhausting, and there were more complications because mothers were in a position where the baby was held back from being delivered.

His initial shock led him to develop his own methods of childbirth, broadly based on traditional midwifery, at Pithiviers in France. Odent believes that, given the opportunity, women in labour return to a primitive biological state, where they function at a new level of animal awareness, lose their inhibitions, and enter a state of consciousness in which they will follow their basic instincts. He believes that the natural pain relievers released by the body, endorphins, are responsible for this.

Pithiviers has the lowest rate in France for episiotomies, forceps deliveries, and Caesarean sections, and all medical interference is kept to a minimum. By no means all of the mothers giving birth there have been low risk. Many were expecting complications (a breech baby, for example), but went on to have successful natural births at Pithiviers.

Sheila Kitzinger

A very highly respected birth practitioner, who has enormous influence in the West, Kitzinger believes that birth is a very personal experience, and that a labouring mother should be an active "birth-giver", rather than a passive patient. She likens the modern, managed birth in a hospital to giving birth in captivity; in essence, to being in a zoo, and however kind that zoo, it still dictates the behaviour of the captives.

She believes that the aim of maternity services should be first to allow parents a real choice, whether for a totally managed birth, a totally natural birth, or somewhere in between, and to respect their wishes about where and how their child is born. Second, she believes that birth is not an illness, and that a labouring mother and her partner should not be treated as patients, but as intelligent adults with a right to have the final say in decisions about the birth of their baby.

The Lamaze method

This method of psychological counselling for childbirth was pioneered in Russia, and was then adopted in France by Dr Ferdinand Lamaze.

More than 90 per cent of women in Russia and 70 per cent of French women are taught variations of the Lamaze method of childbirth. It's become equally popular in the United States, and is the basis of the teaching of the National Childbirth Trust in Britain.

Lamaze believed that no matter how relaxed a woman was, she would almost certainly experience some pain during childbirth, and that she would have to cope with it.

Inspired by Ivan Pavlov's research into stimulus-response conditioning in dogs, Lamaze saw the value of conditioned learning in helping women to cope with the pain of childbirth.

The Lamaze method has three main principles.

■ Fear of labour is reduced or eliminated when you know and understand more about what's happening.

■ You learn how to relax and become aware of your body and how to cope with pain.

■ You consciously use rhythmic breathing patterns through each contraction to take your mind off the pain.

Your experience

When you give birth at home, you'll probably hardly notice the shift from pre-labour (see p.270) into full labour.

■ You'll be able to stay in familiar surroundings with no need to travel while in labour.

■ Once labour is established, the midwife will stay with you throughout – bear in mind, though, that if she reaches the end of her shift and you are still in labour you may have a change of midwife.

■ You'll be encouraged to take your time during labour.

■ Your membranes will usually be left to rupture spontaneously.

■ You'll be encouraged to find ways of easing pain without the aid of drugs (see p.282). If you do want something, pain relief will be available from your midwife in the form of gas and air or pethidine if it is prescribed by your doctor in advance.

■ Your midwife will try hard to help you avoid an episiotomy.

■ Your family as well as your partner can be as involved in the birth as you want.

■ After the birth you'll be free to celebrate as you choose.

Home birth

The big difference between giving birth to your baby at home instead of in hospital is that at home you're in charge and everyone else supports you. The major drawback is that if anything does go seriously wrong, medical backup is not immediately to hand. Fortunately, the chances of this happening are very small because of the more relaxed environment.

What to expect

In the early stages of your labour, you'll probably want to keep active. Use this time to make sure all is ready in your birthing room, gathering sheets and newspapers and preparing all the things you, your midwife, and the baby will need. Once labour is really established, you or your partner should phone the midwife if she isn't already on her way, as well as anyone else you want to be there.

Your midwife will be with you throughout labour and she'll monitor the baby every five minutes with a hand-held ear trumpet or sonicaid (see p.178). She and your partner will encourage you and help you into the most comfortable positions; she can give some pain relief if you need it.

You may find it helpful to squat as the baby is being born. Your partner may "catch" the baby before putting him to your breast so your baby can breastfeed immediately. His cord will be clamped and cut once it has stopped pulsating and he will be quickly checked over (see Apgar score, p.292). The midwife will then help you deliver the placenta before giving your baby a more thorough check and weighing him in a spring scale. You'll be cleaned up and, if necessary, stitched. While this is happening your partner can be holding, cuddling, and looking after your new baby. Then you'll be ready to get to know your new family member.

The advantages

There are obvious advantages to having your baby at home: you'll feel secure in your own familiar surroundings and you can have as much privacy as you want. Your partner can play an important part in the birth and your other children can be there. You'll have the major say in your labour and it's easier to avoid routine medical intervention. You'll probably have the same midwife throughout and there's no danger of being separated from your baby or your partner afterwards. Bonding and breastfeeding usually happen spontaneously after a home birth.

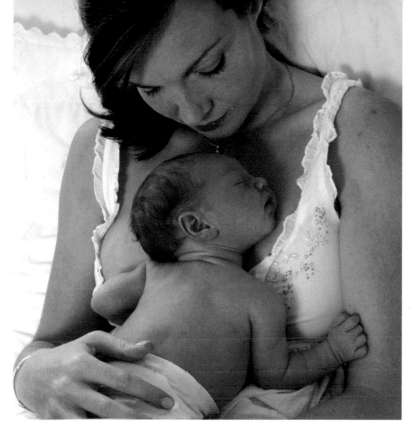

▲ **BIRTH AT HOME** The birth of your baby will be a private moment as he is born into the intimate environment of his family. The absence of hospital hustle and bustle will allow you to greet your baby calmly and gently. If you have other children, they can be there at the moment of birth if that's what you all want.

The disadvantages

Most home births go without a hitch, but there can be problems. Your baby may get "stuck" during the delivery or have difficulty breathing at birth (although breathing difficulties in the newborn are often due to pain-killing drugs given to the mother – one risk that does not usually occur at home). You may retain some or all of the placenta or bleed heavily.

Not all of these problems mean that you have to be rushed off to hospital. Most breathing difficulties, for example, can usually be eased by clearing the airways, giving oxygen, and massage; midwives carry oxygen just in case. But if you have a retained placenta or start bleeding heavily, you and your baby will have to go to hospital and your midwife will go with you. A very few babies may be born too weak or disabled to fend for themselves. They will need the attention of a special care baby unit. If your baby is needy, you and he will have to travel to the nearest obstetrical unit.

Remember, too, that childbirth can be a very messy and noisy business, and a home birth does mean quite a bit of advance preparation to get the room ready and get the supplies you'll need (see p.264).

Your baby's experience

The relaxed atmosphere at home will be good for your baby and he'll have exactly the same care from your midwife as if he'd been born in hospital.

■ Your baby's heart rate will be regularly monitored by a fetal stethoscope or a hand-held sonicaid – you won't have to be attached to a machine.

■ He'll emerge into the skilled hands of the midwife, or be caught by your birth partner.

■ As soon as he's breathing, he'll be given to you immediately after his birth and may suckle spontaneously.

■ His umbilical cord will be clamped and cut once it's stopped pulsating.

■ When you give your baby a welcoming cuddle, the skin-to-skin contact may help start him breathing.

■ The midwife will weigh and examine your baby and there'll be no hurry to clean him up.

Your experience

A hospital birth will vary depending on where you are and who looks after you (see p.120), but may include the following procedures. Talk to your doctor if you want something different.

■ You'll probably travel to hospital while you're in labour.

■ You'll need to go through brief hospital admission procedures.

■ Your membranes may be ruptured and fetal monitoring equipment set in place (see p.275), at least for a short while.

■ If labour slows down, or stops, you'll probably be given oxytocin to stimulate uterine contractions.

■ Pain-relieving drugs of different types will be available if you want.

■ Your birth partner will usually be allowed to stay with you during labour and the birth.

■ You'll probably be attended by different midwives and doctors as shifts change, especially if you're in labour during the night.

■ You may be given an episiotomy to ease the delivery of your baby's head and prevent possible injuries to your perineal or vaginal tissues.

■ You'll probably be given syntometrine (see p.291) to reduce the risk of bleeding after the placenta is delivered.

■ You'll be given your baby to hold after birth and you'll be encouraged to start breastfeeding.

Hospital birth

Even though more and more women are choosing to have home births, most babies are born in hospital. The majority of women choose to give birth in hospital, either because they are encouraged to do so by their medical advisers or because they want to. Most hospitals are now paying much more attention to the mother's wishes so there's no reason why you shouldn't enjoy giving birth to your baby in a hospital setting.

What to expect

You'll probably have been told to leave all valuables at home, and when you get to the hospital you may be asked to remove any remaining personal items such as jewellery. If this worries you, ask if you can keep your personal belongings with you in a bag. If you wear contact lenses, ask about the hospital's policy beforehand as they may prefer you to bring your spectacles instead.

After admission When you arrive at the hospital, your midwife will ask you about how your labour's going – how often you're getting contractions and whether your waters have broken, for example. Then she'll examine your abdomen to confirm the situation, feel your baby's position, and check your baby's heart. (You're unlikely to be examined by a doctor unless the midwives feel they want a second opinion.) Your blood pressure and temperature will be taken and you'll be given an internal examination to see how far your cervix has dilated. You'll probably be asked to wear a fetal monitor for about 20 minutes, but afterwards you should be able to move around as you want.

Giving birth If you've decided that you prefer to manage without drugs for as long as you can during labour, the midwives will usually be more than happy to help you cope using other methods of pain relief (see p.282). Bear in mind, though, that drug relief is available if you want and you can ask to start with smaller doses if you don't feel you need the full measure.

Once your baby is descending, you may be helped to get into a semi-reclining position. If you're in any danger of tearing, you may need to have an episiotomy (see p.109) as your baby's head is crowning. If forceps have to be used, an episiotomy (see p.306) is more likely. Your baby will be delivered on to your abdomen, and while you take your first look at each other you'll be given an injection of syntometrine into your thigh. This is to make sure that your uterus contracts firmly, reducing the chance of severe bleeding after the placenta is delivered. Your baby will be assessed and given an Apgar score (see p.292) while you are cleaned up. If you need to have stitches these are usually done by the midwife at this point.

The advantages

For some mothers a hospital birth gives the best chance of a successful and happy outcome. Having your baby in hospital is the safest option if: you suffer from a medical condition such as heart disease or diabetes; you're expecting twins; your baby is known to be breech; or as a first-time mother your obstetrical history just presents too many unknown factors.

Should anything go wrong during the labour and birth, emergency medical assistance is on hand right away and there's a wide range of pain-relief medication readily available should you want it. You may feel happier knowing that your baby can be given treatment in a special care baby unit straight away if the need arises.

The disadvantages

Once you're in hospital it's easy to feel overpowered by the atmosphere. Bear in mind that hospital staff have to follow rules and routines and you're going to have to fit in with them. But that doesn't mean that you should have to do anything you aren't happy about. It helps to find out as much as you can about the hospital procedures and set-up beforehand, so that you're more prepared once you go into labour.

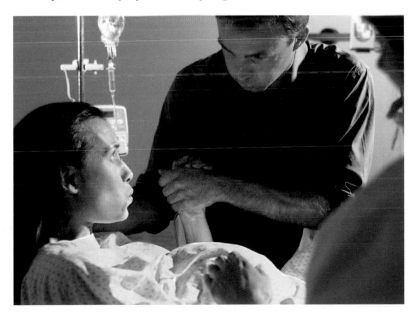

Your baby's experience

Your baby will be born surrounded by medical staff with the expertise to handle any problems that arise.

■ An electrode to measure her heart rate may be attached to her scalp during labour.

■ With the exception of epidural anaesthesia, she'll experience any drugs that you are given, and this can mean that she feels drowsy or is slower to feed once she's born.

■ She'll be handed to you to cuddle and get acquainted for a few minutes right after the birth.

■ Her umbilical cord will be clamped and cut as soon as she's been born.

■ Her mouth and nose may be routinely suctioned to clear them of any mucus.

■ She'll be weighed and examined (Apgar score) by the doctor or midwife (see p.292).

■ She'll be returned to you, possibly cleaned and wrapped in blankets, to begin bonding and breastfeeding.

■ Later on, she'll be more thoroughly examined by a doctor to check for any abnormalities.

◄ **SUPPORT FOR YOU** Your partner can usually stay with you throughout your labour and birth, giving support and helping with your breathing techniques.

What to consider

There are lots of things you'll need to think about or find out when you're choosing your hospital. Here are some questions to ask yourself or others, before you decide.

- What sort of birth do I want?

- What birth facilities are there in my area?

- Am I prepared and am I able to travel for antenatal care? Can I be cared for by my doctor?

- What are the reputations of the hospitals in my area? Have I got as many opinions, from as many different sources, as I can?

- What are the staff at the different hospitals like? What are their views on labour and birth? Do I agree with them? You can sometimes find there's a difference between a hospital's policies and the way the staff actually approach childbirth.

- Do I want a special care baby unit to be immediately on hand?

- How long do I want to be in hospital for, and what sort of rooming-in facilities are there?

- Do I want to feed my baby when and how I feel like it?

- Do I want my baby with me at night? All night?

- What are the visiting hours?

- Can my partner (and children) be with me whenever I want?

- Can my partner stay with me the first night after the birth?

The care on offer

You can ask your doctor, antenatal clinic, social worker, and friends what they know about the maternity care in your area. But really the only way to find out what a hospital or maternity unit can provide and whether it's right for you is to go and have a good look round for yourself and ask questions. There may, of course, be only one hospital or unit in your area, but if you do have a choice, make sure you get satisfactory answers so that you can feel happy and confident about the hospital you choose.

Types of care

In recent years there has been great pressure for change in hospital maternity care, and there are now increasing numbers of midwifery-led units for low-risk births and fewer, but larger, maternity units. Midwifery-led units may be attached to a maternity unit or at a separate location. Epidurals or any other form of interventions (syntocinon drip for slow labour, ventouse, or Caesarean delivery, for example) are not available and if there are problems you would need to be transferred to your nearest maternity unit. Always discuss your preferences with your GP or midwife and remember you have the right to choose where you receive your care.

Visiting hospitals

If you can, tour one or more hospitals with your partner before making your final choice. Most maternity units give a formal tour, sometimes as part of general antenatal preparation classes, otherwise as part of the general welcome made to mothers booking in. Find out about when these tours take place and ask if you can join one before you book in.

Getting to know your hospital

Hospitals can be intimidating, but usually seem less so when you get to know them. Try to visit the hospital of your choice at least once, more if possible. The more time you have to walk around, the more familiar you'll become with the surroundings so you're more relaxed when the big day comes. It's best if you and your partner do this together so that you both get to know the place and the people and will feel confident when you are actually there for the birth itself. Remember, though, that security considerations mean that postnatal wards and maternity units are now carefully monitored, so don't try to visit without an appointment. Any unannounced visitors are likely to be challenged.

It's a good idea for you and your partner to have a look around the outside of the hospital and find the night entrance. Having to search for the entrance in the dark is the last thing you need when you're in labour.

Changing your hospital

If you do have problems and you find that your hospital is not meeting your expectations, you don't have to abandon the system altogether. A hospital is there to serve you; health care is a consumer issue and you do have the right to refuse certain procedures. If you're very unhappy with any aspect of the care, you can arrange to be transferred.

You could also try getting in touch with the head of the clinic or your obstetrician and explain your feelings and what you think is wrong. If you find a sympathetic obstetrician you get on with, you may change your mind about leaving, although it's unlikely that he or she will be there for your delivery. If you feel you must change hospitals, your obstetrician will almost certainly recommend another doctor at a centre of your choice.

Birthing rooms

Most hospitals should have birthing rooms available. These are unclinical and more like your own home, with comfortable chairs, low lighting, soft music, piles of cushions, and drinks and snacks on hand.

The whole aim of a birthing room is to help you relax, overcome fears, and relieve tension. A normal routine before the birth makes for a normal delivery, and once you're in a birthing room you won't be moved unless there's an emergency that needs immediate attention. There shouldn't be any sudden changes in movement, mood, and surroundings. You won't have to lie down to have your baby and you don't need to be surrounded by rather intimidating technological equipment. In a birthing room you can take up whatever position you want for the birth of your baby.

For many women, a birthing room provides the ideal compromise between home and hospital births. It offers comfortable surroundings and facilities, but with emergency expertise on tap if you need it.

Maternity care units

Family-centred maternity care is available at some of the more progressive hospitals and larger medical centres. It's a philosophy aimed at caring for the whole family unit during labour and delivery and after birth. A hospital that adopts this kind of maternity care respects the social, personal, and family importance of childbirth, and is likely to avoid some of the more controversial routine procedures.

Some aspects of hospital maternity care may appeal to you greatly, such as a Leboyer-type delivery, keeping parents and baby together, rooming in, early discharge, and so on. These practices do vary from hospital to hospital, so visit the unit and talk to the staff. A hospital may say that it has family-centred care but this might not meet your expectations, so find out what is offered before committing yourself.

Questions to ask

When you're choosing a hospital, find out as much as you can by asking questions.

■ Will I be able to wear my own clothes and personal effects (rings, contact lenses, spectacles)?

■ Can my partner or friend stay with me all the time? Will they be asked to leave at any time?

■ Will I be able to move around freely during labour, and give birth in any position I choose?

■ Will I be able to have the same carers throughout labour?

■ Can I bring in my own independent midwife to attend to me throughout labour?

■ Are beanbags, birthing chairs, and stools provided?

■ Does the hospital have birthing pools? If not, will I be able to use a hired one?

■ What's the hospital policy on electronic monitoring, and induction?

■ What kind of pain relief is available and is it available at all times?

■ Will I be able to eat and drink if I want to?

■ What's the hospital policy on episiotomies, Caesareans, and the expulsion of the placenta?

■ If I tear or have an episiotomy, are the midwives allowed to stitch me, or will I have to wait for a doctor to attend to me?

Your attendants

Medical professionals can have many different approaches to childbirth. Ask your family doctor, obstetrician, or midwife the following questions to get an idea of their views.

■ What do you think about inducing labour and birth?

■ When would you think it necessary to rupture the membranes?

■ Do you think that electronic fetal monitoring is a valuable aid in every birth?

■ Would you be worried if labour were slower than normal?

■ What do you think about a mother moving around during labour, the use of a birthing pool, and breathing techniques to help relieve pain? What drugs do you normally give to control pain?

■ Would you mind if the lights were dimmed during labour?

■ How often do you perform episiotomies?

■ When would you think it necessary to do a Caesarean section?

■ Will we be able to have some time alone with our baby immediately after his birth?

Professional attendants

You do have some choice about who attends your labour. Most women want to have their partner or a friend with them during childbirth, and hospitals welcome this. You may like to have a birth coach, too – someone who's been through it before and knows what to do.

Your doctor

The first health professional you see will usually be your own general practitioner. You may already know a little about your doctor's views on childbirth – especially if you're thinking about having your baby at home. Some doctors are happy to attend a home delivery of a normal pregnancy, others are not so willing. Some fall somewhere in between, preferring that anyone who wants a home birth should have had at least one straightforward delivery in hospital first.

Many doctors provide antenatal care if you're having the baby in the hospital they've referred you to. Occasionally you may be able to attend your doctor's clinic even if you are booked into another hospital – look at all the options you can and talk to your doctor if you're not happy with what's on offer.

Obstetricians

An obstetrician is a doctor who specializes in medical problems in pregnancy and childbirth. When you book into a hospital you'll be assigned to a particular obstetrician. You can ask to be referred to an obstetrician of your choice, although that consultant is not obliged to take you.

Although the number of women coming into the profession is rising, there are still more male than female obstetricians in most hospitals. If you feel strongly that you'd like a female obstetrician to attend you, find out if there are any at the hospital you're thinking of choosing. If there are, make it clear on your birth plan that you'd prefer to be seen by a female consultant. Of course, there's still no guarantee that the obstetrician you've chosen will be on duty at the time when you go into hospital to give birth to your baby.

You're not likely to see your consultant unless you have any problems during your pregnancy. Most of the routine care is provided by the junior doctors, who work alongside the midwives in the obstetrics team.

Midwives

The modern, professional midwife is a specialist in childbirth. She can care for you through your pregnancy and during labour and delivery, and knows when to call for extra advice and assistance. Unlike an obstetrician, her focus is the normal not the abnormal. She's interested in the whole of you, not just your uterus and how it may misfunction. Midwives working outside hospitals tend to be more flexible than hospital carers.

Domino midwives Midwives working under the "domino" (DOMiciliary IN and Out) scheme are community midwives who come to your house when labour starts, then take you to hospital for the delivery. Your family doctor and hospital staff are rarely involved. If all is well, you may be discharged in a few hours.

Independent midwives These midwives provide continuous care in different situations. They'll deliver your baby at home or in hospital and stay with you throughout the labour and delivery. Independent midwives are private practitioners and very expensive. You have to get agreement from your local hospital for an independent midwife to attend you there.

Hospital midwives In most hospitals midwives now take the lead in the care of labouring women, although the obstetricians are officially in charge. You'll meet most of the midwives during your antenatal care and, if all goes well, they'll deliver your baby with as little obstetric intervention as possible. Your midwife could be a man – there are now over 150 male midwives in the UK and more are being trained.

Independent midwives

Your midwife will be your primary caregiver so you'll want to get to know her. It may help to ask the following questions.

■ What training and experience has she had?

■ Does she work alone, or with other midwives? Will you have a chance to meet them?

■ What are her views about managing labour?

■ What's her back-up system? Does she work closely with any doctors?

■ What equipment, drugs, and resuscitation equipment for the baby does she carry?

■ What antenatal care does she provide? Will she make home visits?

■ Under what circumstances would she transfer you to hospital?

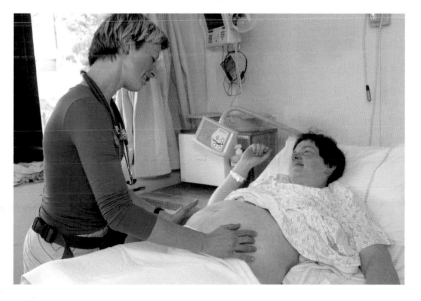

◀ **YOUR BIRTH ATTENDANT**
The professional attendant who assists you to give birth should be someone you've met before and trust, and who'll give you the kind of support and encouragement you and your partner need. Ideally, your attendant helps to create an intimate atmosphere in which you feel happy working with your body to bring a new life into the world.

Looking at the alternatives

Your main birth plan will detail the kind of birth you'd prefer, but it's a good idea to have an alternative plan, just in case.

This alternative plan can set out what you'd prefer to happen if complications should arise. On rare occasions, labour may become unexpectedly prolonged or difficult, or your baby may need special attention. If you think about all the possibilities beforehand, you'll make it easier for your birth attendants to take care of any situation as you wish.

Birth plan

Making your own plan for your baby's birth will help you make sure you have an active involvement in the way he's born and what happens immediately after the birth. Think about all the options available and what you'd prefer and talk them over with your birth attendants and your partner. In this way you'll be able to build a bond of trust with everyone concerned and create a happier, more comfortable labour.

Talk it through

Think about what's most important to you and then find out as much as you can to see if what you want is realistic for your situation (see pp.118 and 120, and column, opposite). There's no point in making a plan that can't be used once you're in labour.

Talk to your family doctor about your birth plan early in your pregnancy. If you're having a hospital birth, ask him to refer you to the hospital that's most in tune with your wishes if possible. It also helps to talk about what you want with your midwife, antenatal teacher, and other members of your antenatal team – they'll be able to give you advice and tell you about the kinds of experiences other mothers have had in your local hospitals. One of the reasons it's good to make a plan is that you have the time to think about everything carefully and discuss issues you're not sure about. When you're in the middle of labour and contractions, you might find you're not feeling up to much discussion!

The hospital view Your hospital team will welcome the preparation you've done for the labour and will encourage you to get involved. Some mothers used to get bad reactions to birth plans from some hospital staff on the grounds that they might interfere with their standard practices. That's unlikely to happen now – in fact there'll be space in your hospital notes for your preferences to be recorded after talking to your midwife.

Working together Cooperation is an important part of a birth plan. Working everything out in detail with all your attendants, including your partner, should ease any anxieties you may have and help you feel more in control of your baby's birth. Check that staff are aware of any alternative plans you've made and keep up a friendly relationship with your carers – they'll want to follow your wishes as far as they can, provided you and

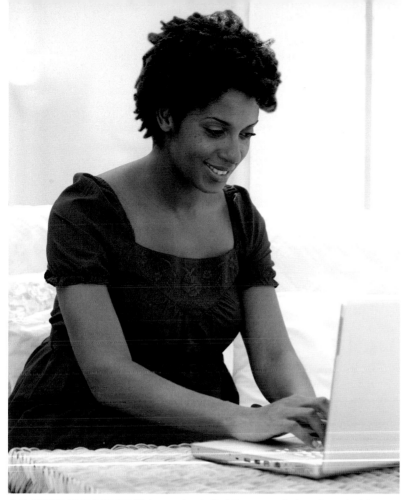

▲ **PLANNING YOUR LABOUR** Make a note of all of the issues that are important to you and talk to your doctor or midwife about them.

your baby are not at risk. Once you've talked about what's important to you, give a copy of the plan that's kept with your hospital notes to each of your birth partners or carers. This could be important if someone who doesn't know your wishes has to attend your labour.

What to put down Note who your birth partners will be; what sort of pain relief you'd like to have; what position you'd prefer for giving birth; how you feel about episiotomy, induction, and your waters being broken; how you'd prefer labour to be managed; and whether or not you want to breastfeed. Once you've made your plan, make sure that everyone who's likely to be involved has a copy and that they're aware of any alternative plans you've made.

Special considerations Be sure to make a note on your birth plan of any particular needs you may have while you're in hospital – for example, if you're vegetarian or you need any other special diet.

It's your choice

Try to be open to all the possibilities. Don't feel the birth has to be totally managed or completely natural; it can be a blend of many things. Here are some alternatives:

■ hospital/home birth

■ medical induction of labour if necessary/spontaneous start

■ amniotomy (artificial rupture of membranes) if necessary/ spontaneous rupture of membranes

■ fetus monitored electronically for a short time only/continuous fetal monitoring

■ nothing by mouth only if high risk of Caesarean/eat and drink as and when desired

■ types of pain relief: pethidine, epidural, gas and air, breathing exercises, TENS, diversion

■ catheterization only with epidural/empty own bladder as necessary

■ commanded pushing/ spontaneous pushing

■ deliberate breath-holding/ no deliberate breath-holding

■ elective episiotomy/episiotomy only if absolutely necessary

■ mother not touching vaginal area/touching baby's head as it crowns, lifting baby out

■ use of syntometrine to speed delivery of placenta/natural expulsion of placenta.

Childbirth teachers

It's a good idea to choose a childbirth teacher fairly early on in your pregnancy; make plans to start classes in your seventh month or earlier.

The quality and approach of classes can vary – some are tightly structured with little question-and-answer time, others allow plenty of time to practise techniques. Some depend mainly on lectures, others on class participation. A good teacher is very often the key to whether a class is successful or not, so do check with other couples you know who've attended classes before you make your final choice.

Try to select a teacher whose philosophy of birth fits in with the type of birth you'd like to have. It can be confusing, and upsetting, if what you learn in class is not reflected in your later experience in hospital or at home.

Find out how many couples are taught in each class. Half a dozen couples is ideal as the teacher will have time to give you all enough attention and you'll be able to get to know the other people in your class.

Childbirth teachers are generally very aware and sensitive to the needs and problems of pregnancy. Yours will probably be more than happy to talk to you – even if you're not yet attending childbirth classes.

Childbirth classes

I'm an enthusiastic supporter of prepared childbirth and I believe that everyone can benefit from going to childbirth classes. These classes are tremendously enjoyable. You'll make friends and you can swap stories and experiences, so you don't feel alone and isolated. It's a great help to be able to share what you're going through, and it helps to relieve tension and anxiety.

Parenting classes

These are designed to give you information that will make you both feel more confident and are particularly useful for first-time parents. They cover three main areas.

First, the classes go through the processes of pregnancy and birth and the changes that are happening to you and the baby throughout your pregnancy. This will help you have a clearer understanding of what's involved and why things are happening. The teachers will also talk to you about the sort of medical procedures that you can expect, and why these will be done. You'll be given plenty of opportunities to ask questions.

Second, you'll be taught relaxation, breathing, and exercise techniques. These will help you to control your own labour, reduce pain, and give you the confidence that only comes with being familiar with what's happening. It's bodies, not brains, that give birth, so try to be open to anything that helps you tune into your body. Your partner will probably be taught how to give you a massage to help relieve your pain (see p.283).

Third, the teachers will talk you through the stages of labour and birth, and give tips on starting to breastfeed. They'll also give you practical advice on how to bathe and dress a baby and change nappies, which will help you feel more confident about caring for your newborn baby.

Exercise classes

Strengthening the muscles used in childbirth can often mean you have an easier and more comfortable delivery. With this in mind, many hospitals hold antenatal classes that include some exercise and relaxation. There are also independent organizations that provide exercise classes for pregnant women – some are even for specific types of birth. Many midwives recommend swimming, as the water supports your weight while you get a gentle work-out. You can attend special aqua-natal classes that offer exercise in water for pregnant women.

Yoga

Practising yoga is an excellent way to prepare for childbirth as it emphasizes muscular control of the body, breathing, relaxation, and peace of mind. But yoga isn't something you can do casually – to be of any benefit, it must be done regularly, preferably starting long before you conceive. There are some special exercises for pregnancy, but it's best to have the guidance of a qualified teacher – particularly if you're pregnant.

Techniques of childbirth classes

Many studies have shown that women who take childbirth classes have shorter labours. In one study, the average length of labour for a group of women who'd been to classes was 13.56 hours, compared with an average 18.33 hours in a group of women who'd had no training. This is probably because knowing how to deal with pain means you have a more relaxed labour. Strategies for dealing with pain taught by childbirth classes include:

Cognitive control You disassociate your mind from the pain by visualizing a pleasant scenario. For example, you'll feel happier about contractions if, every time you have a pain, you imagine your baby moving further down the birth canal, closer to being born. Distracting yourself can also help, although this works best in the early stages. Counting to 20, going through a list of possible names for your new baby, or concentrating on a beautiful picture or piece of music helps you to take your mind off the pain, and keeps it from completely filling your consciousness and over-whelming you. Another way of taking your mind off the pain is to focus your attention on your breathing techniques and think about each breath.

Systematic relaxation You'll learn exercises to relax all the muscles of the body in turn to decrease your fear of pain and increase your tolerance for it. This will help you to isolate pain from your contracting uterus rather than allowing it to spread to other parts of your body.

Hawthorne effect Psychological research has shown how important it is to have positive attention and motivation in any situation. The Hawthorne effect means that if a mother receives extra, focused attention from a birth assistant, she's likely to cope better with labour.

Systematic desensitization You gradually become more tolerant of pain. An example used in many classes is your coach pinching your leg very hard to illustrate how painful a contraction will be. This pinching is repeated every time you go to an antenatal class, and by the end of the course you'll be able to tolerate harder squeezing for longer periods.

Dad's role

Childbirth classes are a good opportunity to show your partner just how central a role he is going to play.

Classes will help make a supportive man a much more effective birth assistant as he will be more familiar with the processes of labour and delivery.

Some courses include father-only sessions when the men can talk freely to the teacher and to other fathers-to-be about any problems or anxieties they have about the coming event.

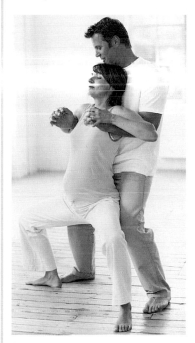

▲ **TEAM EFFORT** Childbirth classes give a couple a unique opportunity to work together as a team towards a common goal – the birth of their baby. This teamwork can often bring a couple closer together.

Food and eating in pregnancy

Eating healthily in pregnancy means having a wide range of the right kind of foods – those rich in essential vitamins and minerals. If you eat plenty of fresh fruit and vegetables, whole grains, fish, organically reared meat, and low-fat dairy produce, you'll be doing the best for your baby.

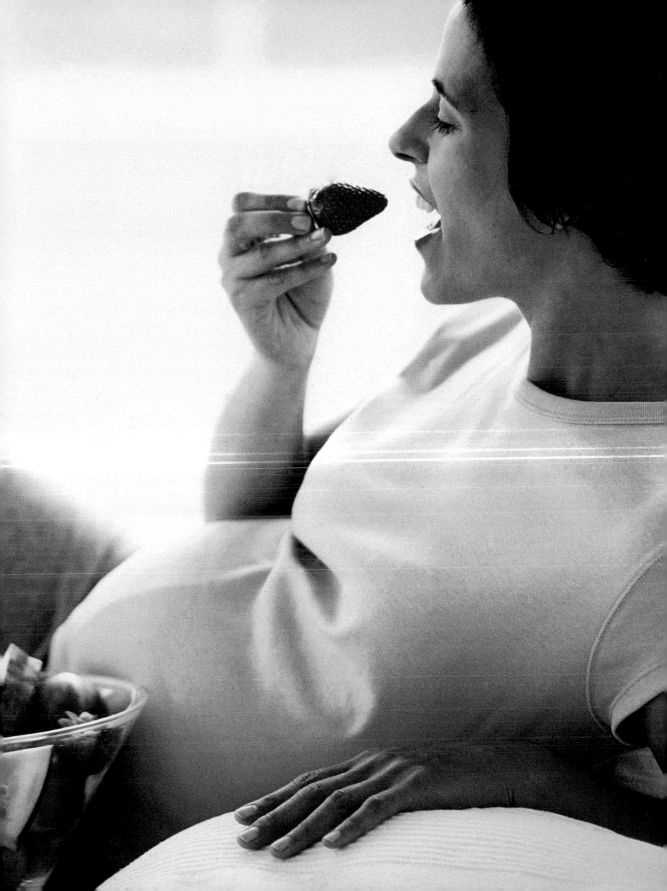

Eating for yourself

Your body works harder when you're carrying and giving birth to a baby than at any other time. You need to eat well to cope with the increased demands on your body and keep up your strength.

- Eat 200–300 calories more than your normal daily intake.

- Eat five or six small meals a day instead of two or three big ones.

- Make sure you eat enough protein and carbohydrates (see p.132). Protein supplies are essential nutrients for your developing baby. Carbohydrates fuel your energy needs.

- Eat foods containing vitamins, such as vitamin C, and minerals, particularly iron (see p.133).

▶ **GAINING WEIGHT** Doctors generally recommend that a woman of average weight, who's having an average pregnancy, shouldn't gain more than 10–12kg (22–26lb) over the 40 weeks, as shown in the chart on the right. About 3–4kg (6–9lb) of this is for the baby and the rest for the baby-support system (placenta, amniotic fluid, increased blood, fluid, fat, and breast tissue). Most women put on very little, if any, weight, during the first trimester, about 450g–1kg (1–2lb) a week between months four and eight, then very little, or none at all, in the last month. A slow steady gain like this means that your body can adapt more easily to your increasing size, and your baby is provided with a continuous flow of nourishment.

Food in pregnancy

When you're pregnant you certainly don't want to bother with measuring portions and calorie counting. And there's no need to do this if you follow some basic guidelines about healthy eating. One golden rule is that the nearer food is to its natural state, the better it is for you. So fresh, unprocessed food is best – it's common sense.

Eating for two?

You'll probably feel hungrier than usual when you're expecting a baby – it's nature's way of making certain you eat enough for both of you. But you certainly don't need to "eat for two" as people used to believe. Most women need to only eat an extra 200–300 calories a day, far less than if you ate twice your normal amount of food. Much more important than the quantity of what you eat is the quality. Everything you eat should be good for you and your baby. Some mothers-to-be, such as those who previously ate an inadequate or unbalanced diet, may be nutritionally at risk and have special dietary needs (see also column, p.138).

Average weight gain during pregnancy

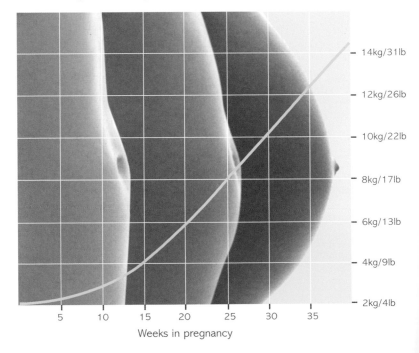

							14kg/31lb
							12kg/26lb
							10kg/22lb
							8kg/17lb
							6kg/13lb
							4kg/9lb
							2kg/4lb

5   10   15   20   25   30   35

Weeks in pregnancy

More problems develop if you eat too little rather than too much. Pregnancy is not the time for dieting. Research has shown that when mothers-to-be eat poor diets, there's a higher incidence of miscarriages, neonatal death, and low birthweight babies than normal.

You owe it to yourself, as well as to your growing baby, to eat a diet that's best for both of you. Try to stick to the healthy eating guidelines on pages 134 and 135, but remember that you can balance your food intake over a 24- to 48-hour period rather than at each meal if you prefer. Just make sure that you don't miss meals – your baby grows all day, every day, and will suffer if you don't eat properly.

Junk food such as chocolate bars and hamburgers and fries contain little other than fat and sugar. They don't do your baby any good, and your body converts these empty calories into fat, so don't eat them.

You'll put on some fat when you're pregnant and your body needs this to convert to milk when you're breastfeeding. Although feeding will help you lose the weight you put on during pregnancy, it's best to avoid really excessive weight gain; fat that's deposited at the tops of your arms and thighs is very difficult to get rid of after pregnancy.

Your baby's needs

While your baby is growing inside your womb, you are her only source of nourishment. Every calorie, vitamin, or gram of protein she needs must come from you. You're in sole charge of your unborn child's nutrition; you, and only you, can make sure the best quality food reaches her.

You'll be doing your best for your baby if you eat lots of fresh fruit, vegetables, beans, peas, wholemeal cereals, fish, poultry, and low-fat dairy products. A Danish study showed that eating oily fish – such as salmon, mackerel, and sardines – may help lessen the risk of premature birth. Make your diet as varied as possible, choosing from a range of foods.

Don't forget mum

The other person to do your best for is yourself. Eating plenty of healthy foods throughout your pregnancy will mean that you have better reserves for coping with, and recovering from, the physical strains of pregnancy and the hard work of labour. Anaemia and pre-eclampsia (see p.224) are much more common in mothers who have a poor diet, and some problems, including morning sickness and leg cramps, may be made worse by what you do or don't eat.

A healthy diet will help to reduce excessive mood swings, fatigue, and many other common complaints of pregnancy (see pp.206–13). And if you cut out or restrict the amount of empty calories you eat, you'll have less excess fat to lose after your baby has been born.

Empty calories

It's best to avoid the following foods when you're pregnant. They're full of sugar or sugar substitutes, and refined flour, so they're no good for you or your baby.

■ Any form of sweetener – and this includes white and brown sugar, golden syrup, treacle, and artificial sweeteners such as saccharine and aspartame.

■ Sweets and chocolate bars.

■ Soft drinks, such as cola and sweetened fruit juices.

■ Commercially produced biscuits, cakes, pastries, and pies, as well as jam and marmalade.

■ Tinned fruit in syrup.

■ Artificial cream.

■ Sweetened breakfast cereal.

■ Ice cream and sorbets that contain added sugar. Freeze fruit juice or puréed fruit instead.

■ Savouries that contain sugar, such as relishes, pickles, salad dressings, spaghetti sauces, mayonnaise, peanut butter, and many others – read the labels.

■ Pregnant women used to be advised not to eat peanuts or peanut butter, but the latest research has shown no link between a mother eating peanuts and her baby developing allergies. However, if you're worried about any particular food in pregnancy, don't eat it – have something else.

Snacks to keep at work

It's not always easy to keep to your healthy diet when you're at work. Planning ahead and keeping some supplies in the office will help.

In the office refrigerator:
- mineral water
- unsweetened fruit juice
- plain live-culture yogurt
- hard cheese
- hard-boiled eggs
- fresh fruit
- "snack" vegetables – carrot and red pepper sticks, tomatoes
- wholemeal bread
- jar of wheatgerm.

In your desk drawer:
- wholemeal crackers, crispbreads, or breadsticks, perhaps with seeds
- dried fruit
- nuts or seeds
- decaffeinated instant coffee and decaffeinated tea bags
- powdered skimmed milk for extra calcium in drinks.

In your handbag:
- wholemeal crackers, crispbreads, or breadsticks, perhaps with seeds
- dried fruit, nuts, and seeds
- fresh fruit or "snack" vegetables
- small thermos of unsweetened juice or milk
- glucose sweets for emergencies.

Make sure everything is securely wrapped and sealed.

The best food to eat

Fresh food that's as close to its original state as possible is best for you and your baby. Eating good-quality food should be your goal throughout, as well as after, your pregnancy.

When you're out shopping, choose fresh produce; seasonal fruit and vegetables are always fresher, as well as cheaper, than imported, out-of-season items. Pick out sound fruit and vegetables and reject any that look tired or are going bad. Buy your meat and fish from shops you can trust – don't run the risk of getting a food-related illness (see p.139). If you can afford it, go for free-range or organic foods grown without pesticides and hormones (used particularly in beef and intensively farmed poultry), but try to check that organic foods have been properly approved (by the Soil Association, for example). Look at the labelling of processed foods to see whether they include any genetically modified (GM) ingredients. Until the scientific research into the safety of these foods has been completed and fully debated, it's sensible to avoid GM foods during pregnancy.

Always keep some packs of frozen vegetables – they're good standbys when you can't get to the shops. Avoid tins, except for plum tomatoes and fish such as sardines. Read the labels on any other packaged foods you buy and remember that the nearer an ingredient is to the top of the list, the more there is of that one ingredient. Sugar has many different names (see p.132) and can appear on a list more than once.

Foods that have been over-refined, such as white flour and white sugar, have had all of the natural goodness stripped out of them and fill you and your baby with nothing but excess calories. Choose wholemeal bread and flour rather than "enriched" refined products; it's highly unlikely that the enrichment puts back in all that's been taken out. The two "waste" products of flour refining are bran (the fibre) and wheatgerm (the heart of the wheat) and these contain most of the goodness. Bran is probably an unnecessary addition for the average pregnant woman (although it will help prevent constipation), but wheatgerm contains lots of vitamins and minerals that are good for everyone. Wheatgerm is crunchy and nutty and can be added to salads and sandwiches, as well as to cooked and baked dishes. You can buy packets of wheatgerm from health food shops and good supermarkets.

Good eating habits

You'll probably need more than willpower if you're going to stick to your healthy regime. The first step is to avoid eating food you know you shouldn't have because there's nothing else available. Keep sugar-free fruit and nut bars, and decaffeinated tea bags with you so you don't give in to temptations like biscuits and a cup of caffeinated tea in the afternoon. If possible, prepare a batch of meals at the weekend that you can store and eat in the week. That will keep you from ringing for a take-away pizza when you're too tired to cook. Banish junk food from your kitchen.

Make the right choices Think before you eat – a chicken and lettuce sandwich on wholemeal bread that's rich in fibre and folic acid is much better for you than fat-rich bacon and mayonnaise on fibreless white! Invest in a healthy-eating cookbook and try some dishes that are lower in fat and sugar but still taste delicious. Get in the habit of snacking on nutritious foods and eat little and often. Towards the end of your pregnancy, you'll find that eating large amounts is difficult anyway.

Vegetarian mothers

Many people prefer not to eat meat; many more limit their intake of meat, particularly red meat. This is fine, but when you're pregnant you'll need to make sure you eat enough protein, vitamins, and iron to meet your own and your baby's needs (see also p.136). Pulses (beans, peas, and lentils), nuts and seeds, and grains, as well as eggs and dairy products, all contain protein and will be good foods for you and your baby.

Combining plant foods Plant proteins need to be eaten in the right combinations to provide you with the necessary amino acids that are found complete in animal proteins. For example, serve peas with rice or corn, or add a handful of nuts to a rice and sweetcorn salad.

You'll also need to make sure you're getting enough iron, as there's relatively little in plant foods and certain substances interfere with how well iron is absorbed by your body (see p.133).

If you're a vegan and you don't eat any animal products at all, you'll have to work even harder to make sure that you're not lacking in any essential nutrients – in particular calcium and vitamins B_6, B_{12}, and D, all of which are provided by dairy products. Although you don't need very much B_{12}, lack of it will eventually lead to pernicious anaemia, so if your diet contains no animal products at all, it's best to take vitamin B_{12} supplements.

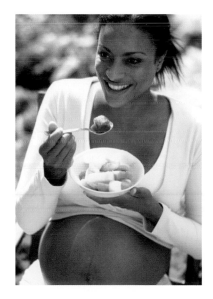

◀ **GOOD FOR YOU BOTH** Eating plenty of fresh fruit and vegetables helps make sure you get the vitamins and minerals essential for your own health and that of your developing baby.

When you're short of time, energy, or money, eating the right foods can seem like too much trouble. Here are some ideas to help you eat well without too much effort:

■ keep a range of frozen vegetables for days when you can't get to the shops

■ buy meat and fish in bulk, and freeze in meal-size portions

■ cook meals ahead and freeze

■ use a microwave – it cooks food quickly and retains nutrients

■ keep meals simple – eat raw vegetables; steam, stir fry, or grill for speed, or bake so you can leave food to cook on its own

■ get help – grandparents-to-be will be keen to give you a hand

■ always have fresh fruit available – the perfect quick snack

■ a big pot of home-made bean and vegetable soup provides you with several meals with little effort.

Choosing proteins

The needs of your growing baby mean that you'll have to make sure that about ten per cent of your calories come from protein foods such as meat, fish, dairy products, eggs, and beans.

Proteins are made up of amino acids, which are vital to body cells and tissues. We need a total of 20 different amino acids. Your body can make 12 of these, the non-essential amino acids, itself. The other eight, the essential acids, must be supplied by food. These are contained in first-class proteins, found only in animal products such as meat, dairy foods, fish, poultry, and eggs. Buy organic produce if you can, especially poultry, eggs, and beef. If you are vegetarian make sure you eat complementary proteins, see pp.131 and 134.

When you're choosing protein foods, think about what else they contain. Meat is the richest source of first-class proteins and contain vital B vitamins. But some meat, particularly red meat, can be very high in animal fat. It's best not to eat liver, or any other offal when you're pregnant as it's high in vitamin A, which may be toxic to your baby.

Fish is a good choice of first-class protein for pregnant women. It's high in vitamins and nutritious fish oils, and is low in saturated fat. Don't eat tuna more than once a week, and avoid shark, marlin, and swordfish as they may contain traces of mercury.

The foods you need

What you eat when you're pregnant is even more important than you might think. Research shows that it not only affects your baby at birth, but also appears to have a long-term effect throughout your child's life. It's important to drink plenty of fluids, too. When you're pregnant you have nearly 50 per cent more blood in your body than usual, so you need to keep up your fluid intake. Water is best. Don't cut down on your fluid intake if your hands and feet swell – it won't make any difference to this type of fluid retention.

Protein

Protein is probably the most essential food for your baby; the amino acids that make up protein are literally the building blocks of the body. The cells and tissues that make up all the muscles, bones, connective tissues, and many of the organ walls are formed from protein.

You need at least three servings of protein foods (see p.134) daily. The type and quality of protein in food varies (see column, left). Meat, fish, and poultry are the best sources, but they can be expensive. Plant foods eaten in certain combinations can be another way of getting enough protein. Wholewheat bread or noodles with beans or cheese; or cornmeal or noodles with sesame seeds, nuts, and milk will keep protein intake high.

Carbohydrates and calories

Carbohydrate foods should make up the bulk of your calorie intake, but eat the best, complex, carbohydrates and avoid empty calories (see p.129).

Simple carbohydrates are sugars in various forms. The most common types and sources are glucose (honey), fructose (fruit), and maltose, lactose, and galactose (milk). These carbohydrates are absorbed quickly from the stomach so are a source of "instant energy", which can be useful when you're in dire need.

Complex carbohydrates are the starches contained in grains, potatoes, and pulses. The body has to break them down into simple carbohydrates before it can use them, so they provide a steady supply of energy over a period of time. Complex unrefined carbohydrates (wholemeal flour and brown rice) are also good sources of vitamins, minerals, and fibre.

Vitamins

Vegetables and fruits are good sources of many vitamins (and minerals). Some are rich in vitamin C; others contain vitamins A, E, and the B group (which includes folic acid), and minerals – all of which you need in your diet. Vitamins are quickly destroyed by exposure to light, air, and heat, and many can't be stored by the body, so you need to top up your supplies every day. Leafy green vegetables, yellow or red vegetables, and fruit supply vitamins A, E, B₆, iron, zinc, and magnesium. Choose broccoli, spinach, watercress, carrots, tomatoes, bananas, apricots, and cherries.

Although we can get some B vitamins from vegetables and fruit, the bulk of our vitamin B intake comes from meat, fish, dairy products, grains, and nuts. Some of the B vitamins are only in animal foods, so vegetarians must make sure that they're getting enough in their diet. If you don't eat dairy products you'll need to take vitamin B₁₂ supplements – ask your doctor for a prescription. Vitamins can be toxic in large quantities – never take supplements without your doctor's advice when you're pregnant.

We can get some vitamin D from food (see p.135), but more important is the action of light on the skin that triggers the body to make vitamin D. Most light-skinned people need about 40 minutes of light (it is not necessary for it to be bright sunlight) a day to make enough vitamin D for their needs. Dark-skinned people living outside the tropics need progressively more sunlight depending on their skin tones.

Minerals

A varied, healthy diet should provide you with enough minerals and trace elements – essential chemicals that help the body function properly, but are not made by it. High levels of iron and calcium, in particular, are important for your baby's healthy development.

Iron The body needs iron to make haemoglobin (the oxygen-carrying part of the red blood cells). When you're pregnant you need to keep up supplies of extra iron to support the large increase in the amount of blood in your body during pregnancy, because your baby's need for iron is constant. Iron can block the body's absorption of zinc, which is essential for the development of your baby's brain and nervous system so you need to eat zinc-rich food, such as fish and wheatgerm, separately from iron-rich food. The amount of iron needed varies from woman to woman. Your doctor will keep a check on your iron levels. If you're lacking in iron when you become pregnant, or develop iron deficiency later, your doctor may prescribe iron tablets or injections to prevent you developing anaemia.

Calcium A baby's bones begin to form between four and six weeks, so you'll need plenty of calcium both before you conceive and while you're pregnant. Dairy products, leafy green vegetables, soya, broccoli, and any fish containing bones (such as sardines) are rich in calcium. If you don't eat dairy products, you may need supplements. Vitamin D is needed for calcium absorption, so try to eat eggs or cheese every day.

Folic acid

One of the B vitamins, folic acid is essential for making red blood cells and plays an important part in the growth of your baby, especially in the first 12 weeks.

Folic acid is vital to the development of the nervous system and research shows that folic acid supplements taken up to three months before conception and for the first 12 weeks of pregnancy significantly reduce the incidence of neural tube defects such as spina bifida. If you haven't started taking folic acid before conception, start as soon as you know you're pregnant. Folic acid is available in tablet form, and it's also in green leafy vegetables, cereals, and bread.

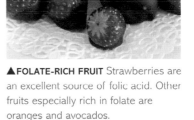

▲**FOLATE-RICH FRUIT** Strawberries are an excellent source of folic acid. Other fruits especially rich in folate are oranges and avocados.

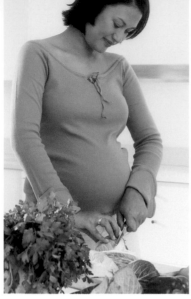

▲ **HEALTHY MEAL** Eat a varied diet and balance your intake of different nutrients over a couple of days, rather than at every meal.

Eating well

There's no need for you to spend lots of time measuring out portions, but you might like some guidelines to help you make sure you're eating well.

Daily needs

So that you and your baby have the best possible diet, try to eat the following each day (each food listed in the table as a single serving).

- First-class proteins – three servings
- Vitamin C foods – two servings
- Calcium foods – four servings in pregnancy, five when feeding
- Green leafy and yellow or red vegetables and fruits – three to four servings
- Other fruit and vegetables – two or three servings
- Whole grains and complex carbohydrates – four or five servings
- Iron-rich food – two servings
- Fluids – eight glasses a day, not coffee or alcohol. Water is best.

What you need	The foods to eat	
Calcium foods	50g/2oz hard cheese 100g/4oz cream cheese 325g/13oz cottage cheese 250ml/9floz yogurt	200ml/7floz milk 75g/3oz tinned sardines, with bones
First-class protein foods	75g/3oz hard cheese 100g/4oz soft cheese 500ml/1pt milk 340ml/12floz yogurt 3 large eggs	100g/4oz fresh or tinned fish 100g/4oz prawns 75g/3oz beef, lamb, pork, poultry, but without the fat
Green leafy and yellow or red vegetables, and fruit	100g/4oz spinach, broccoli florets 100g/4oz carrots 100g/4oz peas, beans 100g/4oz sweet peppers 150g/6oz tomatoes	50g/2oz melon 6 plums 1 mango, orange, grapefruit 2 apricots 4 peaches, apples, pears
Whole grains and complex carbohydrates	75g/3oz cooked barley, brown rice, millet, bulgar 25g/1oz wholemeal or soya flour 1 slice wholemeal or soya bread 6 wholemeal bread sticks	75g/3oz kidney beans, soya beans, chickpeas 100g/4oz lentils, peas 1 wholemeal pitta or tortilla 6 wholemeal biscuits
Vitamin C foods	100g/4oz broccoli florets 225g/9oz tomatoes 200g/8oz blackberries or raspberries 100ml/4floz citrus juice	25g/1oz blackcurrants 100g/4oz strawberries 1 large lemon or orange ½ medium grapefruit

Vitamins and minerals

Foods can provide all the vitamins and minerals our bodies need, except for vitamin D. It is found in some foods, but we get most of our vitamin D from sunlight. The chart below is a guide to the best sources of essential vitamins and minerals. They tend to be easily destroyed so aim to eat foods that are as fresh as possible for the most benefit. Some foods contain a range of vitamins and minerals.

Name	Where it comes from
Vitamin A (retinol & carotene)	Whole milk, butter, cheese, egg yolk, oily fish, green and yellow fruit and vegetables
Vitamin B_1 (thiamine)	Whole grains, nuts, pulses, pork, brewer's yeast, wheatgerm
Vitamin B_2 (riboflavin)	Brewer's yeast, wheatgerm, whole grains, green vegetables, milk, cheese, eggs
Vitamin B_3 (niacin)	Brewer's yeast, whole grains, wheatgerm, green vegetables, oily fish, eggs, milk
Vitamin B_5 (pantothenic acid)	Eggs, whole grains, cheese
Vitamin B_6 (pyridoxine)	Brewer's yeast, whole grains, soya flour, wheatgerm, mushrooms, potatoes, avocados
Vitamin B_{12} (cyanocobalamin)	Meat, fish, milk, eggs
Folic acid (part of B complex)	Raw leafy vegetables, peas, soya flour, oranges, bananas, walnuts
Vitamin C (ascorbic acid)	Rosehip syrup, sweet peppers, citrus fruits, blackcurrants, tomatoes
Vitamin D (calciferol)	Fortified milk, oily fish, eggs (particularly the yolks), butter
Vitamin E	Wheatgerm, egg yolk, seeds, vegetable oils, broccoli
Calcium	Milk, cheese, small fish with bones, walnuts, sunflower seeds, soya, yogurt, broccoli
Iron	Fish, egg yolks, red meat, cereals, molasses, apricots, haricot beans
Zinc	Wheatbran, eggs, nuts, onions, shellfish, sunflower seeds, wheatgerm, whole wheat

Preparing food

Developing some good cooking habits will help you eat healthily.

■ Trim fat off meat before cooking.

■ Skim fat off the surface of casseroles and soups.

■ Bake, steam, microwave, or grill rather than fry.

■ Stir-fry food in a teaspoon of olive oil, plus a little water, or with a stock cube dissolved in a cup of water.

■ Use non-stick pans and as little fat as possible when you make omelettes or scrambled eggs.

■ Use flavoured vinegars, such as raspberry, basil, thyme, or garlic (home-made ones are better than shop-bought), or yogurt for salad dressings, instead of mayonnaise, salad cream, or sour cream.

■ Add dried skimmed milk to milky drinks, or when baking, for extra servings of calcium.

■ Eat fruit and vegetables raw as often as you can.

■ Eat oily fish, but not more than one portion a week. Some fish contain high levels of mercury, which can cause damage to your baby's developing nervous system, so should be avoided altogether (see p.132).

Miriam's casebook

The vegetarian mother

Anne became a vegetarian two years ago, a year after the birth of her second child, Katie, now three years old. Anne's diet includes dairy produce and eggs and she's very healthy, but she's concerned about the extra nutrients her body will need during her pregnancy. We looked at her various worries and, once we'd identified possible protein and calcium deficiencies, I suggested some ways of boosting her diet.

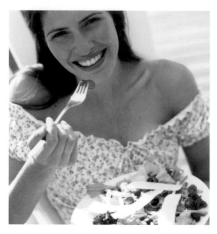

Being vegetarian

Having already had two babies, Anne knew that she might need to make some changes to her diet during her pregnancy, and now she was a vegetarian, she wanted to check a few things.

For example, she'd heard that a vegetarian diet might be short of vitamin B_{12}; if so, would that harm her baby? She'd also read something about folic acid and spina bifida. Was her diet lacking in folic acid, and should she take supplements? She knew that some pregnant women take iron supplements; would she need to?

Anne knew that the main change she had to make to her diet would be to make sure she ate more protein, but she wanted to check what kind of protein would be best and which foods provide it. During pregnancy, the body demands increased calcium intake. Would it be best to take calcium tablets or would she be able to get enough by eating plenty of calcium-rich and calcium-fortified foods?

Differing opinions

Opinions on a vegetarian diet during pregnancy differ widely. They range from those of vegans who believe that women can carry a healthy baby to term without eating any animal protein or even taking vitamin B_{12} supplements, to doctors and healthcare professionals who insist that meat and fish are essential foods for a pregnant woman. In fact, both views are wrong and I'll explain why.

In the case of vegans, if no animal products, including dairy products, are eaten, vitamin B_{12} supplements are absolutely essential. B_{12} is vital to the healthy growth and development of the fetus, as well as that of a breastfed baby. Vegetarian diets often lack B_{12} as it only exists naturally in animal products. A vegetarian woman may need to take supplements to ensure the healthy growth of her baby.

Vegan mothers can opt either to add milk and eggs to their diet, or to take synthetic B_{12}, during pregnancy and while they're breastfeeding.

A vegetarian diet that includes dairy products can support a pregnancy, and later breastfeeding, perfectly well, as long as you have more protein and calcium. All pregnant women should increase their milk intake to 500ml (1pt) a day (skimmed and semi-skimmed milk contain as much calcium as whole milk). Anne can also boost her protein and vitamin intake by drinking vitamin-fortified soya milk and eating lots of other soya and dairy products.

How to meet increasing needs

The simplest way for Anne to increase the protein and vitamin content of her diet would be for her to eat at least four eggs a week. Eggs will provide iron too, although not as much iron as is provided by red meat. While some vegetarians claim that they can get the same amount of iron that red meat provides by eating more green leafy vegetables, they'd have to eat almost 2kg (5lb) of these vegetables per day to do so!

I advised Anne to accept her obstetrician's advice if she is prescribed vitamin, iron, and calcium supplements, but reassured her that if her obstetrician presses her on eating meat, she should contact the Vegetarian Society (see Useful addresses, p.370) for support and further information. The following menu should take care of Anne's needs.

Suggested daily vegetarian menu

Breakfast Two slices of wholemeal toast with yeast extract. Cup of decaffeinated tea with skimmed milk. One banana.
Mid-morning snack Selection of raw vegetables with hummus (chickpea dip) and wholemeal pitta bread.
Lunch Baked potato, topped with cottage cheese, red pepper, tomatoes, and watercress. Glass of tomato juice. Chopped nuts and dried fruit.
Afternoon snack Broccoli and cheese soup (preferably fresh) with chopped walnuts and low-fat fromage frais. Two slices of rye bread.
Dinner Mushroom and tofu lasagna, spinach, steamed mangetout, and wholemeal garlic bread. Fresh fruit with low-fat yogurt. Grapefruit juice.
Bedtime snack Boiled egg and wholemeal toast "soldiers" with yeast extract. Glass of skimmed milk.

Good nutrition for pregnancy

Nature makes sure that a baby's nutritional needs are supplied by the body before the mother's. Anne's baby, therefore, could be better nourished than she is herself. The umbilical cord links Anne's baby with her placenta. All the nutrients necessary for healthy growth and

Miriam's top tips

With a little extra care and attention, it's possible to have a perfectly healthy, nutritional vegetarian diet and a healthy pregnancy. If you're pregnant and vegetarian, you may need to take supplements to ensure the healthy growth and development of your baby as your baby depends entirely on you for healthy nourishment.

■ Make sure you are getting the recommended daily dose of 400mcg of folic acid, either through foods rich in folic acid or by taking a folic acid supplement.

■ If you don't eat any animal or dairy products, vitamin B_{12} supplements, available from your local pharmacy, are absolutely essential.

■ A vegetarian diet that includes dairy products can support a pregnancy, and later breastfeeding, perfectly well, as long as you have more protein and calcium in your diet.

development pass to Anne's baby through the cord. A baby needs plenty of iron for blood formation and organ growth. This can be supplied by eating iron-rich foods such as egg yolks, cereals, and molasses. Calcium is very important as it builds healthy bones and teeth. Anne needs a diet that is rich in calcium to maintain her own needs as well that of her baby. Her diet should also be packed with protein-rich foods that will nourish her baby's fast-growing muscles, bones, skin, and vital organs.

The healthy development of her baby's brain and nervous system depends on sufficient supplies of Vitamin B_{12} as well as on Anne having sufficient levels of folic acid in her blood. The blood sugar of the baby is always lower than that of his mother because it's used so quickly, so a constant supply of calories is needed for healthy growth.

Are you at risk nutritionally?

If any of the following points apply to you, you could be nutritionally vulnerable and your baby may be at risk. You'll need to get special advice and help from your doctor or antenatal clinic before and during pregnancy.

- If you've had a recent stillbirth or miscarriage, or you're having a baby soon after a previous child (at least 18 months between babies is best for your health).

- If you smoke, or drink alcohol heavily.

- If you're allergic to certain foods, such as cow's milk or wheat.

- If you suffer from a chronic medical condition that means you have to take long-term medication.

- If you're under 18, your own body is growing quickly and your nutritional needs will be higher than average when pregnant.

- If you're carrying twins or multiple babies.

- If you've been under a lot of stress or had any physical injury.

- If your job involves physical work or is in a potentially dangerous environment (see p.168).

- If you were generally run-down or underweight before conception, or eating an inadequate or unbalanced diet.

- If you are bulimic, anorexic, or have a BMI (body mass index) of less than 19.

Food-related problems

It's so important to eat enough good food to satisfy your nutritional needs while you're pregnant or you could put yourself and your developing baby at risk. Fresh food rather than processed is best. Take care not to eat food contaminated with bacteria that cause disease; for example, chicken or eggs contaminated with salmonella.

Malnutrition

You need to eat properly for your baby's sake. If you don't, there's a higher risk you could miscarry or have a premature or low birthweight baby, who will be more vulnerable at birth and later in life. (By the way, having a low birthweight baby does not mean labour will be easier.) Being poorly nourished yourself can also slow the growth of the placenta, and low placental weight is related to a higher infant mortality rate. Your baby's brain develops most rapidly in the last trimester of pregnancy (and in the first month of life after birth) so if you're undernourished it can affect your baby's brain function.

A poor diet during pregnancy can continue to affect a child throughout his life, and may mean he's more likely to suffer such middle-aged diseases as high blood pressure, coronary artery disease, and obesity. If there's not enough nutrition getting through to your womb, the baby diverts what's available to those cells that are immediately important, and away from those cells that will not be important until later in life – in effect, your unborn baby trades long life for survival.

On the other hand, if you have enough good food and give birth to a good-sized baby, such a baby will be easier to care for, more vigorous, active, and mentally alert, and less likely to suffer from colic, diarrhoea, anaemia, and infection. If you're on a low income and you can't afford what you need, ask your midwife about free vitamin supplements.

Processed foods Many of these foods contain chemicals to improve flavour and shelf life. As a general rule, it's best to avoid these, especially when you're pregnant – in particular, processed cheese and meats, cheese spreads, and sausages. Check the lists of ingredients on labels for additives – food colourings and preservatives are represented by E numbers. Always make sure that you eat any packaged food well before its use-by date. Avoid highly salted foods, particularly if they contain monosodium glutamate (MSG), which causes dehydration and headaches.

Preserved foods such as smoked fish, meat, and cheese, pickled food, and sausages often contain nitrates. These can react with the haemoglobin in your blood and reduce its oxygen-carrying power so are best avoided.

Drinks Caffeine (in tea, coffee, and chocolate) is a stimulant, so try to cut it down when you're pregnant. The tannin in tea interferes with iron absorption: drink organic herbal teas instead. Soft drinks always contain sugar or sweeteners, so limit your intake of them. Mineral water is fine.

Food hazards

Some foods can be contaminated with large enough numbers of bacteria to cause illness, particularly in vulnerable people – such as pregnant women and babies.

Listeriosis Foods that can contain large numbers of listeria bacteria include soft cheese, unpasteurized milk, ready-prepared coleslaw, cooked chilled foods, pâtés, and meat that hasn't been properly cooked. Listeria bacteria are normally destroyed at pasteurizing temperatures, but if infected food is then refrigerated, the bacteria may continue to multiply. For this reason, you shouldn't eat chilled food after the "use-by" date. Listeriosis can spread through direct contact with infected live animals, such as sheep. Symptoms are flu-like: a high temperature and aches and pains, and also sore throat and eyes, diarrhoea, and stomach pain. An unborn child affected through his mother's blood may be stillborn, and listeriosis may be a cause of recurrent miscarriage.

Salmonella Infection with salmonella is often traced to eggs and chicken meat, so avoid any foods that contain raw eggs, and cook eggs and chicken thoroughly. Choose free-range poultry and look for eggs with the Lion Quality mark, which means they have been produced to the highest standards of food safety.

Symptoms of salmonella, including headache, nausea, abdominal pain, diarrhoea, shivering, and fever, develop suddenly 12–48 hours after infection and last about two to three days. If the infection spreads into your bloodstream, you'll need to take antibiotics.

Toxoplasmosis This common infection can be picked up by eating raw or undercooked pork or beef, or by coming into contact with the faeces of infected cats and dogs (see p.169).

Dysentery This is carried in the faeces of an affected person. It causes dehydration, severe diarrhoea, and abdominal pain and is dangerous for pregnant women. Amoebic dysentery is rare outside tropical areas, but bacterial dysentery is more common. It's usually passed on when an infected person fails to wash his hands properly after going to the toilet and then handles food.

Food safety

Never take unnecessary risks when handling and storing food; bacteria can multiply very rapidly.

■ Always use clean utensils between jobs, or tastings.

■ Always wash hands after going to the lavatory and before touching food, and take good care to seal off any infections or cuts.

■ Defrost and cook food thoroughly, especially poultry.

■ Never let raw meat or eggs come into contact with other foods.

■ Avoid dented and rusty tins and any food that looks or smells "off".

■ Make sure dairy products have been pasteurized.

■ Don't refreeze food that has already been defrosted.

■ Reheat food thoroughly and only once. Throw away leftovers.

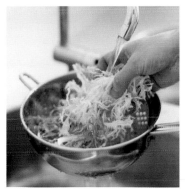

▲ **WASH SALAD LEAVES** It's important to wash all salad leaves under cold running water – even salad marked washed and ready to eat.

Miriam's casebook

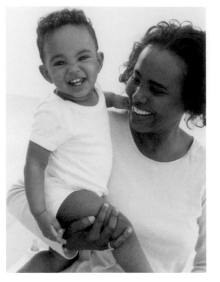

The diabetic mother

Jill developed insulin-dependent diabetes at 25 while she was pregnant with her second child, and has had the disease for a couple of years. She has two healthy sons. Her third pregnancy should be fine, but she's well aware of the importance of frequent antenatal checks. She knows that uncontrolled diabetes would create complications for her and lead to far more serious complications for her baby.

Pregnancy and diabetes

There's no need for women who have or develop diabetes during pregnancy to worry that they'll have a difficult pregnancy or problems giving birth to a normal, healthy baby. As long as diabetes is carefully managed, with an obstetrician and diabetic advisor in close cooperation, the outcome should be good.

As well as being 50 per cent more likely than men to become diabetics, women have a tendency to develop the disease during pregnancy. Certain women are recognized as potential diabetics. They've usually had at least one heavy baby or have a family history of diabetes in parents or siblings. Other women can develop diabetes during pregnancy. Some may remain diabetic after pregnancy but others go back to normal.

Pregnancy can complicate established diabetes, causing the kidneys to function less effectively and changes to occur in eyes and vision. While most sufferers will have been treated with insulin, some women with diabetes may have been treated with diet alone or with diet and blood-sugar lowering (hypoglycaemic) tablets. The extra demands of pregnancy are likely to lead to insulin having to be prescribed so any diabetic who plans to get pregnant should

change to insulin before conceiving. Having been an insulin-dependent diabetic for two years, Jill was meticulous about her pre-pregnancy preparations. She planned this present baby and made sure her diabetes was fully assessed well before she became pregnant. In particular, she was concerned about controlling her blood-sugar levels, the functioning of her kidneys, and the health of her eyes. In the months before conceiving she kept up careful control of her diabetes. She also took folic acid supplements in the period before conceiving.

Controlling diabetes

Jill knows that diabetes can mean a greater risk of her baby having cardiac and skeletal problems but that good control of her diabetes during the first trimester should greatly reduce this risk (see Possible health considerations, p.18). She came to ask my advice very early in the pregnancy.

I explained to Jill that now she's pregnant, she may need less insulin for the first three months. Then her body will start to produce hormones with an anti-insulin effect, so she'll need more insulin than before. Jill will need to test her blood sugar and adjust her dosage of insulin accordingly.

Possible complications

Pregnant women with diabetes usually go to an antenatal clinic where there is an obstetrician and a specialist in diabetes. Diabetic women usually have extra scans at 28, 32, and 36 weeks to check their baby's growth. As an established diabetic, Jill may have a number of disorders while she's pregnant because of fluctuations in her blood-sugar levels. She may suffer from urinary tract infections, thrush (see p.212), high blood pressure, pre-eclampsia (see p.224), and polyhydramnios (an excess of amniotic fluid). She could go into premature labour.

How diabetes affects her baby

If a mother's blood-sugar levels get high, sugar crosses the placenta and is converted into fat, muscle, and enlarged organs. The baby then becomes overweight. The baby produces large quantities of insulin to cope with the high sugar levels. At birth, when he's suddenly cut off from the source of sugar, the baby experiences a sudden, severe drop in blood sugar, while his insulin production remains high. If left untreated, this causes profound hypoglycaemia (shortage of blood sugar), which can ultimately result in coma and death but this is prevented with good antenatal care.

A preterm baby of a diabetic mother can be prone to respiratory distress syndrome, as the diabetes prevents the baby's lungs from producing the surfactant they need to aid breathing. The good news for Jill is that her careful control of her diabetes will make a big difference. Unless there are complications, such as high blood pressure or pelvic disproportion, and as long as her diabetes remains under control, Jill can hope for a normal vaginal delivery. She'll probably be advised to have an induction at 38 weeks if her baby isn't born by then, so he doesn't grow too big. I advised her to have a glucose and insulin intravenous drip to control the diabetes during labour, and continuous fetal heart monitoring and fetal blood sampling to detect any fetal distress. After the birth her baby will be checked in a neonatal special care unit in case he needs any immediate treatment, he'll be given to Jill so he can be breastfed.

As long as diabetes is closely managed during pregnancy, with help from your obstetrician and diabetic advisor, the outlook for mother and baby is good. Keep in mind the following:

■ have a full assessment of your diabetes before becoming pregnant and start taking 400mcg folic acid daily.

■ consult your doctor about changing to insulin before conceiving because the extra demands of pregnancy are likely to lead to insulin having to be prescribed.

■ watch your diet very carefully during your pregnancy.

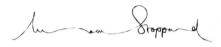

Jill's baby

Jill's doctor will be aware that her baby may be very large so he may have to be delivered with forceps or by Caesarean section. It is also possible that he may suffer from mild hypoxia (low oxygen supply to the tissues) shortly before birth, and this can lead to neonatal jaundice (see p.342) – a condition that can be treated after birth.

Jill's baby will be carefully checked after birth for any complications. In some hospitals, all babies of diabetic mothers are taken to special care so their blood-sugar levels can be closely checked, and Jill will be advised to breastfeed as soon as possible in order to counteract any trace of hypoglycaemia (shortage of blood sugar) her baby may have after birth.

Some diabetic mothers tend to have bigger and bigger babies, and they can be very heavy at birth: 4–5kg (9–11lb) for instance. While such a large baby may of course be delivered without a hitch, some obstetricians prefer to induce before term (at around 36 weeks, say) or opt for a planned Caesarean section before the baby has reached its full size or outgrown its food supply.

A healthy pregnancy

Keeping both your body and mind fit during
pregnancy is so important. Exercising will help
you do both. Everyone gets stressed and anxious
sometimes, and you may even be faced with some
potentially risky situations and substances. If you
find ways of coping with and avoiding any problems
that come up, you'll have a truly fit pregnancy.

Good for you

Taking some regular exercise helps you feel happier as well as keeping you fit. It's an enjoyable way of getting ready for the months of change ahead.

■ Hormones called endorphins, which your body releases when you exercise, will lift your spirits.

■ You'll feel more contented and relaxed after you exercise as the endorphins released have a tranquillizing effect.

■ Your self-awareness will improve as you learn how to use your body in new ways.

■ Regular exercise helps to ease backache, leg cramp, constipation, and breathlessness.

■ You'll find you have more energy.

■ You'll be better prepared for the work of labour.

■ After delivery you'll get your figure back more quickly.

■ You'll meet other mums at antenatal exercise classes so you'll make more friends.

■ Share your exercise routine with your partner or other members of your family and they'll get fitter too.

Stay active for a fit pregnancy

Regular exercise will build up your stamina and improve your suppleness and strength. This will help you cope with the extra demands made on your body as it adapts to pregnancy and childbirth. By exercising you can also develop a better understanding of what your body can do and learn different ways of relaxing.

Exercising helps you feel positive so you're less likely to think of yourself as clumsy, fat, or ungainly, particularly in the last three months. Your circulation will improve and that can help to ease tension. Labour may be easier and more comfortable if your muscle tone is good, and many of the exercises you learn in antenatal classes, combined with relaxation and breathing techniques, will help you trust your body during labour. And if you keep in good shape during pregnancy you'll get your figure back more quickly after your baby's birth.

Your exercise routine

You might think it's impossible to fit some exercise into your already busy schedule every day. But many of the exercises that it's good to do when you're pregnant, as shown on the following pages, can be done while you're getting on with something else: you can do pelvic floor exercises while you're cleaning your teeth; foot and ankle exercises when sitting at your desk or on the bus; and tailor sitting (see p.150) when you're reading or watching television.

Whatever type of exercise you choose, start your routine gently and gradually build up to what feels right for you. Before each exercise, take a few deep breaths. This gets the blood flowing around your body and gives all your muscles a good supply of oxygen. If you feel any pain, cramping, or shortness of breath, stop exercising, and when you start again, make sure you go more slowly. If you're out of breath, your baby won't be getting enough oxygen either.

Doing a little exercise several times a day is better than a lot of exercise all at once and then none at all. Normally a woman can restore her energy by lying down for half an hour, but when you're pregnant it can take half a day to recover properly from fatigue. So be kind to yourself and choose a way to exercise that you enjoy and find relaxing.

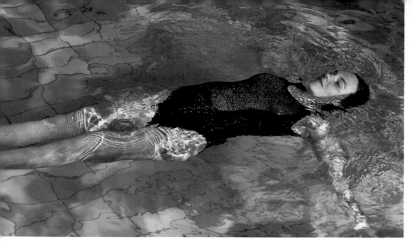

▲ **START SWIMMING** Exercising in water is safe during your pregnancy, even in the last trimester, because your weight is well supported.

Good ways to exercise

Most sports are fine, as long you've been doing that sport regularly before your pregnancy, and you keep it up consistently once you're pregnant so that you stay in shape.

Swimming is an excellent way to exercise when you're pregnant. It tones most of your muscles and is a good way to build up your stamina. Your body weight is supported by the water, so you're unlikely to strain or injure any of your muscles and joints. Many sports centres offer special swimming classes and aqua-natal exercise classes for pregnant women.

Yoga is good too, helping to increase your suppleness and reduce tension. It also teaches you to control your breathing and concentration, which are useful skills during labour. Or try a Pilates class for pregnant women, which will improve your posture, stability, and breathing.

Walking helps your digestion, your circulation, and your figure. Even if you're not usually very active, you'll be able to manage some regular walks of a mile or more. Try to walk tall, with your buttocks tucked under your spine, your shoulders back, and your head held up, not hanging down. Towards the end of pregnancy, though, you may find that the cartilage in your pelvic joints has softened so much that you get backache if you walk more than a short distance. Always wear well-cushioned flat shoes when you go out for a walk.

As long as you're not too energetic, it's fine to dance as often as you like throughout pregnancy.

Go carefully

It's safest not to continue cycling, skiing, and horseback riding once you're in the third trimester, because your balance is thrown off by the extra weight out in front. Other activities to avoid in the last months are jogging, backpacking, and sit-ups, which can put your body under unnecessary stress that could harm you and your baby.

Good for your baby

Every time you exercise within your limits, your baby gets a surge of oxygen into her blood that sets her metabolism alight and gives her a real high. All her tissues, especially her brain, function on top form.

■ The hormones that your body releases when you exercise pass across the placenta and reach your baby. So when you start to exercise, your baby receives an emotional lift from your adrenaline.

■ While you're exercising, your baby also feels the positive effect of your endorphins. These are your own natural morphine-like substances, released while exercising, that make us feel extremely good and happy.

■ After exercise, endorphins have a profound tranquillizing effect that can last up to eight hours, and your baby experiences this too.

■ The movements you make when you exercise are very soothing and good for your baby. She feels comforted by the rocking movements.

■ As you exercise, your abdominal muscles exert a kind of massage on your baby that she'll find comforting and soothing.

■ During exercise, your blood flow is at its highest and so your baby's growth and development benefit.

Why warm up?

A gentle warm-up routine gets your body ready for more demanding exercises and is easy to fit into your daily life.

Warming up helps to relieve tension. It gently warms up your muscles and joints and prevents muscles from overstretching, so reducing the risk of injury. You may suffer from stiffness and cramp if you don't warm up before you start exercising.

Stretching

Before beginning any exercise routine, always warm up gently with these stretching exercises. They'll stimulate your blood circulation, giving you and your baby a good supply of oxygen. Repeat each of the exercises five to ten times. Make sure you're comfortable while you stretch and that your posture is good.

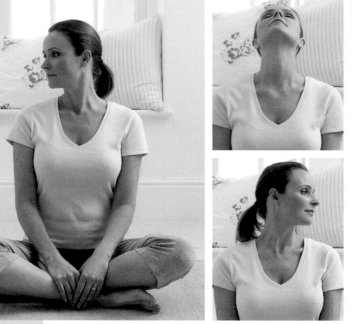

Keep your neck and back straight

Place your hand on your knee to help control the stretch

▲ **HEAD AND NECK** Gently turn your head to one side, then lift your chin and rotate your head back and gently over to the other side and down. Repeat, starting from the other side. Keeping your head straight, turn it slowly to the right, back to the front, and then back to the left. Return to face the front and repeat.

◀ **WAIST** Sit comfortably with your legs crossed and your back straight. Breathe out and turn your upper body to the right, placing your right hand behind you. Place your left hand on your right knee and use this hand as a lever to twist your body a little further, gently stretching the muscles of your waist. Repeat in the other direction.

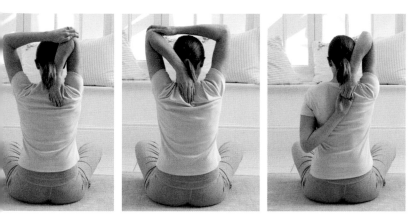

ARMS AND SHOULDERS Sitting on the floor, lift your right arm up and slowly stretch it to the ceiling. Bend it at the elbow and drop your hand down behind your back. Put your other hand on your elbow, and push the arm down your back (above left). Hold for 20 seconds, then relax. Repeat with other arm (centre). Bend your right arm again and drop your hand down your back. Put your left arm behind your back and reach to grasp the right hand. Hold for 20 seconds, then repeat with the opposite arms.

Take care

- Work on a firm surface.

- Always keep your back straight. Support your back against a wall or with cushions, if you need to.

- Start your routine slowly and gently and don't strain.

- If you feel pain, discomfort, or fatigue, stop at once.

- Always remember to breathe normally – otherwise you'll reduce the flow of blood to your baby.

- Never point your toes – always flex your foot to prevent cramps.

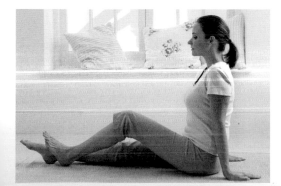

LEGS AND FEET Sit with your back straight and your legs stretched out in front of you. Place your hands on the floor next to your hips to support your weight. Bend one knee slowly and then straighten. Repeat with other leg. This will tone your leg muscles and help to ease cramp.

IMPROVING CIRCULATION Raise your foot off the floor and flex it outwards. Then draw large circles in the air with your foot, only moving your ankles. Keep your back straight and your weight central. Repeat with the other foot.

Bend your foot towards you to make the muscles work harder; take care not to strain

Your pelvic floor

Your pelvic floor muscles form a funnel that supports your uterus, bowel, and bladder, and closes the entrances to your vagina, rectum, and urethra.

The pelvic floor muscles lie in two main groups, making a figure of eight around your urethra, vagina, and anus. Muscle fibres come from back and front, high up on your lower back and pubic bones. The layers of muscle overlap so are thickest at the perineum.

When you're pregnant, the extra progesterone in your body softens and relaxes your muscles, and pressure from your enlarging uterus can stretch and weaken your pelvic floor. Half of all women who've had babies find they have a weakness in their pelvic floor. As a result they may feel uncomfortable or suffer so-called "stress" incontinence – leaking a little urine when laughing, coughing, or sneezing.

To counter this, physiotherapists have developed exercises you can do to keep your pelvic floor toned.

Pull in and tense the muscles around your vagina and anus. Hold as long as you can without straining. Relax. Repeat 25 times or more each day.

Do this exercise during pregnancy and start again as soon as you can after your baby's born. Early exercise will tone up your vagina for sex, too. Try to make the exercise part of your daily routine.

Body exercises

If you do some exercises for your whole body, you'll relieve the strain caused by your extra weight and strengthen important muscles. Also, if you learn to move your pelvis easily during pregnancy, you'll find it's easier to get into a comfortable position during labour. These pre-natal exercises are based on yoga positions and will help to increase your suppleness and reduce tension.

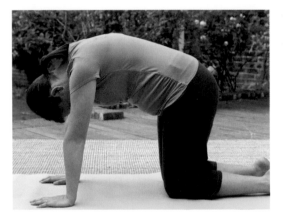

◀ **PELVIC TUCK-IN** Kneel down on all fours with your knees about 30cm (12in) apart. Clench your buttock muscles and tuck in your pelvis so that your back arches upwards into a hump. Hold for a few seconds, and then release, making sure you don't let your back sink downwards. Repeat several times.

Forward bend

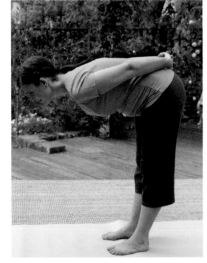
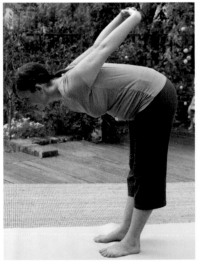

1 **BEND SLOWLY** Place your feet 30cm (12in) apart, keeping them parallel. Clasp your hands behind your back. Bend slowly from your hips, with your back straight. Breathe deeply for a few breaths, then rise slowly.

2 **RAISE YOUR HANDS** You should only do this step if you are able to do Step 1 comfortably. After bending forwards from your hips, slowly raise your hands until you're holding them as far above your head as possible.

Lower back release

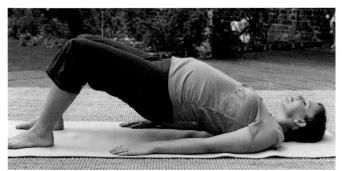

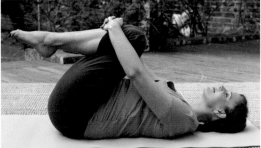

1 LIFT YOUR PELVIS Lie flat with your arms by your sides, palms down. Press your feet into the floor. Lift your pelvis so that your spine rises as high as you can. Come down one vertebra at a time.

2 HUG YOUR KNEES Keeping your lower back in contact with the floor, gently hug your knees. Hold for a few minutes, breathing deeply.

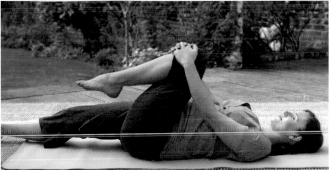

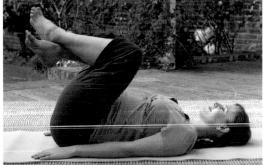

3 ALTERNATE LEGS Straighten your right leg on the floor and gently hug your left knee. Repeat with the other leg.

4 ROTATE YOUR HIPS Bend both knees and cross your feet at the ankles. Then rotate your hips clockwise, making tiny circles with your lower back on the floor. Repeat the movement in the other direction.

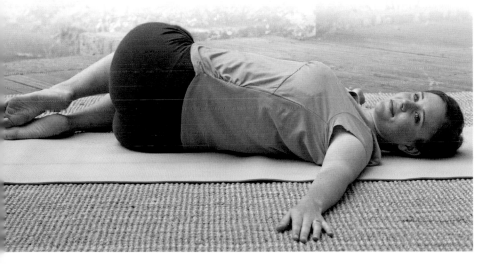

◄ **SPINAL TWIST** Keep your shoulders and arms flat on the ground and, as you breathe out, slowly turn your knees over to the right and your head over to the left. This gently twists your spine. Hold this position for a few seconds. Come back to the centre, keeping your knees bent, and then relax. Then slowly roll your knees over to the left and your head to the right. Repeat the exercise.

Shaping up for labour

▼ TAILOR SITTING Sit on the floor, and stretch your legs out in front. Make sure your back is straight. Bend your knees and bring the soles of your feet together, then pull them as close as you can to your groin. Open out your thighs and lower your knees towards the floor. Relax your shoulders and the back of your neck. Breathe deeply. Concentrate on breathing down towards your pelvis resting on the floor, relaxing as you breathe out. As you breathe in, lift up and stretch your spine while keeping your pelvis on the ground.

If you prepare your mind and body beforehand, you're more likely to have a comfortable labour. You'll find the following exercises very useful during pregnancy. You may want to give birth while squatting, and tailor sitting will strengthen your thigh muscles and increase circulation to your pelvis, making your joints more supple. This exercise also helps to stretch your pelvis and relax the tissues of your perineum.

After exercising, spend 20–30 minutes relaxing, and, if possible, try to arrange to have a regular break during your day. You don't have to sleep – spending five or ten minutes with your eyes closed and your feet up is enough to refresh you. Learning breathing and relaxation techniques will be a great help during labour, when tension can make the pain worse. If you're able to concentrate on the rhythm of your breathing, you'll feel less anxious and save your energy.

If you find it difficult to pull your feet close to your groin, you can start with them about 30cm (12in) away from your body and gradually bring them nearer. With practice your muscles will loosen

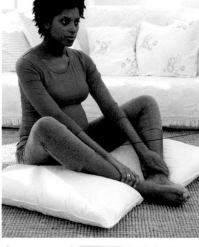

Support your thighs with some cushions or blankets, or sit against a wall at first if you find it easier

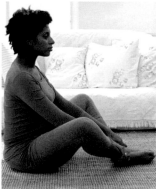

◄ STRAIGHT BACK Sit up straight and don't round your back or slump. Look straight ahead, not down at your legs.

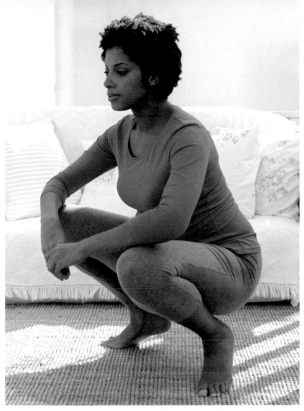

▲ **SQUATTING** Stand with your back lengthened and straight, and your feet 45cm (18in) apart. Squat down as low as you can and spread your knees apart. Try to get your heels on the ground with your weight evenly distributed between heels and toes, but don't worry if you have to raise your heels. Hold the squat for a few minutes or for as long as you like if you're comfortable. Then come forwards to kneel or stand up.

▼ **HOLD ON** If you need to, hold on to something steady, such as a chair, low stool, or window ledge, to support your back as you squat, and place a towel underneath your heels. You can also lean against a wall.

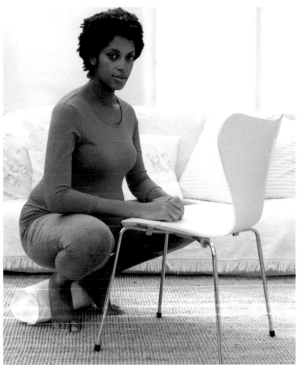

Relaxation

It's comfortable to lie with your legs up on a chair or a bed, but as you get bigger, avoid lying on your back for too long. You may find it helps to prop your shoulders up with pillows so you don't feel dizzy. When your pregnancy is advanced it may be more comfortable to lie on your side.

▼ **LYING DOWN** Lie on your side with a pillow under your head. Bend your upper leg upwards and place a pillow under this knee; keep your lower leg straightened. Close your eyes and concentrate just on your breathing.

Clear your mind and breathe in deeply. Hold to a count of five and breathe out. Relax all parts of your body

Lying this way eases pressure on your major blood vessels and your abdomen

Massage extras

A few extras can make your massage even better. Have everything ready before you start so you don't break the mood.

■ Scented oils will help hands glide over your skin, and leave it soft and smooth. The fragrance of the oil will add to the atmosphere, making each occasion special.

■ Try rubbing feathers, fabric, and other soft-textured materials against the skin to leave it tingling.

■ Cover any exposed skin with some warm, fluffy towels so you don't get cold.

■ Use spinal rolls for firm, smooth counter-pressure (see p.296).

■ Gently brushing your hair with light strokes of a soft bristle hair-brush can be very relaxing.

Massage for relaxation

Being massaged by your partner, or doing it yourself, is a wonderful way to relax and unwind at the end of a long day. Massage stimulates the nerve endings in your skin, improves your circulation, and soothes tired muscles, giving you a sense of peace and wellbeing. Your baby will enjoy the sensation of your body being caressed too, and find the movements comforting.

Soothing touch

Use some good-quality massage oil (one with a vegetable oil base) to smooth your skin and make your massage more pleasurable. To create a comfortable, relaxing atmosphere: dim the lights, put on some soft music, and put some pillows or cushions around and underneath yourself. Later on in your pregnancy, you may find it's more comfortable to lie on your side supported by pillows, or to sit astride a chair.

You can massage most parts of your body, apart from your back, quite effectively yourself. Using the palms and fingers of one hand, work clockwise around each breast, stroking from the base towards

Self massage

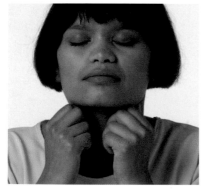

▲ **FIRM YOUR NECK** Make gentle pinching movements around your jawbone. Softly squeeze the skin between your thumb and the knuckles of your index finger. Don't drag your skin.

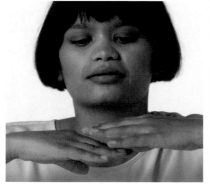

▲ **TONE YOUR CHIN** Stimulate the blood circulation under your chin with brisk movements. Using the backs of both hands, gently slap upwards with one after another.

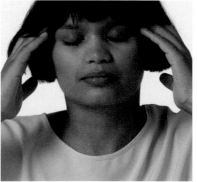

▲ **SOOTHE YOUR FOREHEAD** Put your fingertips on your forehead and the heels of your hands on your chin. Leaving your fingertips on your forehead draw your hands away from your face.

your nipple; gently knead your nipples between your fingers and thumb. Massage your abdomen, hips, and thighs, with the palms of your hands, using smooth, circular movements.

If your partner or anyone else is giving you a massage, make sure that their hands are warm before starting and that they've taken off any rings, bracelets, or watches. When you're both comfortable, take a few deep breaths to help you relax. It's best for the masseur to begin massaging you gently. The pressure can gradually be increased if it's comfortable for you, but always keep the movements slow and gentle.

If you should decide to go for a professional massage, always make sure the therapist knows that you're pregnant.

Circling Using the palms of both hands at once, make circling strokes in the same direction away from the spine. Lighten the pressure when massaging over the abdomen and breasts.

Effleurage Make light, feathery, circular movements with the fingertips as though tickling the skin. This type of massage can be done all over the abdomen during pregnancy.

Gliding Place the palms of both hands on either side of the lower back, with the fingers pointing to your head. Push the hands up to the shoulders, without exerting body weight on to the hands. Slowly glide the hands down the sides of the body back to the starting point.

Massage by a partner

Essential oils

Using aromatic oils in your massage can help you feel relaxed and refreshed. Their scents also help conjure up wonderful images.

These oils are distilled from flowers, trees, and herbs, and are said to have healing qualities. For example, lavender oil relieves headaches and insomnia. Be careful, however. There are some essential oils, such as camphor, aniseed, and fennel, that shouldn't be used in pregnancy, so always check with an experienced aromatherapist before using anything. Use only a small amount of essential oil – about two drops to 10ml (½floz) of carrier oil.

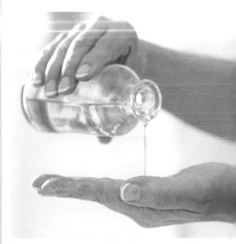

▲ **SOOTHING SCENTS** Blend any essential oils with a carrier oil such as almond or olive before applying it to your skin. Never use undiluted essential oil.

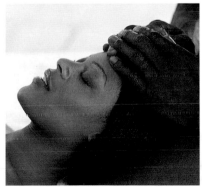

▲ **TENSION SOOTHER** Place your hands on her forehead so that your fingertips just meet in the middle and hold lightly. Press gently, release, and hold lightly again before lifting your hands away.

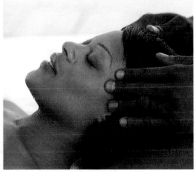

▲ **FOREHEAD MASSAGE** This also helps to soothe away tension. Using your fingertips, make tiny circular movements all over her forehead, working from one side to the other and then back again.

Will my moods affect my baby?

You may worry that your changing moods will somehow affect your baby.

Your baby does react to your moods and may start kicking when you're angry or upset, but your different emotions don't seem to have any harmful effect on your baby (see also A mother's influence, p.192).

Dreams and nightmares can be very vivid, and you may find that you wake up suddenly, feeling hot, drenched in sweat, and with your heart racing. Don't worry – this won't harm your baby.

On the other hand, your baby enjoys your good moods, when you're excited and happy. When you feel good, your baby feels good. When you're relaxed, your baby also feels tranquil.

If there's something that makes you feel content and happy, such as listening to music, dancing gently, painting – do as much of it as you can and share the good feelings with your baby.

Emotional changes

It's not only your body that alters during pregnancy. Your emotions will change rapidly, too, and you'll experience feelings you've never had before. It'll help if you accept that you will feel upset from time to time – all pregnant women do – and that there are things you can do to help you cope with your mood swings.

It's the changes in hormone levels that are making your moods change so suddenly, making you weepy and sad one minute and on top of the world the next. On top of that we all occasionally feel anxious about how good we're going to be as parents. Your changing body shape can disturb your self-image, too. Emotionally, pregnancy can be very difficult.

Hormonal changes

There are enormous changes in your body during pregnancy and, because of this, your mood is likely to change often. You might find yourself being hypercritical and irritable, you might have exaggerated reactions to minor events, you may feel unsure of yourself and panicky sometimes, and you may have bouts of depression and crying.

It's normal to go through all of these things because you're less in control of your feelings than usual. The swinging levels of hormones have taken over and are controlling your moods the way a conductor controls an orchestra. So don't feel guilty or ashamed if you show your irritation, anger, or frustration. If you explain what's happening, most people will understand. At work, you may have to struggle to keep up an appearance of calm. This effort will definitely pay off, especially if you plan to go back to your job after the birth of your baby.

Worries about pregnancy

However positive you are about your pregnancy, it's normal to have worries sometimes. One moment you're thrilled at the prospect of your new baby, the next you're feeling terrified of the new responsibilities to come. Becoming a parent is a time of reassessment and change, of worries and fears.

The first and most important thing you have to do is to accept your pregnancy. This may sound obvious, but there are some women who blithely sail through the early months of pregnancy giving it as little thought as possible, which is especially easy until the baby begins to show. You and the baby's father have to come to terms with the pregnancy and begin to think about the reality. Until now your thoughts about a baby and parenthood may always have been in soft focus, a pastel picture of a loving threesome.

Conflicting feelings are sure to surface once you begin to accept the realities to come. Don't worry – it's good to have conflicting feelings. It's normal to feel this way so don't feel bad about it. It means that you're genuinely coming to terms with the situation. You won't have the shock some people do, who wait to face all this when they bring their baby home.

Your changing shape

You might also be troubled by the changes in your body shape and might worry that you look unattractive. You may feel strange, even unrelated to the body in which you find yourself. Don't worry about your shape – a pregnant woman looks sensuous and beautiful. Thinking of pregnant women as fat, and therefore ugly, is essentially a Northern European attitude: many other cultures see pregnant women as sensuous and beautiful. Don't look at your increasing curves with despair, think of them as a reaffirmation of life. See your roundness as ripeness, and glory in your body's fertility. Feel confident and proud of your shape.

Practical problems

Everyday difficulties that you'd normally deal with quite calmly can turn into dramas during pregnancy. Keep a level head, and try not to overreact.

Finances Financial problems are always one of the main causes of stress between a couple, and they can become especially troubling during pregnancy. You may find it difficult to cope with a reduction in income, even if you plan to return to work, but remember that you're in this together. Work out before the birth how you're going to manage on your income once your baby has arrived.

Housing Moving or expanding your home may be something that you have to think about – perhaps extra space will be needed, or there may be a lack of facilities for babies and children in your area. All this can be stressful, and tends to be worse when you're pregnant. If you must move – and it's not the best idea from a physical point of view – do it before your pregnancy is too advanced.

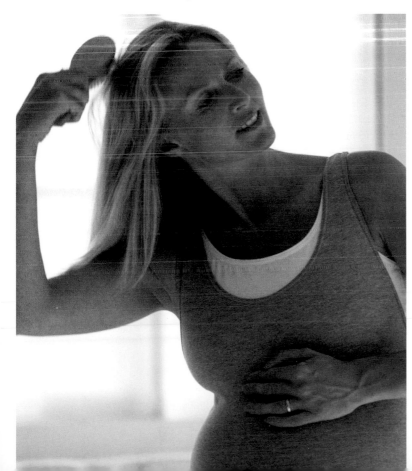

◀ **YOUR CHANGING SHAPE** The more positive you are about your body and the way you look while you're pregnant, the better you'll feel.

Dreams

You may find your dreams become more frequent, and even frightening, in the last trimester.

Many pregnant women report common themes and all express deep feelings and concerns that are entirely natural – everybody worries at one time or another that something will be wrong or go wrong with their baby. You may have dreams about losing your baby; and this is usually an expression of fear about miscarrying or having a stillborn baby. Dreams like these may be the brain's way of preparing for an unwanted outcome and also help to bring these feelings to the surface. Dreams can act as a release for your anxieties.

Dreams, nightmares, and thoughts in general may also be a way of expressing hostility to your unborn child. She's going to take over your life, disrupting your privacy and comfortable routine. They may express feelings you may not be able to cope with or even be consciously aware of. Again, don't make the mistake of taking dreams literally and then feeling guilty or frightened.

Fears

Perhaps you worry about labour – whether you'll be able to cope with the pain, whether you'll scream, lose control of your bowels, or need an episiotomy or an emergency Caesarean? Most of us do get anxious about these things, but there's no need. Labour is usually straightforward and it doesn't really matter how you behave. You may be surprised at how calm you are or you may not be calm at all, and both are okay. Just remember that your birth attendants have seen it all before, so there's nothing for you to feel embarrassed about.

You may worry about how good a parent you'll be, whether you'll hurt or harm your baby, or not care for her properly. These are normal feelings and represent very reasonable fears. Many people don't know much about baby care and worry about doing a good job. The answer is to get some hands-on experience – handle and care for a newborn baby if you can. Perhaps you could babysit for a friend's baby, or spend some time with her? If you change and cuddle someone else's baby, it'll give you some confidence. Try to get your fears into perspective – you probably had similar worries about starting a job.

Superstitions

You may find you're more superstitious than usual. In the past, old wives' tales and superstitions were ways of explaining an inexplicable world. But with the excellent medical care available today, your chances of having a damaged child are very low. Something you see as a bad omen certainly doesn't mean that anything will go wrong with your baby.

Coping with emotional changes

If you can, look on the emotional turmoil you're going through as a positive force as you adjust to being pregnant and becoming a mother. Don't imagine that having second thoughts or fears means you've made a mistake. You're just tossing this around in your head the way one wrestles with any big life decision. Yet social conditioning can make us feel guilty if we don't walk around with a madonna-like expression and saintly attitude to everything. That's absurd. Being pregnant isn't all fun. Accepting the reality is the best thing you can do for yourself and your child.

Spend time daydreaming Imagining and thinking about your baby helps you to build your relationship with her even before she's born, so don't feel silly if you find yourself spending a couple of hours doing nothing but thinking about your baby. Making that connection with the tiny person growing inside you is the first step in accepting your child. Many mothers find they have an undisguised preference for a girl or a boy in their daydreams. Although it isn't usually a problem if your newborn turns out to be the opposite sex from the one you wanted, it can mean you have to readjust, so try not to get too carried away with your plans!

Think about your parents Your parents are about to become grandparents, perhaps for the first time. They may be delighted, they may be upset, or they may feel a combination of both reactions. In other words, they might be feeling confused about their new role too. Some people see becoming grandparents as meaning that they're getting old, and this can be unsettling for someone who perhaps feels only just middle-aged. Try to be understanding and loving with your parents. Include them in your pregnancy and share your feelings with them.

Talk to other mums A pregnant woman can feel isolated. You may find that you're the first in your circle of friends to start a family, and that you don't know any other pregnant women or mums. It can be lonely. There's so much that you want to know and talk about. You may have little niggles and worries that you feel are too irrelevant or silly to talk about at your antenatal clinic, and you may wish you knew someone who was going through the same thing or who already had a child. If you feel like this, find someone you can talk to – join parent groups, make friends with other pregnant women in your childbirth classes, and ask your friends or family if they know any pregnant women, or parents whom you could get to know. You may find these relationships go on long after your baby is born. And don't forget your partner – if you're feeling isolated, the chances are he is too, so include him and expand your social circle together. There are also a number of websites (see p.370) for pregnant women and mums where you can log on and discuss all sorts of worries and questions, and share your experiences.

Share your feelings Wanting to talk through and share what you're feeling and thinking during your pregnancy is natural. Your partner is an obvious first choice, and he'll probably be anxious to talk to you. There are bound to be things that he'd like to talk about: worries, things that he may have not wanted to discuss with you because he thought that he might upset you or you might think him silly, or because you were too busy, or too tired. Keep talking. You need each other more now than ever before. Denying or ignoring your fears and feelings won't make them go away. Suppressed feelings have a very nasty way of festering and then surfacing when you're least able to deal with them, so turning into full-blown problems. If you bring these problems out in the open when they first come up, you'll be able to deal with them and get on with your lives.

Grandparents

A new baby means a new role not only for you but maybe for your parents, too.

Once your baby's born they're bound to revel in their roles as doting grandparents, but they may feel they're still too young when you first tell them the good news.

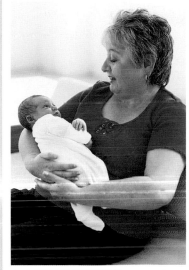

▲ **A SOURCE OF HELP** Your parents may provide practical help and can be invaluable sources of expertise and reassurance when you have a new baby to care for.

Make-up tips

The tone and colour of your skin can alter when you're pregnant so you may want to change your usual make-up routine. Have a facial and treat yourself to some new products.

Fine lines or wrinkles If your skin gets drier than usual, any lines look more obvious. Stop using shiny or glittering eye shadows, heavy foundations, and coloured powders – they draw attention to lines and wrinkles.

Extra greasy skin To combat this, use an astringent lotion, oil-free foundation, and finish your make-up with translucent powder.

Extra dry skin If your skin becomes so dry that it flakes, it's best to stop wearing make-up. Keep on moisturizing your skin well. Otherwise, use an oil-based film of foundation and some powder to help to slow water loss. Thick, creamy moisturizers will also act as a barrier to water loss on dry patches.

High colour and spider veins Stipple a thin, light coat of matt foundation on to your cheeks – use a beige colour that's free of any pink. When it's dry, cover with your regular foundation and some translucent powder.

Dark circles Put on a thin layer of foundation, stipple on an under-eye cover-up cream, and leave to dry. Cover with another thin layer of foundation and blend well. Finish with translucent powder.

Body care

Pregnancy hormones can affect almost every part of your body, including your breasts, skin, hair, teeth, and gums. To keep your body in good shape, you'll probably need to make some changes in your daily routine. Your growing abdomen may affect your posture, too, so check the way you stand and move (see p.160).

Skin

Your skin will probably "bloom" during pregnancy. All the extra hormones encourage the skin to hold moisture that plumps it out, making it more supple, less oily, and less prone to spots. The extra blood circulating round your body also makes your skin glow. But there can be problems, too. Red patches may get bigger, acne may worsen, areas may become dry and scaly, and you may notice deeper pigmentation across your face.

Skin care Here are a few general tips for looking after your skin during pregnancy. Soap removes natural oils from the skin, so use it as little as possible. Try using baby lotion, or glycerine-based soap and body wash. Always add some oils to your bath to lessen the dehydrating effects of hard water, and don't lie in the bath for too long as this dehydrates the skin. Make-up can help cheer you up and it helps moisturize the skin as it prevents water loss.

Deeper pigmentation This happens to nearly every woman, especially on areas of the body that have pigmentation already, such as freckles, moles, and the areolae of the breasts. Your genitals, the skin on the inside of your thighs, underneath your eyes, and in your armpits may become darker too. A dark line, called the linea nigra, often appears down the centre of your stomach. It marks the division of your abdominal muscles, which separate slightly to make room for your expanding uterus. Even after you've had your

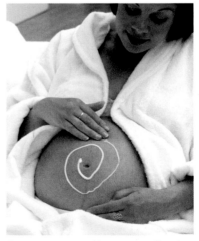

▲ **STRETCH MARKS** No creams will make much difference to stretch marks, but they do moisturize the skin and you'll enjoy the feeling as you rub them in.

baby, the linea nigra and the areolae usually remain darker for a while, but will gradually fade. Sunlight intensifies the colour of areas of skin that are already pigmented, and many women find that they tan more easily when they're pregnant. Since ultraviolet A (UVA) rays can lead to skin cancer, and the effect they have on the unborn baby is unknown, it's important to avoid sunburn. If you're out in the sun use a sun block. Keep your skin covered up in hot sun, and don't use sunbeds. Don't use fake tan products during pregnancy as these can cause skin allergies.

Brown patches Some women develop brown patches on the nose, cheeks, and neck during pregnancy. This is called chloasma, or the mask of pregnancy, and is a special form of pigmentation. You can make it less noticeable by using concealer or the cover-up cosmetics used for birthmarks. Don't try to bleach the marks – they'll fade after the birth.

Spider veins Your blood vessels are very sensitive when you're pregnant and you may find tiny broken blood vessels called spider veins on your face. Don't worry – they'll fade soon after delivery and will probably have disappeared by three months after the birth.

Pimples If you've always been prone to coming out in spots before your period you may get them when you're pregnant, particularly in the first few months. Keep your skin really clean and use a cleanser two or three times a day. Never squeeze spots as this only spreads the infection into deeper layers of skin.

Stretch marks Most women get some stretch marks during pregnancy. These are usually on the tummy, but may also appear on the thighs, hips, breasts, and upper arms. They're caused by the breakdown of protein in the skin by the high levels of pregnancy hormones and there's not much you can do about them. Whatever you rub into your skin or eat doesn't really make much difference, although putting on weight gradually should help. Don't worry – they'll fade soon after delivery and will probably have disappeared by three months after the birth.

Teeth

When you're pregnant your gums tend to become soft and spongy so more likely to bleed and become infected. This is because of the extra blood in your body and the high levels of hormones. Be very careful about cleaning and flossing your teeth, and make sure you eat a good diet with plenty of calcium-rich foods to help keep your teeth healthy. Avoid sweets and sugar.

Your hair

During pregnancy, many women find that their hair changes in quality, quantity, and manageability.

The high levels of hormones stop your usual cycle of hair growth and loss. Usually some hair grows and some is lost every day. When you're pregnant, your hair is arrested in the growth phase.

After delivery, the cycle passes into a resting phase and you might lose masses of hair. Hair loss can go on for up to two years and may be alarming, but don't worry, it will stop – pregnancy never causes baldness. The hair you lose once your baby is born is simply the hair you would normally have lost throughout the whole of the nine months of pregnancy.

If your hair is more difficult to manage, think about changing to a simpler hairstyle that's easier to care for. Choose the mildest shampoo you can find. When you wash your hair, use only one application of shampoo, massage gently to a lather, leave for 30 seconds, and rinse off.

Body and facial hair may increase in quantity and it may even become darker in colour.

Check your posture

Making sure your posture is good should help you suffer less of the backache and fatigue that can happen later in your pregnancy.

Bad posture, caused by the increasing weight of your baby, is common in pregnancy. Your growing abdomen thrusts your centre of gravity forwards and to balance this you may arch your back. This puts your back muscles under strain and can cause backache. When you're standing, sitting, or walking, check that your posture is correct, with your neck and back in a straight line.

Avoiding problems

Pregnancy hormones stretch and soften your ligaments, particularly those in your lower back, so they tend to strain more easily. If you're careful, though, you can avoid the unnecessary back problems and tiredness that many women suffer during their pregnancy.

▶ **DON'T BEND DOWN** When you're doing jobs at home or in the garden and you need to work on something at ground level, sit or kneel down so it's in easy reach. Whenever you can, avoid bending or stooping.

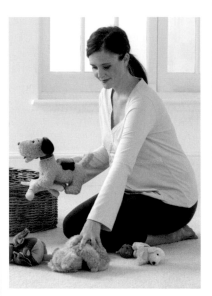

◀ **LIFTING AND CARRYING** When you want to lift something from the floor, reach down to it by bending your knees, keeping your back as straight as you can. When you pick it up, hold it close in to your body, and lift it by straightening your legs, so that you use the strength of your leg and thigh muscles to do the actual lifting. Never struggle to lift any objects that are too heavy – get someone to help you. Don't try lifting heavy things to or from high shelves or upward. If you're carrying heavy bags, try to divide the weight equally between both your hands.

Getting up without strain

1 TURN ON TO YOUR SIDE When you want to get up after lying down on the floor – after exercising, for instance – take it in easy stages. First, turn on to your side.

2 MOVE TO SITTING Keeping your back straight, use your hands to support yourself as you move yourself into a sitting position.

3 STAND UP FROM KNEELING Still with your back straight, use your thigh muscles to push yourself up into a kneeling position. From here, you can stand up without straining your abdomen.

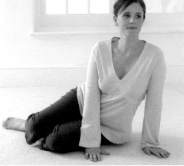

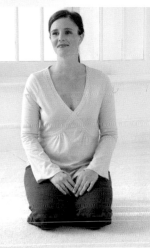

Nail and skin problems

POSSIBLE PROBLEM	WHAT TO DO
Itching or chafed skin The skin of your extended abdomen may become quite itchy when you're pregnant, and the area between your thighs may become chafed.	Massage your skin with baby lotion to stimulate the blood supply and soothe irritation. Keep the skin on your thighs dry, dust with powder, and wear cotton underwear.
Rashes A rash in your groin and under your breasts can be caused by excess weight gain and the sweat that gathers in the folds of your skin. Not washing often enough increases the risk.	Keep your groin area and the skin under your breasts clean, and apply calamine or other drying lotion. Wear a good bra that supports your breasts properly.
Pigmentation Many women find that their skin pigmentation changes when they're pregnant; this particularly affects areas that already darker, such as moles and the areolae of your breasts.	Use a sun block to protect your skin from the ultraviolet rays in sunlight. The extra pigmentation will disappear after the birth.
Nails Your fingernails grow faster than usual when you're pregnant. They may also become brittle and split, or break more easily than they did before your pregnancy.	Keep your nails short and well trimmed. Wear gloves when you're washing dishes or working in the garden.

What to wear

Comfort is the main thing where clothes are concerned when you're pregnant. As you get bigger, try to stay one step ahead – there's nothing worse than clothes that are too tight for you. You'll probably feel warmer than usual during pregnancy because your blood is circulating round your body at a faster rate. Your feet and legs may tend to swell, so choose your shoes and tights with extra care.

Clothes

You don't need to buy lots of expensive maternity clothes. Many high street shops now have excellent ranges at good prices. If you have a few specially bought basics, such as a pair of maternity jeans with an expandable front panel, a selection of properly fitted maternity bras, some maternity cotton or wool tights and leggings with expandable gussets, and one or two maternity dresses for special occasions, you can add a few inexpensive items, such as ethnic dresses, drawstring cotton trousers, and comfortable tops and jumpers – some of which you can wear after your pregnancy. Lots of pregnant women no longer want to wear tent-like clothes, preferring to show off their new shape.

Before you splash out on any special outfits, find out if any of your friends or neighbours have pregnancy clothes that you could borrow. In some areas you'll find shops that specialize in nearly-new maternity clothes, where you can buy clothes at bargain prices. It's best to avoid synthetic fabrics if you can – natural fabrics will be far more comfortable.

Work clothes If you wear a uniform to work, let your employers know that you're pregnant in good time so they can provide you with new clothes when you need them or give you financial help to get a uniform for yourself. If you normally wear heels to work, change to flat shoes.

Underwear

Bra A good bra is essential when you're pregnant. Your breasts will get bigger, particularly during the first three months, and if you don't support them, they're likely to sag later. This is because the sling of fibrous tissue to which they are attached never gets its shape back once it's stretched. A well-fitting bra will help to prevent stretching in the first place. When you buy a bra, it's best to have it properly fitted. A large department store or a shop specializing in maternity clothes or lingerie will have trained staff to

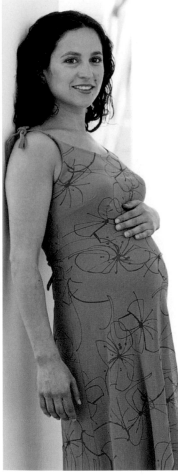

▲ **MATERNITY OUTERWEAR** Choose clothes that are comfortable, practical, and look good too. Bear in mind that the seasons will change as you grow bigger.

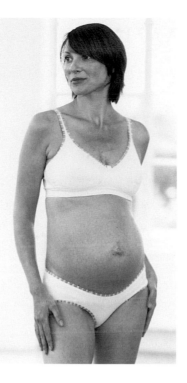

▶ **MATERNITY UNDERWEAR** A well-fitting bra that gives you good support is vital for comfort during pregnancy – and for your figure afterwards.

Shoes

The bigger you get, the more unstable you become, so it's best to wear flat or low-heeled, comfortable, easy-fitting shoes.

Make sure they support your foot well, are roomy enough, and preferably have a nonslip sole for safety. Trainers are ideal – choose a pair with a Velcro fastening because later in your pregnancy you might find it hard to bend down to do up laces. You'll find there are plenty of smart, flat shoes in the shops that are versatile and hard-wearing. Your feet will swell during pregnancy, so choose a size bigger than normal. Best of all, go barefoot whenever you can

help fit one for you. Look for a bra that gives you good support with a deep band underneath the cups and wide shoulder straps that don't cut deep into your skin. Back-fastening bras may be better than front-fastening. Only buy a couple of bras to begin with as your breasts will continue to get bigger, and you'll have to get a larger size later in pregnancy. If your breasts become very big, it helps to wear a light bra in bed at night to give them extra support.

Just before your due date, buy two or three front-opening feeding bras so that you can breastfeed your baby easily. You can buy feeding bras at any maternity shop or department store.

Briefs There's a range of different types of maternity briefs available that provide light support for your tummy. You can also buy bump support belts which relieve your back of strain and help prevent backache.

Socks Choose cotton socks that are loose fitting. Synthetic materials don't have any give and can cut really deeply into swollen feet. In addition, they don't let you sweat, so the skin becomes waterlogged and soft. It's best to avoid knee-high socks – they can form a restricting band around the top of your calf, and encourage varicose veins (see p.212).

Tights and stockings Even sheer maternity tights will give you a lot of support. You'll find lots of different types in plenty of colours in maternity shops and most department stores. If you have a tendency to suffer from thrush (see p.212), you might prefer to wear stockings instead of tights. You'll probably find that support stockings, or ones containing a high percentage of lycra, are the most comfortable, although they don't give you as much support as maternity tights. Suspender belts that fit on your hips under your abdomen will be most comfortable, so find a belt that's big enough and shorten the straps if you need to.

A working pregnancy

There's no reason why you can't carry on working well into your pregnancy if you want to, unless your working environment could be dangerous for your baby. If you do want to go on working and return to your job after your baby is born, make sure you've all the information you need to protect both your health and your job.

When you're pregnant your body does change and you may be rather uncomfortable at times, but carrying on working can help you feel more normal. By continuing to work, you can keep up this important and stable aspect of your life at a time when you may be feeling disorientated in other ways because of the physical and emotional changes of pregnancy.

Putting your rights into play

Most employers will be keen to help you continue working during your pregnancy and after your maternity leave, but it's up to you to tell them what you want to do. You need to let them know when you plan to stop work before your baby's born and when you'll be coming back afterwards.

Protect your job Make sure you know what maternity leave and pay you're entitled to (see p.64) and talk to your employer, manager, or trade union representative. Don't forget you're allowed paid time off for antenatal care, and this includes time to go to relaxation classes.

Protect your health If there's any chance of an aspect of your work causing harm to your baby – for example, exposure to X-rays, doing heavy lifting, or handling harmful chemicals – your employer must find you another job while you're pregnant, or, if this isn't possible, you should be suspended on full pay. This is your right, no matter how many hours you work or how long you've been employed by the company.

Adapting your routine

Working long hours may leave you feeling very tired, and bouts of morning sickness can make the situation even more difficult. Overtiredness can make feelings of nausea worse, and you might also find yourself losing concentration and falling asleep. Added to this, travelling to work, especially if you use public transport, can be absolutely exhausting, particularly in the later stages of your pregnancy.

Making changes If there's anything about your job that worries you, find out if you can make changes until your baby is born. You may be able to start and finish work at a different time to avoid travelling in the rush hour, for example. If your job involves a lot of standing or walking, find out if there's something you can do that allows you to spend more time sitting.

Take it easy Don't push yourself too hard. Be more relaxed about household tasks – your health and that of your baby are far more important. Relaxation is vital and it's important to make time to look after your body with an exercise routine and massage. Have a rest when you get home from work and make sure your partner shares the chores.

Deciding when to stop

Some women happily continue working until they near labour. But towards the end of your pregnancy your heart, lungs, and other vital organs have to work harder, and a great deal of physical stress is placed on your spine, joints, and muscles. When you stop work depends a great deal on your health and circumstances, but it's best to allow yourself a few weeks' rest before your baby is due.

Deciding when to return

Think carefully about when you want to return to work, and talk to your employer about your plans. If you want to change the date of your return later you can, but you must give your employer eight weeks' notice of the change. You may want to go back under different working conditions, and you'll need to talk to your employer about this. For example, you might want to try working part-time or try a job share, flexible working, or some freelance activity that allows you to work from home. Bear in mind that both you and your partner are entitled to take a year's extra parental leave (unpaid) during your child's first five years, provided you've worked for your employer for at least a year (see p.64).

Sharing responsibilities

If you've agreed between you that one of you will go back to work and the other partner will care for the baby at home, the carer will need a lot of support, especially in the early days. Try to share the responsibilities; don't assume your partner will always sort out problems or be the one to cope when, say, your baby is ill. If you're both working, share the household jobs and the daily routine, including collecting your baby from the childminder or getting home first to take over from the nanny. Far from being a chore, these precious moments alone with your baby will be something you'll come to cherish.

Your baby's safety

Watch out for any chemicals in your workplace that could damage your baby. If you're worried, talk to your doctor and employer about the risks and take steps to avoid any dangers.

Many pregnant women working in offices are worried about the dangers of exposure to radiation from copying machines and computers. However, research shows that these very low levels of radiation won't harm your baby.

Smoking is now banned in nearly all workplaces and other enclosed public places in the UK. Don't allow anyone to smoke in your home or near you because passive smoking (inhaling cigarette smoke in the atmosphere) is just as bad for you and your baby as smoking cigarettes yourself.

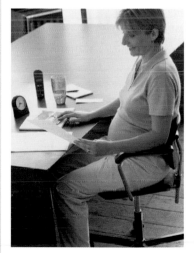

▲**SAFETY AT WORK** Employers are obliged by law to protect the health and safety of pregnant workers and ensure there is no risk to their babies.

Miriam's casebook

Choosing single parenthood

A barrister specializing in family law, Ros, 38, is now 14 weeks pregnant. Ten years ago, Ros made the decision to abort an 11-week pregnancy because she didn't want to interrupt her career and didn't want to make any form of long-term commitment that meant giving up her independence. As she got older, Ros began to yearn for a baby, but she still hadn't found a man to whom she wanted to commit.

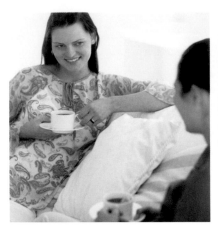

Finding a father

During a recent passionate and rather whirlwind affair with a younger man, Ros decided that she'd be more than happy if her lover, Timothy, was to become the father of her baby. Although she felt very fond of Timothy, she couldn't see the relationship lasting, though, and didn't particularly want it to.

She talked the idea over with Timothy, who agreed that he didn't want to make any long-term commitment to Ros either, although he was happy to father her baby. The affair has now ended, but they've remained firm friends, and Ros has just begun the second trimester of her pregnancy.

A healthy baby

This will be Ros's only child and she wants to do everything she can to make sure her baby will be healthy. She went to a genetic counsellor before getting pregnant because a cousin on her father's side suffers from haemophilia (see p.25). As her father hadn't suffered from the disease, the counsellor reassured Ros that she wasn't carrying the gene.

After she'd talked to Timothy about the possibility of him fathering her child, Ros asked him about his family health background. Happily, everything seemed to be normal. On her first antenatal visit, Ros found out that her lifestyle was more important than her age in determining the smoothness of her pregnancy. She's being very careful about her diet (see p.128) and exercise (see p.144), and she's not smoking, drinking, or taking any medication.

All of her medical tests have proved normal and she knows that she shouldn't put on too much weight, that her blood pressure will be carefully checked, and that she must be on the look-out for signs of water retention (tight rings, swollen ankles) as this could be a warning sign of pre-eclampsia (see p.224). At her last antenatal visit Ros had a scan to check for any obvious abnormalities in the baby, among other things. Everything was normal. Although ultrasound scanning revealed no abnormality, Ros is keen to have the added check for genetic or chromosomal diseases provided by amniocentesis (see p.185).

A working pregnancy

Ros hopes that by cutting down her workload and working flexible hours she'll be able to work right up until labour. Although she's allowed up to 52 weeks maternity leave by law, she intends going back to the office part-time two weeks after the birth. Given her tough working schedule, Ros knows how important it is to rest. Already she puts her feet up for

20 minutes at lunchtime and tries to snatch a nap in chambers or in the car during the afternoon. She's rigorous about getting enough sleep, has stopped socializing except at weekends, and is in bed by 9.30pm. I advised her to learn deep muscle and mental relaxation and to keep doing yoga.

Ros is determined to have the very best medical care available during labour and has chosen to have her baby at a large teaching hospital that's at the forefront of technology. She wants to have an active birth and she's pleased that she'll be attended by a team of midwives – she won't have a birth partner and so will depend on her carers for emotional support during labour. She's made a birth plan (see p.122), which has been added to her hospital notes.

After the birth

Ros plans to hire a full-time nanny who will live in with her and the baby as soon as she returns from her hospital delivery. The nanny will be on night duty from the end of the first two weeks so that Ros can get a full night's rest in preparation for returning to work.

Ros wants to breastfeed her baby for as long as she can and she's prepared to express her milk and store or freeze it so that her baby has the benefits of breast milk even when Ros herself is at work.

I mentioned to Ros that one of the hardest things about being a single parent is that she won't have anyone to share great moments with – when her baby first smiles or says her first words, for example. I also warned her that although her baby won't suffer in any way from having only one parent, it does mean that the demands, both emotional and practical, on Ros herself will be very high.

Ros's work will continue to give her great satisfaction but I encouraged her to have as active a social life as she can too. It's all too easy to become isolated when you're working hard and bringing up a small child by yourself. I suggested that Ros start finding out about local activities where she'll probably meet other working mothers as well as looking into hobbies or exercise classes at a local gym or health club with crèche facilities.

Ros's baby

Ros's baby will have only one parent right from the start, so her experience of life will be somewhat different from a child who has two parents caring for her. Ros will be able to give her baby just as much care as two parents would. Her baby will also become very attached to her nanny, who'll be a very important person in her life, but there's nothing wrong in this. Ros's baby won't see her mother all the time, but when she is with her, it will be special time. She'll be breastfed, even though Ros is going back to work, but will need to adjust to being given a bottle of defrosted breastmilk by her nanny and being breastfed by her mother.

Ros and her child will tend to be everything to each other, which may lead to a rather intense one-to-one relationship. Babies do need and thrive on having plenty of contact with people other than their parents, so it's important that Ros's baby has a chance to interact with a wide range of children and adults. Both mother and baby will gain a great deal from having this broad network of support and loving care.

Drugs and your baby

Check with a doctor before taking any drug – prescription or non-prescription. Always tell the doctor that you're pregnant.

It's best not to take anything while you're pregnant unless your doctor confirms that the benefit to you outweighs any risk to your baby. The long-term effects of some drugs on the unborn child are still unknown. Other drugs are known to be dangerous to the fetus and should be completely avoided, others can only be taken in small doses (see below).

Avoiding hazards

Many activities that are normally harmless may pose risks when you're pregnant. Cleaning out a cat litter tray, being in contact with harmful chemicals at work, passive smoking while socializing, or having immunization for travelling all may affect the development of your unborn baby, and it's wise to take precautions.

At home

You can't live in a perfect hazard-free environment while you're pregnant, but you can do your best to avoid risks. For example, don't handle raw meat, touch other people's pets, clean out pet litter trays, or work with pesticides in the garden. Don't drink alcohol, and avoid coffee, and teas containing caffeine as far as possible. Herbal teas are generally safe (although don't drink raspberry leaf, which is said to trigger contractions).

Drugs to avoid

DRUG	USE	POSSIBLE SIDE EFFECTS FOR YOUR BABY
Amphetamines	Stimulant	May cause heart defects and blood diseases
Anabolic steroids	Body-building	Can have a masculinizing effect on a female fetus
Tetracycline	Treats acne and other infections	Can colour both first and permanent teeth yellow
Streptomycin	Treats tuberculosis	Can cause deafness in infants
Antihistamines	Allergies/travel sickness	Some cause malformations; check with your doctor
Anti-nausea drugs	Combats nausea	May cause malformations, but there are some that can be used safely to treat morning sickness
Diuretics	Rid body of excess fluid	Can cause fetal blood disorders
Narcotics (morphine, etc)	Painkillers	Addictive; baby may become addicted to morphine and suffer withdrawal symptoms
Paracetamol	Reduces fever	Safe in small doses
LSD, cannabis	Recreational	Risk of chromosomal damage, and miscarriage
Sulphonamides	Treat infections	Can cause jaundice in the baby at birth
Anti-inflammatories (ibuprofen, etc)	Relieve pain and inflammation	Can cause premature closing of an important valve in baby's circulatory system

Harmful chemicals Try not to use aerosol spray products at home – you can get alternatives. Although modern aerosols contain halogenated hydrocarbons (rather than CFCs), which have not been shown to harm either the fetus or mother, my feeling is that we're all exposed to invisible sources of potentially harmful chemicals, and it's wise to take every possible precaution.

Avoid substances that give off vapours, such as glue and petrol. These may be toxic and should never be inhaled, whether you're pregnant or not. Read the label of any material you use, and don't handle any that could be harmful. Some common examples are cleaning fluids, contact cement, creosote, volatile paint, lacquers, thinners, some glues, and oven cleaner. Colouring your hair is probably safe, but I'd suggest waiting until after the first three months, when the most crucial organs in your baby's body have formed, just in case.

Hot baths It seems that saunas and hot whirlpools can be involved in fetal abnormalities, particularly those of the baby's nervous system, in exactly the same way as fever. When your body is subjected to extreme heat over a lengthy period, you can become overheated, which may affect your baby. Don't use saunas and whirlpools, especially in the first trimester, and have warm, rather than hot, baths.

Immunizations When you're pregnant, your entire immune system is changing and may be weakened, so you may have unpredictable reactions to immunizations. If you've been in contact with infectious diseases, or you have to travel somewhere that requires immunizations, talk to your doctor and find out what is best to do. Generally, doctors advise against giving vaccinations prepared with live viruses – rubella, measles, mumps, and yellow fever. And it's best not to have the flu vaccine when you're pregnant, unless you have a high risk of heart or lung disease.

At work

When you find out that you're pregnant you may have worries about your job. How safe is my workplace? Will the demands of my job put my pregnancy at risk? How long can I go on working? If your job is strenuous, involving a lot of standing, walking, lifting, or climbing, it may be hard for you to have enough rest during your pregnancy and you may get very tired. Your doctor may suggest that you reduce your working hours, transfer to less strenuous work, or stop working several weeks before your expected delivery date (EDD). In all circumstances, pregnant women must not do anything that exposes them to physical danger, including some police work, motorcycle racing, and so on.

Toxoplasmosis and your baby

This parasite normally produces only mild flu-like symptoms in an adult, but it can seriously damage an unborn child.

It can cause brain damage and blindness in a baby, and can even be fatal. It's most dangerous during the third trimester.

Toxoplasma is carried in the faeces of infected animals, particularly cats, but most people get it from eating undercooked meat. About 80 per cent of the population have had it and have antibodies, but the younger you are, the less likely you are to be immune. You can ask your doctor to do a blood test.

Guidelines to follow:
- don't eat raw or undercooked meat, especially pork, rare steak, or steak tartare

- don't feed raw meat to your cat or dog. Keep their food bowls away from everything else

- don't empty your cat's litter tray or use your dog's poop-scoop. If you have to, wear gloves and wash your hands in disinfectant immediately afterwards

- don't garden in soil used by cats, and wear gloves when gardening

- do wash your hands after gardening, or petting your animals

- do cook meat to an internal temperature of at least 54°C/129°F – at which bacteria are killed. Use a meat thermometer to be sure.

Your risk of infection

In the first 12 weeks of pregnancy, try your best to avoid contact with anyone, especially a young child, who has a high fever, even if the fever is not thought to be caused by German measles (see p.19).

If you get mumps when you're pregnant it'll run the same course as if you weren't pregnant. There's a slightly higher risk of miscarriage if you get the disease in the first 12 weeks.

You won't be vaccinated against mumps during pregnancy because it's a live vaccine, so could affect your baby.

Chickenpox is rare among adults, so it's uncommon in pregnancy. There's some evidence that the disease can cause fetal malformations.

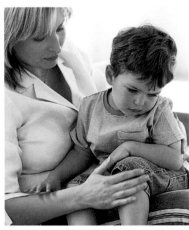

▲ INFECTION If you have young children, there's not much you can do to keep away from them if they're ill. If you're a school teacher, be fairly strict about sending home any feverish child.

Your doctor may also suggest it's safest for you to stop working if you have certain diseases, such as a heart condition, if you have a history of more than one premature baby or miscarriage, or if you're expecting more than one baby. Women who are suffering from pre-eclampsia or placenta praevia will also be advised to stop work.

At work, watch out for anything potentially harmful and make sure your employer transfers you to a hazard-free working place or job. Avoid:

■ Chemicals used in manufacturing and other industries – for example, lead, mercury, vinyl chloride, dry-cleaning fluids, paint fumes, and solvents.
■ Animals, which present a risk of toxoplasmosis.
■ Exposure to infectious diseases, especially childhood rashes.
■ Exposure to toxic wastes of any kind.
■ Unacceptable levels of ionizing radiation (these are now strictly monitored by government regulation). It's generally accepted that day-to-day exposure to ultraviolet or infra-red radiation given off by equipment such as printers, photocopiers, and computer screens is not dangerous to you or your baby. But just to be extra careful, if you make photocopies every day it's a good idea to keep the top of the photocopier closed when the machine is copying.

Otherwise, if you're a healthy woman, with a normal pregnancy and working in a job with no hazards greater than those you meet in everyday life, you can usually work until close to your expected delivery date.

Socializing

Infections are caught from the people we come into contact with in our daily life. Although you don't want to become a hermit when you're pregnant, or wear a gauze mask when talking to people, it does pay to be careful – especially around children (see column left), or adults who are running a temperature.

Colds and flu won't harm your baby, but do your best to avoid fevers. If your temperature is very high, ask your doctor which medications are safe to take – paracetamol is usually recommended as safe in pregnancy in small doses. You can try using a fan to cool your skin down. Don't take cold or flu medicines that contain antihistamines. There's some evidence that particularly virulent flu viruses can cause miscarriage.

Travelling

There's absolutely no evidence that travel brings on labour, or leads to miscarriage, or any other complication of pregnancy. It is wise, though, to be extra careful about travel if you've miscarried before or have a history of premature labour. Ask your doctor for the name of an obstetrician in the area you're visiting and, in the last trimester, limit yourself to trips within easy reach of home.

Trains Book a seat if possible, and check that it's not next to the buffet car as the smell may make you feel nauseous. Eat lightly to lessen the risk of travel sickness. Don't lean on, or stand close to, carriage doors as they have been known to fly open – this obviously applies even when you're not pregnant.

Cars Travelling by car can be exhausting, so limit your journeys. Stop and get out of the car at regular intervals so you can have a short walk to keep your circulation going. Always fasten your seat belt, but buckle it low, across your pelvis, and use a shoulder harness if you have one. Keep on driving as long as you're comfortable behind the wheel, but you must stop as soon as you begin to feel at all cramped. This may seem obvious, but don't drive yourself to the hospital if you're in labour!

Air travel Travelling by plane isn't a good idea after your seventh month, because of pressure changes in the cabin. If you must fly at this time, check with the airline about whether they'll need to see a doctor's letter before letting you on the plane. If you sit over the wings or towards the front of the plane you'll feel less of the plane's motion. Don't fly in small private planes that have unpressurized cabins.

While flying, eat lightly because pregnancy makes you more prone to motion sickness. Make sure that you empty your bladder before you board the plane in case there's a delay in taking off, or the seat belt sign stays on a long time. When fastening your seat belt, make sure that you buckle it low across your hips.

Foreign travel Always follow the guidelines I've given to protect against listeria and other food-related diseases (see p.139). Drink bottled water when in doubt.

Check with your doctor about immunizations you may need for travel to some places (typhoid vaccinations, for example, could harm your baby). Even if you've been exposed or are in a typhoid epidemic, the bad effects of the live vaccine will have to be weighed against the risk to your baby. Refuse to have a yellow fever vaccination unless you've had direct exposure. You may need rabies and tetanus vaccinations, particularly if you've had any risk of exposure. Chloroquine may be used for malaria, but only if you're going to an area where the disease is common. The polio vaccine may be given during pregnancy if you're not already immune.

Good travelling

A little extra care will make travelling when you're pregnant a more comfortable experience.

■ Leave more than enough time for your journey.

■ Aim to leave more time than you normally would between any connections you have to make so you don't have to rush.

■ Travel in short bursts rather than a long stretch.

■ Travel safely (see main text).

■ Carry a drink, such as milk or fruit juice, in a flask.

■ Take some easy to-carry food with you, such as wholemeal crackers, cold hard-boiled eggs, raw fruit or vegetables, and nibbles like dried fruit, nuts, and seeds.

■ Have some glucose sweets to help prevent nausea caused by low blood sugar.

■ Wear an eye mask and some ear plugs so that you can get some sleep when travelling by train or plane.

Your antenatal care

Excellent antenatal care should be rewarded with healthy mothers and babies. The routine tests you'll have usually pick up any problems as soon as they arise, and there are special tests for mothers and babies with particular needs. At your antenatal clinic you'll also have the chance to ask questions about your pregnancy and to meet other women going through the same experiences as you.

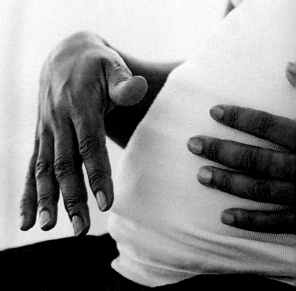

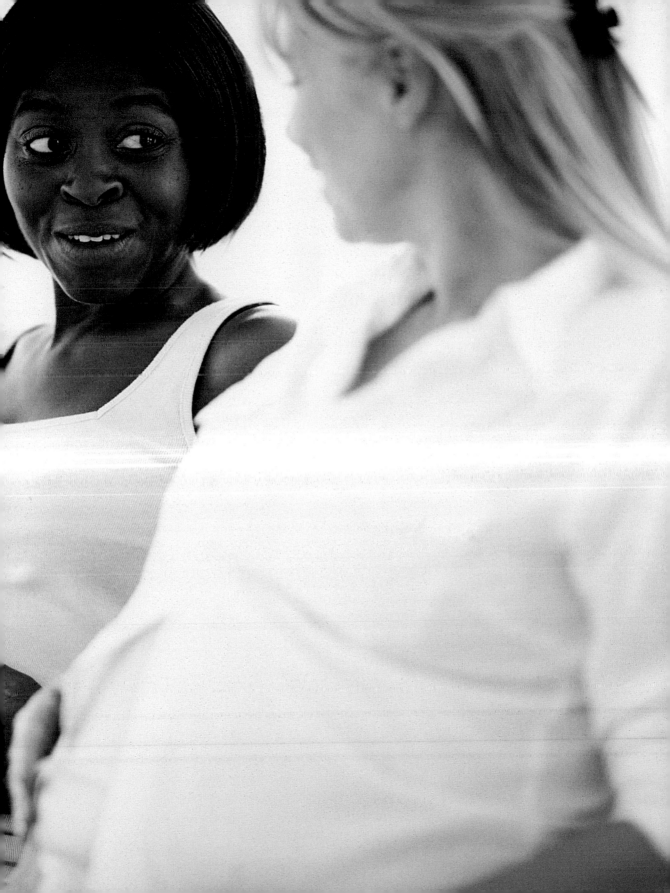

Your first visit

When you make your first visit to the antenatal clinic, you'll probably be asked questions about the following:

■ your personal details and circumstances

■ childhood illnesses or any serious illnesses you've had

■ illnesses that run in your family, or in your partner's family

■ if there are twins in your family

■ your menstrual history – when your periods started, how long an average cycle is, how many days you bleed, and the date of your last period (see p.62)

■ what symptoms of pregnancy you have, and your general health

■ details of previous births, pregnancies, or problems in conceiving

■ if you take a prescription medicine or suffer from any allergies.

Antenatal care

You'll have consultations, check-ups, and tests throughout your pregnancy to make sure you and your baby are doing fine. Most pregnancies are perfectly normal, but it's vital to have these checks to make sure all is well and to spot possible problems early before any harm is done.

The antenatal clinic

Your antenatal check-ups may be at your doctor's surgery, the local health centre, or the hospital. You'll probably have a "booking-in" appointment at between eight to 12 weeks, and you can expect about ten further visits if it's your first pregnancy and about seven if it's not. The exact number and timing of antenatal checks varies from area to area. If you have any complications, such as a multiple birth, a medical condition you had before you became pregnant, or you're at risk for some other reason, you'll have checks more frequently.

Most antenatal care is now handled in the community, so appointments are much less stressful than when most women had to go to hospital clinics. There's a more relaxed atmosphere, and if you do need to go to a hospital clinic, you'll probably find it less crowded than it used to be. There'll be times, though, when you have to wait around, especially if you're having an ultrasound scan or a blood test. Take something to read or to do while you're there, and have some food and a drink with you in case you have a long wait but don't want to risk going to the café and missing your appointment. Ask your partner to go with you if he can. If you have other children, it's best to ask someone to look after them if possible, rather than take them with you.

The clinic can be a good place to start making friends with other expectant mothers, so chat to whoever's there.

Talking to your carers

Midwives at a hospital-based antenatal clinic may find it hard to find time to talk to you as much as you'd like. Community clinics should be more relaxed and you'll be able to find out what alternatives are open to you, talk about your preferences, and get reassurance about any worries and fears. If you feel that you're being hurried through your appointment, ask your midwife for some more time. Don't let yourself be browbeaten, but do bear in mind that many women feel very emotional and weepy when pregnant, so you may cry much more readily than usual in any stressful situation. If you have strong preferences but worry that you won't be able to stand up for yourself, take your partner along for moral support. It'll help to make a list of points you want to talk about beforehand and rehearse them together.

Understanding your notes

When you go for your first antenatal visit you may be given your "hand held" antenatal notes or these may be given to you when all the results are available. Your midwife or doctor will record details here of routine tests and your pregnancy's progress, as well as any special tests. You may find your notes difficult to understand because many of the medical terms are abbreviated. Compare these with those listed below. If your notes still don't make sense, ask your midwife or doctor to explain.

Take your notes when you go to the clinic. In fact, it's best to carry them all the time, so that if you need medical attention, the information is at hand. And take them with you to the hospital when you go into labour.

Understanding the terms on your notes

NAD or nil or a tick No abnormality detected

BP Blood pressure

FH Fetal heart

FMF Fetal movements felt

Ceph Cephalic, baby is head down

Vx Vertex, baby is head down

Br Breech, baby is bottom down

LMP Last menstrual period

EDD/EDC Estimated date of delivery/confinement

Hb Haemoglobin levels (to check for anaemia)

Eng/E Engaged (baby's head has dropped down into the pelvis ready for birth)

NE Not engaged

Para 0 Woman has had no other children

Para 1 (etc) Woman has had one or more children

Fe Iron has been prescribed

TCA To come again

TOS Trial of scar (expected normal delivery after Caesarean section)

Height of fundus The height of the top of the uterus. The baby pushes this up as he grows and often the height is used to work out how many weeks you are. The height of the fundus (from the top of the pubic bone to the top of the uterus) is measured with a tape measure in centimetres

IUGR Intrauterine growth restriction

SFD Small for dates

IOL Induction of labour

ARM Artificial rupture of membranes

SRM Spontaneous rupture of membranes

PET Pre-eclamptic toxaemia

Long L Longitudinal lie (the baby is lying parallel to your spine in your uterus)

AFP Alpha-fetoprotein

CS Caesarean section

LSCS Lower segment Caesarean section

VBAC Vaginal birth after Caesarean

H/T Hypertension (high blood pressure)

MSU Midstream urine sample

Primigravida First pregnancy

Multigravida More than one pregnancy

VE Vaginal examination

1/5–5/5 Indicates extent of head engagement

Baby's position

In your notes you'll see certain abbreviations used to describe how the baby is lying in your uterus. They refer to where the baby's spine and occiput (back of head) are in relation to your body. For example, in ROA, the baby's spine and occiput (O) are on the right (R) side of your uterus towards the front (or anterior/A).

Key to abbreviations: L: left side of uterus; R: right side of uterus; O: occiput, or back of baby's head; A: anterior, or towards front of uterus; P: posterior or towards back of uterus; L: lateral, or at right angles to the mother's spine.

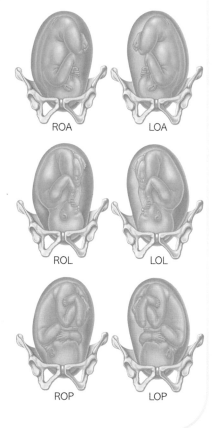

ROA   LOA

ROL   LOL

ROP   LOP

Routine checks

While you're pregnant, you'll have some routine checks to make sure both you and your baby are doing well. Some may be done at every visit, or at different times during your pregnancy. Other tests only need to be carried out once. If the tests show that there is, or may be, a problem, you'll be monitored closely and prompt action will be taken if necessary.

Height Your height will be measured at your first visit. If you are petite, your midwife may suspect that you have a small pelvic inlet and outlet. The chances are, though, that your baby will match your particular physical build.

Weight Women used to be weighed at every visit, but many units now only weigh you at the booking-in appointment. If you lose weight in the first trimester it's usually because of nausea and vomiting due to morning sickness and so it's nothing to worry about. Maternal weight gain used to be taken as a reliable indicator of the growth of the baby. Recent research, however, shows that external examination, blood and urinary tests, and especially ultrasound scans, are much more accurate in measuring fetal growth. A sudden weight gain could mean you have fluid retention, a sign of pre-eclampsia (see p.224).

Legs and hands In the third trimester your legs will be checked for varicose veins, and your ankles and hands will be examined for signs of swellng and puffiness (oedema). A little swelling in the final weeks of pregnancy is normal, particularly in the evening, but excessive puffiness may give an early warning of pre-eclampsia (see p.224).

Breasts Your breasts will be checked for lumps and the condition of your nipples at your first visit. They won't usually be checked again but if you're worried about anything, ask your midwife.

Urine When you go for your first antenatal visit you'll be asked for a sample of midstream urine to test for any underlying bladder or kidney infection. To collect a midstream sample, you'll be given a sterile pad to clean your vulva and a sterile container. You pass the first few drops of urine into the toilet bowl and collect some midstream urine in the container. You then finish urinating into the toilet.

You'll be asked to bring a morning sample of urine with you on other visits. This will be tested for urinary infection; for sugar, to check you're not developing diabetes; and for ketones, which are the classic sign that

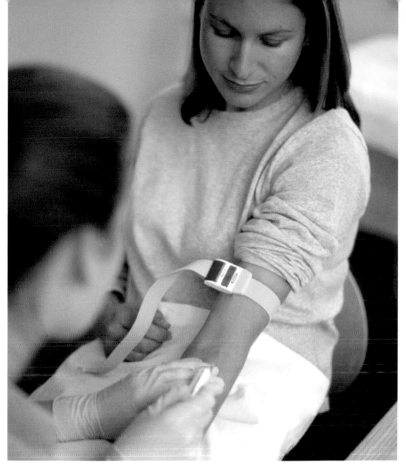

HIV and hepatitis B

Hepatitis B All pregnant women should have a blood test for hepatitis B. Infected women can then be given treatment to prevent the disease being passed on to their baby.

HIV Screening for HIV is now recommended and offered to all pregnant women. Treatment is available for women who test positive to lessen the risk of the disease being passed on to the baby. It's important to diagnose HIV early as this improves the likelihood of having a healthy baby.

▲ **TAKING A BLOOD SAMPLE** Blood tests are important for finding out if you have, or are likely to have, any problems during your pregnancy.

diabetes is established and needs urgent treatment (see p.140). A rare cause of ketonuria (raised levels of ketones) is very severe vomiting in pregnancy, called hyperemesis gravidarum, which means that you must go to hospital right away. If you do have diabetes, it may disappear completely once your baby is born but come back in future pregnancies. Protein in your urine in late pregnancy may be a warning of pre-eclampsia. This will be looked into at once because of the risks of intrauterine growth restriction, premature delivery (see p.298), or seizures.

Blood tests

Also at your first antenatal visit, you'll be asked for a blood sample, usually from a vein in your arm. This is used to check your basic blood group (A,B,O), and also your Rhesus (Rh) blood group (positive or negative), in case a blood transfusion becomes necessary. If you are Rh negative, you'll be tested for Rhesus antibodies later in your pregnancy as well.

Your haemoglobin level will also be checked. This is a measure of the oxygen-carrying power of your red blood cells. The normal level is between 12 and 14 grams; if yours falls below ten grams, you may be

Your baby's heartbeat

Your baby's heartbeat will be monitored at every visit from week 14. Your baby's heart beats almost twice as fast as yours (about 140 beats per minute compared with 72 beats per minute), and sounds just like a tiny galloping horse.

Pinnard stethoscope The doctor or midwife may listen to your baby's heartbeat using a traditional ear trumpet known as a Pinnard stethoscope, although these are now rapidly falling out of use.

Sonicaid It's more likely that a sonicaid will be used. This is a small portable instrument (about the size of a telephone). It's placed on your stomach and uses Doppler (see also p.187) to listen to the baby's heartbeat. The sonicaid magnifies the sound of your baby's heartbeat, so you can hear it too.

Electronic monitor There are two kinds of electronic monitor. In one type, an external monitor is strapped around your abdomen and sensors record the baby's heartbeat. The other, an internal monitor, has a tiny electrode that is clipped to the baby's scalp and records the heartbeat more accurately. This can only be used once your membranes are ruptured during labour. The latest monitors use radio waves so you can walk around while being monitored.

given treatment for anaemia. Iron and folic acid raise the oxygen-carrying power of your blood, so it's essential to eat a healthy diet with plenty of vitamins and minerals (see p.128).

The blood test will also show whether or not you've already had German measles (rubella) (see p.19) – if you have, you're immune. Also, any sexually transmitted diseases, such as syphilis, will be revealed and some genetic disorders, such as sickle-cell anaemia and thalassaemia (see pp.24 and 25), are detectable in blood. You may also have a special screening blood test to help rule out certain types of fetal abnormality.

You can also ask to have your blood tested for toxoplasmosis (see p.169). The toxoplasma is a parasite that can be picked up from cat faeces and from poorly cooked meat. Toxoplasmosis is harmless to adults, but it can cross the placenta and cause blindness, epilepsy, and developmental delay in the baby. You won't necessarily be given this test, so if you're worried – particularly if you have pets that hunt outside – ask for the test. Only about 20 per cent of women in the UK are immune to the disease.

External check

At every visit the midwife will gently feel your abdomen for the top of the uterus (fundus) to check the size of your growing baby. This gives a good idea of whether your baby is about the right size for your dates. Before ultrasound scans became routine, women were measured at intervals through pregnancy to monitor the baby's rate of progress. Now, scans at about 12 weeks and 18–20 weeks provide an accurate picture of how your baby is growing, and if there's any doubt you'll be scanned more frequently (see p.180). After 26–28 weeks the doctor or midwife will also feel for your baby's "poles" (head and rump) so they can assess which position your baby is lying in (see p.175).

Your blood pressure

You'll have this taken at every visit. As always it measures the pressure at which your heart is pumping blood through your body. The reading is made up of two numbers: the upper one is the systolic pressure – when the heart contracts, and "beats", as it pushes out blood. This is measured when the arm band is tight. As the pressure is released, the lower, or diastolic, reading is made. This is the resting pressure between beats.

The statistically average blood pressure reading in pregnancy is 120 over 70, although blood pressure differs with age, and there's a range of blood pressures that are considered normal. A higher reading than normal during pregnancy may be a sign of pre-eclampsia (see p.224) and you'll probably be advised to go into hospital for bed rest. Constant checks are made so that changes are quickly noted.

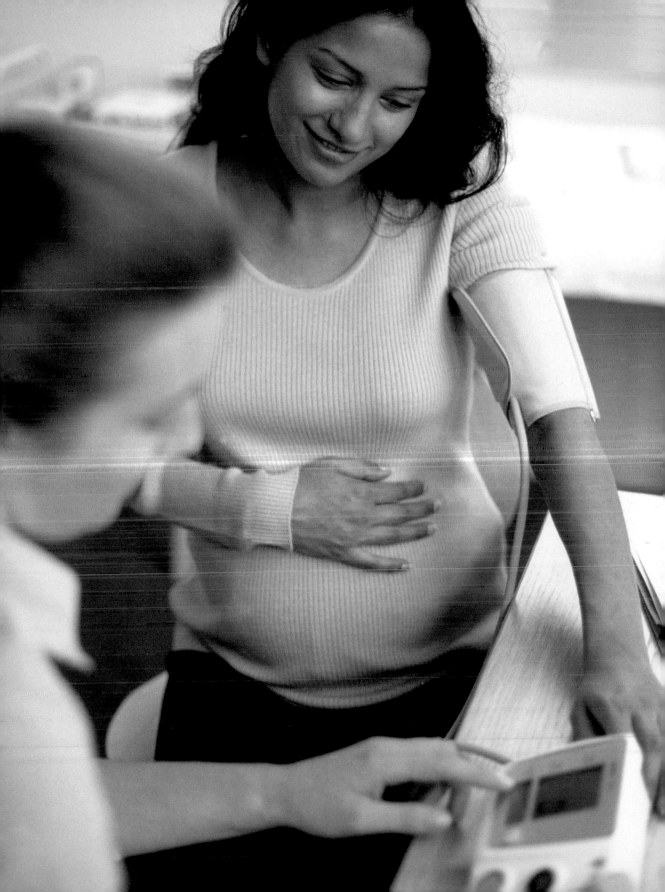

Why you have scans

Ultrasound scans are done routinely twice during your pregnancy to check that your baby is developing normally. Sometimes you may need to have extra scans. Main reasons for these are:

■ to identify abdominal problems such as an ectopic pregnancy

■ if your doctor suspects an imminent miscarriage

■ to check for a multiple pregnancy

■ to check the position of the placenta

■ to check the growth of your baby and the amount of fluid around her.

Ultrasound scan

Scans are used during pregnancy to check your baby's general wellbeing and position, or guide doctors when they're carrying out any special tests and operations. You'll be given two scans – the first at around ten to 13 weeks, to confirm dates and check whether you're expecting more than one baby. Between 18 and 22 weeks you'll have another scan to check that your baby is growing well and there are no abnormalities.

How it works

The process is based on a sonar device that reveals objects in fluid, which was first used by the US Navy to detect submarines during World War II. A crystal, inside a device called a transducer, converts an electrical current into high-frequency soundwaves that the human ear can't detect. The soundwaves form a beam that penetrates the abdomen as the transducer is moved back and forth. The beam reflects off material in its path, and the transducer records these "echoes". The echoes are converted into electrical signals, which produce an image that can be displayed on a screen. The beam can only penetrate fluids and soft tissue such as the amniotic sac, kidneys, and liver. It cannot pass through bone, or register gas. An ultrasound scan is increasingly used to assess

▶ **HAVING A SCAN** You'll be asked to lie down on a bed and lift up your top to expose your abdomen. An oil or jelly, which acts as a conductor of the soundwaves, is rubbed on your abdomen, and the transducer is passed over this area in different directions. You can just lie back and enjoy your first view of your baby as the image appears on the screen.

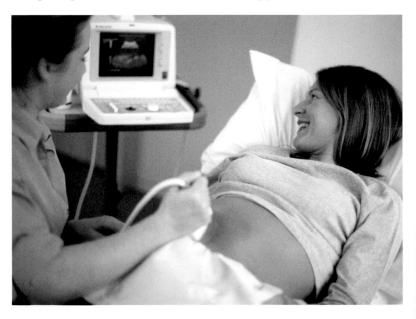

threatened miscarriage, check you're not having an ectopic pregnancy, and in infertility treatments, such as IVF, and for fetal surgery (see p.200).

Your first scan

The first ultrasound scan can be a thrilling moment for you and your partner – a chance to see your baby for the very first time. Scanning equipment has been improved and refined over the years, and the technique is not intrusive. Having an ultrasound scan usually takes about 15 minutes and doesn't hurt. You'll probably be asked to drink about 600ml (20floz) of water, and not empty your bladder before arriving at the clinic. This may be a little uncomfortable, but it's worth it – a full bladder provides a clearer picture of your baby on the screen.

You should be able to hear your baby's heartbeat, and to see the gentle movement of her hands and feet, waving and kicking, as she floats in the amniotic fluid. Ask the ultrasound operator to explain the image on the screen to you as some details may be difficult to make out. Some clinics will offer you a print of the image of your baby as a memento to cherish, although they may charge you for this.

Is it safe?

There are no known risks to your baby from ultrasound scans. There have been some worries about long-term effects, such as hearing impairment caused by the impact of soundwaves, but recent research suggests that ultrasound is not harmful to mother or baby. The waves are of a very low intensity, and so it's safe for the scan to be performed repeatedly.

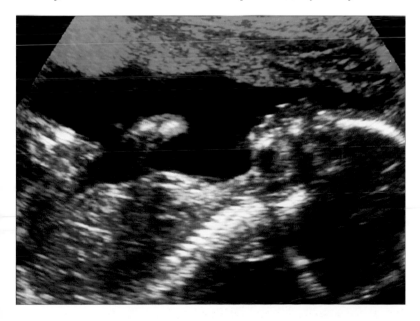

Why your baby needs scans

A routine ultrasound scan shows if your baby is healthy. It may also be used for the following reasons:

■ to check on her growth rate, particularly if you're not sure about the date of conception

■ to check how she's lying and the development of the placenta

■ to find out whether she's ready to be born if she's overdue

■ to confirm that she is in the usual head down position, and not bottom down, after week 38

■ to detect certain fetal abnormalities, such as spina bifida

■ to monitor her during tests such as amniocentesis or fetoscopy

■ to assist in operations performed on her in the uterus.

◀ **20-WEEK ULTRASOUND SCAN** A scan of your baby will show that she's healthy, how she's lying – and whether you are expecting more than one. This scan shows a baby in her mother's uterus. The baby is floating in the amniotic sac, moving around all the time. At the scan you may be able to see your baby doing things such as sucking her thumb, yawning, blinking, and urinating.

Miriam's casebook

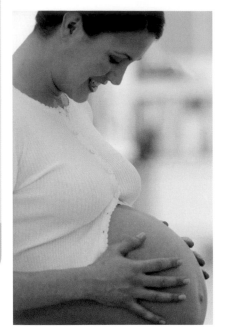

Twins

Karen was told she was expecting twins when she had an ultrasound scan at 14 weeks. Mother of two, she knew from the beginning that there was something different about this pregnancy. For one thing, she was constantly sick in the first couple of months, which she hadn't been with her previous two pregnancies. She also looked huge – at three months she looked about five! Both previous pregnancies had been normal, except for oedema (swelling of feet and ankles) in the last month.

Suspecting a multiple pregnancy

Once they'd got over the initial surprise of finding out that they were expecting twins, Karen and her parnter, Joe, were delighted, if a little apprehensive. Their first concerns were for the wellbeing of Karen and the twins throughout the pregnancy, and then how they would manage to cope with the extra responsibilities that having two babies would bring.

Many women guess early on that there's something different about their pregnancies when they're carrying twins. Size is often a clue, as well as the shape – twins tend to push the abdomen out sideways as well as forwards. Twins can be diagnosed by week six of the pregnancy with an ultrasound scan.

Experiencing a twin pregnancy

Some women sail through a twin pregnancy with very few or no side effects. Some don't. The extra physical stress of carrying two babies can increase feelings of tiredness and sickness as your body adjusts. Also, twin pregnancies need to be watched carefully for raised blood pressure, anaemia,

oedema (swelling of feet and ankles), and pre-eclampsia (see p.224). Like all expectant mothers of twins, Karen will go to her antenatal clinic more often than a woman expecting one baby. Her doctor will watch for oedema happening again, and may get her into hospital if she seems likely to develop pre-eclampsia. She needs a good, high-protein diet.

Sheer size can be a problem in later pregnancy, and it can be hard to get comfortable. I suggested to Karen that she might find that being in water helps as it will support her weight. Gentle swimming would be fine as long as her doctor agrees. She might also like to hire a birthing pool (see Useful addresses, p.370) as an extra large bath in which she can relax. Making love is usually fine, although Karen should follow her doctor's advice and check straight away if she has any discharge or bleeding or if she has contractions.

A twin labour

I suggested to Karen that she get as much rest as she can during her pregnancy. Among women expecting twins those who don't have enough rest are much more likely to go into premature labour than those who've had more rest from the fifth month. Whatever work you do during a twin pregnancy, including caring for young children, make sure it isn't too strenuous. I advised Karen to try to arrange some extra help with her older children when she can, and have at least three hours' bed rest a day.

A twin labour is always managed in hospital because of the potential risks involved. Doctors and midwives are highly sensitive to the difficulties that can occur, so 30 minutes is the most they'll allow between births. The second twin is always monitored closely for any signs of distress. There may have to be an emergency Caesarean section if a twin appears to be in danger.

Identical or not?

One-third of all twins are identical. They are always the same sex and usually share the placenta, although this depends on how late the egg splits. Half of non-identical (or fraternal) twins are boy–girl pairs and half are same sex. Their placentas are separate, but may be fused together. The incidence of identical twins appears to be completely

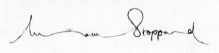

Miriam's top tips

Every twin pregnancy is different, but there's no doubt that a multiple pregnancy puts an extra strain on a woman's body. My advice is to:

■ ask your doctor for an early scan if you experience symptoms early on in your pregnancy that lead you to suspect you might be carrying twins

■ make sure that your diet is nutritious and high in iron and protein (see p.134)

■ rest when you can during your pregnancy, especially after the fifth month. The more daily rest you manage, the less likely you are to go into premature labour.

Miriam Stoppard

random, while non-identical twins often run in families, inherited through the mother's side. The likelihood of having non-inherited, non-identical twins rises until a woman is in her mid-30s, then drops again. It also seems to be higher if she's tall, well built, and conceives easily. The chances of having non-identical twins also appear to increase with each subsequent child.

Birth of twins

A twin pregnancy and birth is different in several important ways. Twins have a shorter gestation period than single babies – they're normally born at 37 weeks rather than 40 weeks. This is mostly because there's just not enough space in the mother's womb, although other external factors are also important. Because they have a shorter gestation period, twins weigh less than single babies.

There are extra risks for the second-born: she has to go through the intense contractions of expulsion twice over. The second twin may also suffer from a lower oxygen supply to the placenta because the mother's uterus will start to contract once the first twin has been delivered.

Single fertilized egg divides in half

Two separate eggs are fertilized

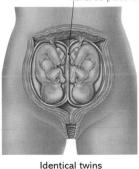

Shared placenta

Two placentas

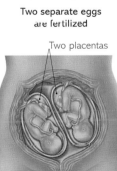

Identical twins

Non-identical twins

▲ **TWIN BABIES** Identical twins occur when a fertilized egg divides in half; non-identical (or fraternal) twins occur when two individual eggs are fertilized and two placentas develop.

Special tests

During your antenatal care you may have a number of special screening and diagnostic tests to check for various complications or defects that can affect the baby. These tests can be reassuring if they rule out something you're worrying about, but they may reveal a problem that makes you question continuing with your pregnancy. This can put an enormous strain on parents-to-be. It's important to talk to your doctor beforehand about the risks of the tests and the implications of the results.

Screening tests

Most maternity units now have a number of tests available that screen for a variety of fetal abnormalities. These tests can't tell you for certain whether anything is wrong, but will give a probability. If a test shows that there may be a problem, a diagnostic test can confirm it or rule it out.

Nuchal scan The risk of having a Down's syndrome baby (see p.24) can be assessed at around 11–14 weeks using a special ultrasound scan called a nuchal scan that measures the fluid at the back of the baby's neck. ("Nuchal" means neck.) All babies have some fluid, but a greater amount than normal may indicate a higher risk of chromosome defects such as Down's syndrome, especially in the older mother (see column, opposite). If the scan shows there is a risk of Down's, amniocentesis can confirm the diagnosis. Many centres now carry out amniocentesis only after a nuchal scan has been done. Chorionic villus sampling (CVS) may be suggested as a way to detect problems (see p.186).

Serum screening This is also known as the Bart's triple test. A sample of the mother's blood is taken between 14 and 20 weeks to measure the levels of three substances – oestriol, human chorionic gonadotrophin, and alpha-fetoprotein. The results are assessed in relation to the mother's age to predict the chance of her baby suffering from Down's syndrome. If the chances seem high (more than one in 250), doctors may suggest you have amniocentesis. If you're not offered this test, you can ask to have it.

Combined test Many units now offer the combined test either to all pregnant women or selectively to women over 35 years old as their risk

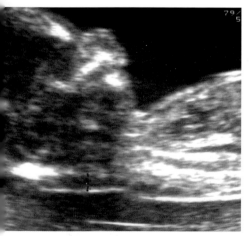

▲**NUCHAL SCAN** This scan measures the fluid accumulation in the neck of the developing fetus. The scan above is of a 12-week-old baby and shows a relatively high measurement, indicating a greater risk of Down's syndrome and the need for further diagnostic tests.

of having a baby with Down's syndrome is statistically higher. With the combined test a nuchal scan is performed and a blood test is taken on the same day for the triple screening. The combined results are given to you about a week later, with an estimated overall risk of abnormalities.

Diagnostic tests

These tests are used to confirm abnormalities in the fetus, and are generally only used after screening tests or ultrasound scans have shown that you may be at a high risk. The main diagnostic tests are amniocentesis and CVS. Amniocentesis is the most common diagnostic test; although CVS can be carried out earlier, it is not available in all centres, and it carries a higher risk of miscarriage.

You and your partner will need to think very carefully about the implications of these tests and talk them through together and with your doctor. Ask for specialist counselling if you want it.

Amniocentesis

Amniotic fluid contains cells from the baby's skin and other organs which can be used to diagnose his condition. Amniocentesis is the name given to the procedure that withdraws this fluid from the uterus.

Why it's done You'll probably want to have amniocentesis if you are over the age of 37, as the risk of chromosomal abnormalities (such as Down's syndrome) increases with age (see column, right). It may also be suggested after serum screening (Bart's triple test), or if a nuchal scan shows a risk of Down's syndrome (see opposite). Amniocentesis can also reveal other important information, which may be sometimes helpful in determining the care and progress of your pregnancy.

At one time amniocentesis was used to check for metabolic disorders, but most of these are now diagnosed by CVS. It was also used to check the bilirubin content of the fluid to help work out if a Rhesus-positive baby had fetal anaemia and needed a blood transfusion while still in the mother's uterus, but this is now done by a Doppler scan (see p.187).

What amniocentesis can reveal Where there is cause for concern, this test may show the following:

■ The sex of the baby: cells sloughed off by the fetus accumulate in the amniotic fluid. Under the microscope, male cells can be distinguished from female cells and the baby's sex determined. In gender-linked genetic disorders such as haemophilia, a male child will have a 50 per cent chance of being affected.

Older mothers

Your age is just one of several factors that can affect the outcome of your pregnancy. Your diet is much more important.

If your general health is good, you shouldn't be treated any differently from younger women during your pregnancy. Age is a factor, though, in certain fetal abnormalities, and an older mother may have a higher risk of maternal diabetes and placental insufficiency. You may be screened for these more frequently.

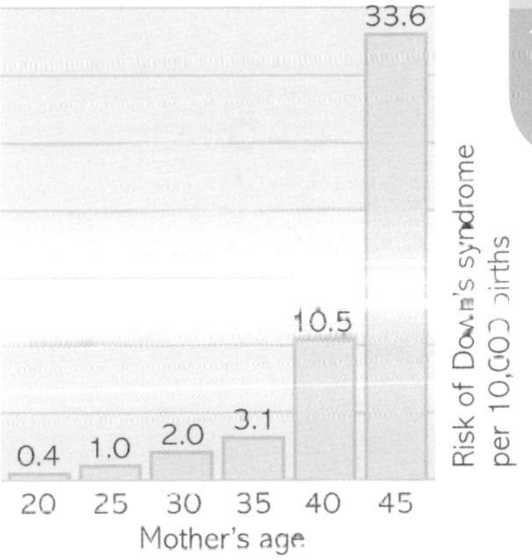

▲ **DOWN'S SYNDROME AND YOUR AGE**
Maternal age seems to be a factor in Down's syndrome. As you can see in the graph, the risk of having a baby with this condition rises as you get older, but isn't really significant until after 35 years of age. As most babies are born to women under 35 who don't have screening, there are more Down's babies in the pre-35 age group than in the post 35 age group.

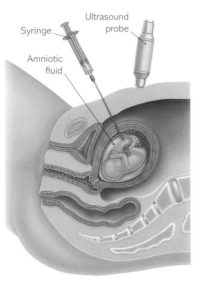

▲ **AMNIOCENTESIS** Amniotic fluid is extracted only after an ultrasound scan has determined the position of the fetus and the placenta. Using ultrasound as a guide, the doctor passes a needle through the abdominal wall and into the uterus. A small amount of amniotic fluid is withdrawn.

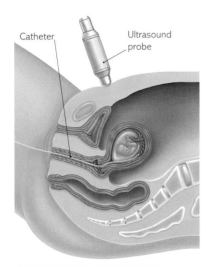

▲ **CHORIONIC VILLUS SAMPLING THROUGH THE CERVIX** A small amount of chorion (placental tissue) is taken from the uterus via the cervix with the aid of a catheter. As in amniocentesis, the ultrasound guides the procedure, which usually takes around 20 minutes.

■ The chemical composition of the amniotic fluid: this can reveal metabolic disorders caused by missing or defective enzymes.
■ The chromosome count. This is determined by examining discarded cells. Any deviation from the normal chromosomal structure usually means that the baby has a disability.

How is it done? Amniocentesis is usually carried out at 16–18 weeks. Guided by ultrasound, the doctor inserts a hollow needle into the amniotic sac through the abdominal wall. About 10ml ⅓ floz) of amniotic fluid is usually withdrawn. This is spun in a centrifuge to separate the cells shed by the baby from the rest of the liquid. The cells then have to be cultured and it takes about three weeks for the results to come through, which can be a very stressful period for couples. Many women talk about putting their pregnancies "on hold" during this time, until the results confirm that the baby is unaffected.

Amniocentesis is always undertaken with ultrasound monitoring to guide the needle into the amniotic sac, so that neither the placenta nor the fetus is harmed. The risk of the procedure inducing a miscarriage is small – about two in 100. There's also the possibility of a small risk (less than one per cent) of respiratory difficulties in babies after amniocentesis.

Amnio PCR In many centres an amnio polymerase chain reaction (PCR), or rapid result test, is now offered. Although not quite as accurate as the cultured cells method, the results are available in 24–36 hours. The cultured cells result backs up the PCR findings in 99.8 per cent of cases.

Chorionic villus sampling (CVS)

Chorionic villi, finger-like outgrowths on the edge of the chorion, are genetically identical to the fetus. They develop earlier than amniotic fluid, so examining a sample of chorionic villi provides valuable information about your baby's genes and chromosomes before it's possible to carry out amniocentesis.

What it can reveal The most important group of mothers needing CVS are those at risk of having a Down's syndrome baby. An abnormality of haemoglobin, such as sickle-cell disease or thalassaemia, can also be diagnosed with CVS. Inborn errors of metabolism are fortunately rare, but if a family is afflicted, the incidence may be as high as one in four of their children. The basic defect is an enzyme deficiency, and direct enzyme analysis on the chorionic tissue gives a diagnosis within two days. Single gene disorders, such as cystic fibrosis, haemophilia, Huntington's chorea, and muscular dystrophy, can be detected with the use of CVS.

How is it done? CVS is also carried out under ultrasound control, usually between ten and 12 weeks of pregnancy, before the amniotic sac completely fills the uterine cavity.

Two routes are used: the trans-cervical and the trans-abdominal. For the former, the cervix is first examined using a speculum. A plastic or metal catheter is then introduced through the cervical canal, across the uterine cavity, and then into the outside edge of the placenta. A small amount of chorionic villi tissue is then removed for analysis.

The second method of chorionic villus sampling is similar to that of amniocentesis, but with a sample being taken of the placental tissue rather than of the amniotic fluid. The risk of miscarriage following CVS is about one per cent higher than the spontaneous miscarriage rate (see p.218). The advantage of CVS is that it gives an initial result within 24–48 hours, with full results in about a week. This is helpful if the risks are high and you don't want to have to wait until your pregnancy is at a more advanced stage for the results of amniocentesis.

Umbilical vein sampling (cordocentesis)

This procedure is used to check the makeup of fetal blood and, in cases of fetal anaemia, for intrauterine blood transfusion. It's also used to check for infections and to assess your baby's levels of haemoglobin. Umbilical vein sampling is no longer used in cases of suspected slow growth. Instead, Doppler scans (see right) provide the necessary information and these are available in most units.

Infection detection Rubella, toxoplasmosis, and the herpes virus may be detected by performing a specific radio analysis of certain proteins that are present in a baby's blood.

Rhesus iso-immunization In cases of Rhesus incompatibility (see p.202) assessing the baby's haemoglobin is the best way to determine the severity of blood-cell destruction and whether a blood transfusion for the baby in the womb (also done through the umbilical vein) needs to be carried out.

How is it done? Under ultrasound guidance, a hollow needle is passed through the front wall of the mother's abdomen and uterus into a blood vessel in the umbilical cord, about 1cm (½in) from where it emerges from the placenta. A small quantity of blood can then be removed for testing. The risk to the fetus appears to be only about one to two per cent. In theory, umbilical vein sampling can be used to undertake any investigation performed on a blood sample.

Doppler scan

Now available in most units, the Doppler scan uses black and white or colour images to look at the blood flow between the placenta and your baby through the umbilical cord.

Doppler uses a slightly different sort of soundwave from a normal ultrasound scan. It bounces off moving red blood cells and shows how fast they're moving through the fetus's blood vessels. Doppler is used to check when a baby is small for dates or seems not to be growing as fast as it should. Doppler can be used to assess whether the developing fetus has anaemia. An anaemic baby will show an unusual pattern of blood flow around the body. Doppler is also used in place of a bilirubin count (the pigment formed from the breakdown of red blood cells) to find out whether a Rhesus-positive baby needs a blood transfusion in the womb. A baby with an unusual blood flow revealed on the scan is more likely to need a transfusion.

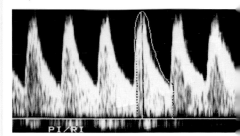

▲ **DOPPLER SCAN** This umbilical Doppler scan shows that the baby's blood flow is normal. The scanning process is painless and there are no associated risks.

Miriam's casebook

Testing for abnormalities

At 26, Daniella was particularly keen to have her babies while she was young and fit. After Daniella had missed two periods and a home pregnancy test had proved positive, she and her partner Will visited their doctor, who referred them to the antenatal clinic at the local hospital. They both found this visit off-putting, particularly when they realized how many screening and diagnostic tests they would be offered.

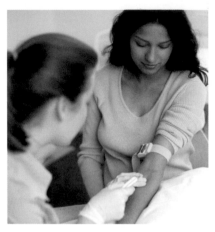

Why screening is offered

Today's technology allows doctors to investigate the health of the fetus before birth at earlier and earlier stages. Like Daniella, most pregnant women are now offered routine screening tests. These sometimes lead to much more invasive diagnostic tests for confirmation with little discussion of the implications of the tests and what they might discover about the health of a baby in the womb.

At the clinic Daniella and Will were given a list of routine screening tests that would be carried out during Daniella's pregnancy. As a young, healthy first-time mother, Daniella hadn't expected to be screened for fetal abnormalities. They both found the idea frightening and it started them thinking about the implications of screening tests. They were both keen to have a natural birth and were resistant to the technological approach they met at the hospital.

Routine screening tests

Daniella and Will were told that she would start having tests to screen for abnormalities in her baby at 11–12 weeks with the first ultrasound scan. Then at 14-plus weeks, a blood test (known as the serum screening test, see p.184) would be taken to look for Down's syndrome, spina bifida, and

hydrocephalus. At 18–22 weeks, she'd have her second ultrasound scan, possibly after an amniocentesis (a diagnostic test, usually carried out at 14–18 weeks) if either screening test suggested a risk of abnormality in her baby.

I explained to Daniella that a screening test is by definition a blunt instrument. It doesn't give any precise information. It can do no more than pick up a tendency for something to happen. The way doctors express this tendency is in terms of probability.

So if a blood test gave a one in 500 chance of the baby having Down's syndrome, it would mean that if Daniella had 500 babies, one of them would have Down's. By any criteria this is a very small risk, but as Daniella said, any risk of Down's syndrome seemed a big risk to her. Like all mothers, she wanted the test to come back entirely negative. As I pointed out, on the scale of probability, one in 500 is exceedingly low. There'd be little cause for concern until the risk rose, to say, one in 250, the probability threshold at which amniocentesis would be offered to every pregnant woman. The next step would be a precise diagnostic test to detect a specific abnormality. This is normally only done if a screening test is positive.

How diagnostic tests work

Such tests are precise enough to give the answer "yes" or "no"; "present" or "absent"; "normal" or "abnormal". Unfortunately, they're quite invasive, and the most widely used, amniocentesis (see p.185), involves a specimen of amniotic fluid containing cells from the baby being drawn out of the uterus – a delicate operation requiring skilled guidance with ultrasound. The cells are then examined for chromosomal or genetic damage in a specialist laboratory. I told Daniella that amniocentesis itself carries a risk of miscarriage of about two in 100 (two per cent).

I explained that in most centres, the definitive test takes three weeks, as it takes that long for enough of the baby's shed cells to multiply sufficiently to be safely analyzed. The newer polymerase chain reaction (PCR) results, however, are available much sooner and are regarded as being highly reliable. Daniella then asked what would happen if amniocentesis confirmed Down's. I explained that she and Will would then be counselled about whether or not to terminate the pregnancy. Of course hearing this upset Daniella as she had never even thought about the possibility of terminating the pregnancy.

Other available tests

I went on to explain that a nuchal scan, which can be done as early as 11 weeks, would alert Daniella and Will to the possibility of a chromosome defect in their baby. This would be followed immediately with a diagnostic test, such as chorionic villus sampling (CVS) (see p.186), which can be done much earlier in pregnancy than amniocentesis and results can be obtained in as little as 24–48 hours. Like amniocentesis, CVS carries a small risk of miscarriage.

Screening tests aren't compulsory, they're optional. I suggested to Will and Daniella that they asked to see the obstetrician in charge of the clinic to talk further, before deciding their approach to tests. In the event, they had a healthy baby girl, born at their local hospital under the care of a team of local midwives, and the family is thriving.

Miriam's top tips

Try to think of screening and diagnostic tests as a means of drawing you closer to your baby and giving you a better understanding of her health and wellbeing in the womb.

■ Find out as much as you can about the tests you are likely to be offered during your pregnancy. Discuss their implications with your partner and your healthcare professional.

■ Ask your partner to accompany you to scans and routine tests. It's comforting and reassuring to have another person to support you at these times.

■ Take advice at every stage and seek a second opinion if you feel you need further clarification.

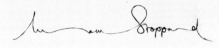

Checklist of specialist tests

Screening tests

■ **Nuchal scan:** An ultrasound scan at 11–14 weeks that screens for high risks of chromosomal defects (see p.184).
■ **Serum screening test:** A sample of the mother's blood at 14–20 weeks screens for hormone levels that indicate a higher risk of Down's syndrome (see p.184).

Diagnostic tests

■ **Chorionic villus sampling (CVS):** Cells from the developing placenta are examined at ten to 12 weeks to check the baby for chromosomal abnormalities (see p.186).
■ **Amniocentesis:** Fetal cells from the amniotic fluid are removed at 14–18 weeks and checked for chromosomal abnormalities such as Down's syndrome (see p.185).
■ **Cordocentesis:** Fetal blood from the umbilical cord is tested for abnormal chromosomes or infection (see p.187).
■ **Doppler scan:** A special scan that looks at the blood flow between the placenta and your baby through the umbilical cord (see p.187).

Caring for your unborn baby

If you're observant and aware, you and your partner can be in touch with your unborn baby throughout pregnancy. Your baby can hear you, and can feel you touch him through your abdominal wall. And while not all babies have a trouble-free development, modern medical techniques mean that even those babies who do not have the best possible chance.

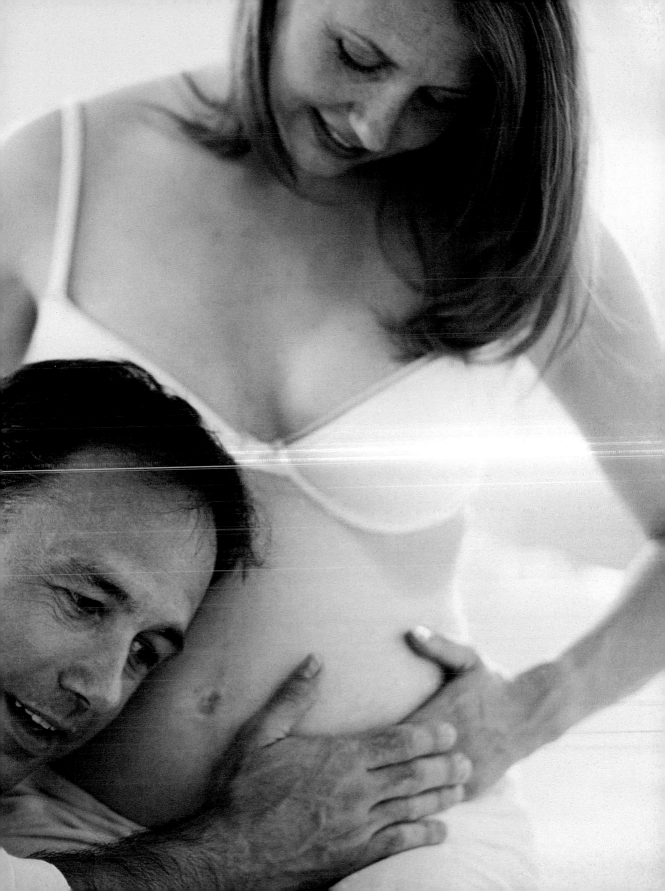

What you can do

It's never too early to start getting in touch with your baby. What you say, do, think, or feel, even the way you move, may be carried through to your baby in your womb.

Talk and sing Get in the habit of talking out loud to your baby, and singing to her. Some children have recognized lullabies played to them when they were in the womb. Play music to your baby.

Touching Stroking your baby through your tummy is another way of keeping in touch. It will usually quieten her, and stroking her may continue to do so after she is born. In the final months you may be able to feel her foot or hand through your skin.

Thinking Be aware of your baby. Think positive, happy thoughts about her. If you're upset about something, don't shut her out.

Moving Keep your movements as relaxed as you can. The gentle movement of your womb as you walk soothes her. Rocking and swinging will remain a favourite relaxing activity after she's born.

Feeling When you feel happy and excited, so does your baby. When you feel depressed, so does she – so reassure her that you still love her. Share feelings with her consciously.

In touch with your baby

Being aware of your unborn baby at all times is the first stage in bonding with her and making sure you have a good relationship in the future. Keeping in touch means you'll be aware of what's best for your baby's physical and emotional health.

What your baby experiences

Even while she's in your womb, your baby feels, hears, sees, tastes, responds, and even learns and remembers. She's not, despite what doctors used to think, an unformed, blank personality. She has firm likes and dislikes. She enjoys soothing voices, simple music with a single melody line (lullabies, flute music), rhythmic movements, and the feeling of you stroking her through your skin. Dislikes include loud voices, strong flashing lights, and rapid, jerky movements.

Sight Although your baby is protected by the walls of your womb and abdomen, very strong light can get through to her; she can detect sunlight if you're sunbathing, for instance. What she sees is probably just a reddish glow, but from about the fourth month, she'll respond to it, usually by turning away if it's too bright. The limits of her sight at birth (she'll be able to see faces within 20–25cm/8–10in of her own) may be a result of the limits of her "home" before she was born.

Sound Your baby's sense of hearing develops at about the fourth month, and by midterm she's able to respond to sounds coming from the outside world (see above). She's suspended in amniotic fluid that carries sounds well, although what she hears will be muffled just like sounds are when you're under water. She's also able to make out the emotional tone of voices and moves her body in rhythm to your speech. She'll be soothed if you use a soft, reassuring tone.

A mother's influence

Your unborn baby first experiences the world through you, her mother. A baby senses not only things happening outside the womb (see above), but also your feelings. She can do this because our emotions trigger the release of different chemicals into our bloodstream – anger releases adrenaline, fear releases cholamines, stress releases cortisol, and elation releases endorphins. These chemicals pass across the placenta to your baby within seconds of you feeling that particular emotion.

Babies don't like their mother feeling negative emotions, such as anger, anxiety, or fear, for long periods. But short bursts of intense anxiety or anger (caused by a moment of panic or an argument with your partner), don't appear to have any long-term effect on your unborn child. They may even be good for her as they may help her start to learn how to cope with stressful situations in the future.

On the other hand, research suggests that long-term festering anger or anxiety, such as you might feel if you have relationship problems or an unsupportive partner, or you're living in difficult conditions, can be harmful for your baby. These effects may include a problematic birth, a low birthweight, being a colicky baby, and future learning problems. Fortunately, studies also show that if a mother is generally happy and positive about being pregnant and doesn't shut out her unborn baby, any periods of negative emotions seem to have far less effect.

A father's influence

As the expectant father, you are the second most important influence in your unborn baby's life. Your attitude towards your partner, the pregnancy, and your child is crucial. If you're happy and looking forward to your baby being born, your partner is much more likely to be content and to enjoy her pregnancy. Your baby, in turn, is much more likely to be a happy, healthy child. Try to talk to your unborn baby as often as you can because research has shown that newborn babies can recognize the voices of their fathers as well as their mothers.

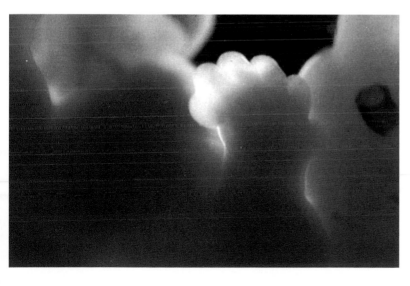

What your baby does

Even while still in the womb, your baby is a little personality, with many ways of interacting with her world.

Movement She moves constantly while she's awake. She'll kick and wriggle her body in response to what's happening outside – for instance, if you sit in a position she finds uncomfortable.

Hearing From week 18 your baby responds to sounds. She moves in rhythm to your voice and may kick when you raise your voice.

Seeing She doesn't like bright light, especially if it flashes. She'll move away, put her hands up to her face, or become agitated.

Feelings She'll have changes in mood to match yours when the chemicals your emotions release into your bloodstream cross the placenta into her body.

◀ **YOUR HEARTBEAT** The sound of your heartbeat is a constant presence in her world and this seems to have a lasting influence on her. In one study, newborn babies who were played a tape of mothers' heart sounds gained more weight and slept better than babies who did not hear the tape.

Sensing the movements

You can feel your baby's movements because they're transmitted through the wall of your womb to the sensitive nerve endings in your abdomen.

The reason you don't feel any of your baby's movements until several weeks after they actually begin is partly because they're very weak at first, and partly because your womb doesn't transmit them. Only when your womb has grown enough to touch the wall of your abdomen are you able to feel any of the movements that occur inside it.

If your baby is kicking or squirming more than usual, sit down in a comfortable, quiet place and calm her down. Playing her gentle, relaxing music, singing her a lullaby, or humming to her will often help. The sound will be pleasant to her and you'll become more relaxed yourself so she'll tend to do the same. Reading to her, or just talking, is also soothing, as is gently stroking your stomach.

Your baby's movements

The moment you feel your baby move inside you for the first time is a huge thrill – proof that she actually exists. Even though you may have had an ultrasound scan, which showed your baby moving about in the womb, she'll seem much more real when you feel her for yourself. If she's your first baby, you'll probably first notice her movements inside your womb at about 18–20 weeks. If you've already had a child, you may feel movements at 16–18 weeks or even before. The earliest noticeable movements of the baby – known as the "quickening" – cause a delicate sensation that's been likened to the fluttering of wings. First-time mothers often mistake this feeling for indigestion, wind, or hunger pangs, but the experienced mother knows what to expect, so is quicker to identify these feelings as movements of her baby.

Why your baby moves

Your baby stretches and flexes her growing limbs as they develop. This activity is vital to help her muscles grow properly and starts around the eighth week, when she begins making tiny movements of her spine. In those early weeks you won't notice her movements, but by about the end of the sixteenth week, you may feel the vigorous kicking of the now fully formed limbs, although you might not recognize them.

Your baby will kick, push, punch, squirm, and turn somersaults, and you'll often see as well as feel her movements. She'll move more and more as she grows, and is at her most active between weeks 30 and 32. The typical baby averages 200 movements a day at week 20, rising to 375 a day at week 32, but the number of movements a day can range from 100 to about 700 over a period of several days.

After week 32, it will become harder for your baby to move as she grows to fill the uterus. Although restricted, she'll still be able to give plenty of sharp kicks. When her engaged head bounces on your pelvic floor muscles, you'll feel a jolt.

Changing position and emotional reactions Your baby needs to exercise and coordinate her growing muscles but she also moves around for other reasons.

She may, for instance, shift her position because she feels like a change, or perhaps because you're sitting or lying in a position that's uncomfortable for her. Or she may be trying to find her thumb that she'd been happily sucking before she moved.

She may also be moving around in response to your emotions. Hormones, such as adrenaline, are released into your bloodstream when you're physically or emotionally stimulated. Pleasure, excitement, anger, stress, anxiety, or fear also stimulate the production of chemicals that will pass across the placenta and into your baby's bloodstream. These hormones affect your baby, so if you get angry or very anxious, she may become agitated and start kicking and squirming. If you can, sit down in a quiet place and practise your relaxation techniques (see p.258). This will help to calm both you and your baby.

Playing games with your baby

Your unborn baby responds to everything she experiences in her womb environment. You can even start bonding with your baby in the womb by playing with her and teaching her games through your pregnant tummy. This is how you do it. Whenever your baby kicks, touch your tummy at that point and say, "Kick, baby, kick!" As soon as she responds, touch a different part of your tummy and repeat: "Kick, baby, kick!" Very soon she'll join in by kicking wherever you invite her to. This is called "spaced repetition" and it's a great way to interact with your little one. In a way, it's an early form of the to-and-fro – of taking turns and sharing conversation – that she will experience as she learns to talk.

Counting the kicks

Just like the rest of us, your baby will feel and be more active on some days than on others, but her daily pattern of movements will become more consistent after about week 28. If you like, you can keep a check on your baby's movements. On average, most women can feel around nine out of every ten of their baby's movements, although for some women the proportion is only six out of every ten.

Whether you feel a movement or not depends on its direction and strength, and the position your baby is in when she makes it. For instance, if she's facing and kicking in towards your spine, you won't feel the sort of short, sharp jab that you get if she kicks out towards your belly or up towards your ribs.

Monitoring your baby's movement

If you notice any significant change in the pattern of your baby's movements as your due date approaches, tell your doctor. If you feel fewer than ten movements for two days in a row, ring your doctor or the hospital. If you don't feel any movements at all in one day, get in touch with your doctor or the hospital immediately. But even if your baby's movements seem to have stopped, don't panic. Your doctor or midwife can quickly assess your baby with ultrasound and electronic fetal monitoring and decide whether anything needs to be done.

Diagnosing heart problems

A congenital condition is one that's present from birth. Congenital heart disease can be diagnosed by chest X-rays or a form of ultrasound scanning called echocardiography.

A congenital heart condition, such as hole in the heart (ventricular septal defect – see main text), sometimes isn't detected until a baby is about four weeks old. Both chest X-rays and echocardiograms are used to confirm the diagnosis and how serious the problem is so the right treatment can be given.

▲ **ECHOCARDIOGRAM** This scan shows a baby's heart with a ventricular septal defect. Echocardiograms are produced using ultrasound and displayed as a series of lines on the screen. The flow through the septal defect is shown as the coloured area. Normally, the right ventricle pumps blood into the lungs to be oxygenated; the left ventricle pumps reoxygenated blood back to the body. When there is a hole, some of the oxygen-rich blood passes back to the lungs instead of out into the body through the aorta.

Fetal problems

I know this is something that every mother worries about, but I can't stress strongly enough that such problems are very, very rare, so please try not to be too anxious. The cause of many fetal defects is still unknown. Some may be caused by a defective gene (see p.24) while others could be due to the harmful effects of drugs, radiation, infections of the baby in the womb, or metabolic disturbances.

There are a number of different kinds of defects – most are very rare. The parts of a baby's body that are most actively growing at the time when the damaging factor happens are the most likely to show the defect. Some malformations are incompatible with life, and no treatment is possible. The defects that are especially important to recognize just after birth are those that endanger life but, with prompt intervention, can be treated successfully. The good news is that an increasing number of problems are now picked up by ultrasound scans before birth (see p.180) and many can be treated just after birth or later in infancy.

Imperforate anus This means that the anus is sealed, either because there's a thin membrane of skin over the anal opening, or the anal canal that links the rectum with the anus has not developed. The rectal pouch may be connected to the vagina, urethra, or bladder, and a baby with this problem will need immediate surgery. This condition is rare, but every baby is carefully checked at birth, so treatment can be given if necessary.

Umbilical hernia In most babies, the gap in the muscle sheath in the abdominal cavity, where the umbilical cord entered his abdomen, normally closes up in time. Sometimes, though, a soft swelling called an umbilical hernia forms when the abdominal contents bulge through this weak spot in the abdomen. The hernia usually disappears eventually, although a few babies may need surgery later in childhood.

Congenital heart disease Hole in the heart (ventricular septal defect) is the most common form of congenital heart disease. In this condition there's a hole in the baby's septum, the thin dividing wall between the right and left ventricles (pumping chambers) of the heart, so the ventricles are connected instead of being divided. A newborn baby doesn't usually show any signs of the problem. It may take as long as four weeks for the blood vessels in the lungs to relax sufficiently to allow pressure differences to develop between the ventricles and this means that there may not be much left-to-right shunt of blood through the hole for a month or so. Until then, there probably won't be any symptoms. Signs to look out for are a bluish tinge to the skin especially round the mouth, floppiness, and breathlessness. One of the first signs may be breathlessness while feeding. Not all babies need surgery; in some, the hole seals of its own accord.

Some types of congenital heart disease can be picked up by an ultrasound scan before birth. If your baby is found to have a serious heart problem, your doctors may advise you to give birth in a hospital that's equipped with special facilities for dealing with such conditions.

Congenital hip dysplasia In this condition the ball at the head of the thighbone doesn't fit snugly into the socket of the hip joint. It ranges in severity from mild loosening to complete dislocation of the thighbone. In the newborn infant this is a potential, rather than an actual, problem. It's twice as common in girls and following breech births.

When your midwife does a routine check of your newborn baby (see p.293), she'll check the hips for excessive mobility, or for a characteristic "clunk" felt when the baby's legs are spread apart and the thighs are flexed. If there's any doubt, she'll get specialist advice. Early follow-up and treatment such as manipulation and splinting may prevent trouble later, but some babies with severe dislocation need surgery.

Spina bifida In this condition the vertebral bones of the spine do not fuse at some level in the spinal column and the meninges (the coverings of the brain and spinal cord) bulge through the gap. The area may be covered with skin or only by a bluish membrane, and may contain nerve roots, or the spinal cord itself may be exposed. In mild cases, the place where the vertebrae are not fused is covered with skin and is only marked by a small, dark, hairy mole. Happily, spina bifida is becoming less common. There's careful monitoring of those more at risk and we know much more about the importance of taking folic acid before conception and during the early weeks of pregnancy (see p.20).

As the various coverings that normally protect the cord aren't there, meningeal infection can happen easily, but can be prevented by immediate surgery to cover the defect. Spina bifida can be picked up by ultrasound and babies with a good prognosis can be sent to a special centre where surgery can be performed without delay. For babies with severe defects the outlook is not encouraging. Problems may include paralysis, incontinence, mental retardation, and hydrocephalus (see p.198).

Cleft lip and cleft palate

These conditions happen when the upper lip or the palate, sometimes both, don't develop completely.

In a cleft lip, sometimes known as a harelip, the halves of the upper lip fail to join properly as the baby is developing. In a cleft palate, similarly, the halves of the baby's palate fail to join.

Babies with these problems can usually breastfeed, but bottlefeeding may be more difficult. It may be necessary to use a cup and spoon. You also have to be careful when feeding a baby who has a cleft palate, because the cleft may allow milk to enter his nose. This is best avoided as he may gag.

It's important to see a plastic surgeon as soon as possible to plan treatment, although some hospitals are now performing immediate closure of the cleft lip at birth. If a cleft palate is closed too early, though, it may mean a major operation during early adulthood, as the palate might not be able to develop fully.

Trisomies

Trisomy is a chromosomal disorder. There are three chromosomes where normally there would only be a pair, and this defect exists in all the cells of the affected person.

The most common trisomy is Down's syndrome (see p.24), or trisomy 21, in which there are three number 21 chromosomes.

The baby is born with small features, a tongue that tends to stick out, and slanting eyes with folds of skin at their inner corners. The head is flat at the back, and the ears are unusual. The baby may be floppy, with hands and feet that are short and wide, and have a single transverse crease across the palms and soles. The baby may also have congenital heart disease.

Down's syndrome sufferers usually have learning dificulties, although the degree of difficulty varies, and many Down's syndrome children are near normal.

Children with Down's syndrome are very rewarding. They're affectionate, outgoing, and have a great sense of humour. With careful attention and early education many do well and some manage to live independently.

Other trisomies include trisomy 13 (Patau's syndrome) and trisomy 18 (Edwards' syndrome), both of which produce a number of severe physical and mental abnormalities. Both these conditions are much rarer than Down's syndrome.

Hydrocephalus (water on the brain) Hydrocephalus means there's too much cerebrospinal fluid inside the baby's skull. It often accompanies other neurological defects, such as spina bifida, and it's caused by restricted circulation of cerebrospinal fluid in the brain. Hydrocephalus is most common following brain haemorrhage in an unborn baby. The baby's head swells, and as the skull bones are not yet fused, the soft tissues between them (fontanelles) become wide and bulging. If this happens before birth, due to congenital malformations, it will obstruct labour, or cause a baby's head to get very large after birth. Neural tube defects such as spina bifida and hydrocephalus are usually diagnosed by ultrasound (see p.180) well before a baby is born.

Cerebral palsy This is caused by damage to the brain before, during, or after birth – for instance, because of a poor supply of oxygen to the brain in late pregnancy or a difficult labour. Other causes include infection of a mother's uterus, meningitis, or a severe injury to the baby's head after birth. Premature babies are particularly vulnerable.

Cerebral palsy causes muscular paralysis, stiffness, and coordination problems. It cannot be detected before birth and the symptoms aren't usually obvious until a baby is several months old and his development appears to be delayed. He may not be walking, sitting, or making normal progress as expected; he may have stiffness in his arms or legs, or a persistent abnormal posture. The degree of disability varies widely.

Cerebral palsy is incurable, but it is not progressive – it doesn't get worse as the child grows older. And it's quite common for children with cerebral palsy to have normal intelligence and social capabilities. Physiotherapy will help to prevent deformities caused by stiffness and spasms and to develop muscular balance and control; speech therapy will help to ease communication problems. As with all disabled children, the emphasis should be on what the child can do, not on what he cannot do.

Respiratory distress syndrome (RDS) In this condition, a baby's lungs are lacking in surfactant, a substance that keeps open the minute air sacs in the lungs through which oxygen is absorbed into the blood. It happens because the baby's lungs are immature, or because crucial lung cells arc tcmporarily not working properly because of a lack of oxygen. RDS is most common in small premature babies and in babies of mothers with diabetes whose condition is not sufficiently well controlled. It's very rare in full-term babies.

Now that doctors are better able to detect immaturity of a baby's lungs before birth and the management of early deliveries and resuscitation has improved, RDS happens more rarely. It can also sometimes be prevented or made less severe by treating the mother with corticosteroids before delivery. Infants born with RDS need to be cared for in an intensive care unit and are given surfactant to mature their lungs.

Pyloric stenosis In this condition the ring of muscle (the pylorus) linking the stomach to the small intestine thickens and narrows. It's much more common in boys, but the cause is unknown.

Symptoms begin when the baby is two to four weeks old. Milk builds up in the stomach, which contracts powerfully in an attempt to force the fluid through the narrow pylorus. Because this is impossible, milk is vomited up violently after a feed. This is known as projectile vomiting because the vomit may be thrown for some distance (up to 2m/6½ft). The baby may also suffer from constipation and dehydration. A simple operation widens the pylorus, giving a complete cure.

Epispadias and hypospadias About one in 1,000 male babies has an abnormality of the penile opening of the urethra. In epispadias, the opening is on the upper surface of the penis; the penis may curve upwards. In hypospadias, the opening is on the underside of the glans (head) and the penis may curve down. Surgery is straightforward and usually successful. Neither epispadias nor hypospadias cause infertility.

A baby with club foot is born with the sole of one foot, or both feet, facing down and inward or up and outward.

The exact causes of the many kinds of club foot are not fully understood, but the condition can run in families. On rare occasions sufferers spontaneously recover.

Most babies, though, need treatment to correct the defect. The usual remedy is for the child's foot to be manipulated regularly over a period of many months. Between manipulations, the foot is held in place by some form of bracing such as a splint or a plaster cast. Some babies may need to have surgery and this is usually successful.

Fetal defects per 10,000 births

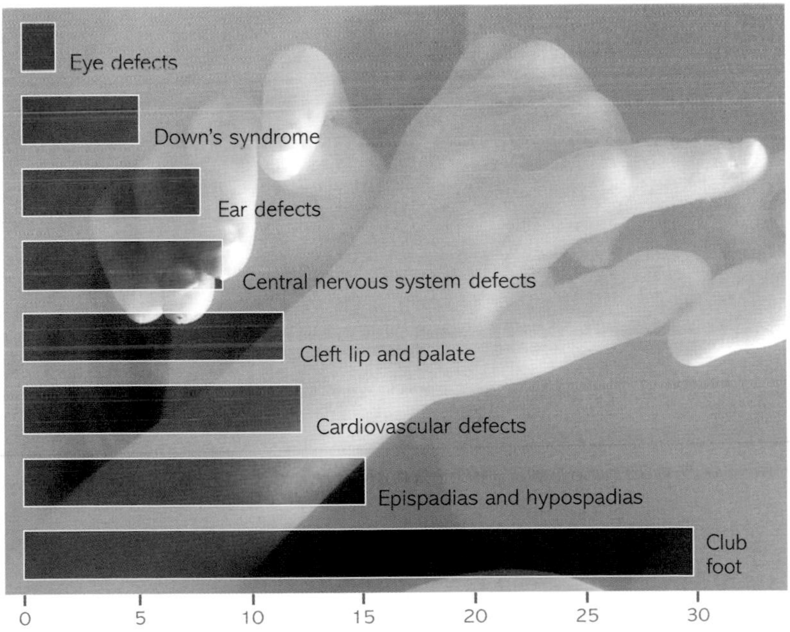

Eye defects

Down's syndrome

Ear defects

Central nervous system defects

Cleft lip and palate

Cardiovascular defects

Epispadias and hypospadias

Club foot

0   5   10   15   20   25   30

◀ **INCIDENCE OF FETAL DEFECTS** This chart shows the typical incidence of birth defects in babies born in England and Wales. It may be worrying to think about, but the chart shows just how rare most of these defects are. The most common is club foot, which affects both boys and girls. Epispadias and hypospadias, the second most common, are defects of the urethra and affect only boys. Cardiovascular defects affect the heart and circulatory system, and include congenital heart disease. Defects of the central nervous system include spina bifida and hydrocephalus.

Effects on parents

If your unborn baby has to have surgery it's going to be a very stressful time. But most parents cope extremely well.

When an unborn baby is diagnosed as having a serious illness or defect, doctors may suggest fetal surgery. This is a hard decision for parents and they'll be given expert counselling to help them decide whether or not to go ahead. Fetal surgery is advancing rapidly but is still very much at the experimental stage. In some experienced centres, simple procedures like exchange transfusions are performed routinely. The most complicated techniques, though, are only attempted if there's nothing to lose.

If the surgery is successful, the rewards are immense, and the mother's fertility doesn't seem to be affected much. Many women conceive again and have normal pregnancies. With less successful surgery, a woman could suffer miscarriage or premature birth, or need to have a Caesarean section. She may also have complications after the operation, which can be very stressful for all concerned.

Fetal surgery

Thanks to the development of specialized surgical techniques, it's now possible to correct some defects when a baby is still in the womb. Some procedures are still experimental, but they may be the baby's only chance, and many parents see this as a risk worth taking.

Ultrasound-guided surgery

In the more straightforward types of fetal surgery, thin needles are inserted through a mother's abdomen and womb and into the amniotic sac. Ultrasound allows the surgeon to see the baby and manipulate the needles (only one at a time is used) to take blood or tissue samples or give the baby drugs or blood transfusions as necessary.

Using ultrasound-guided techniques, surgeons are able to treat a growing number of life-threatening conditions. Rhesus and other incompatibilities between the immune systems of mother and baby may be corrected through intrauterine blood transfusions. Drugs to correct fetal heartbeat irregularities and destroy tumours may be injected into the baby; minute drainage tubes (shunts) that prevent further build-up of fluids may be inserted to drain excess fluids from the baby – for instance from the brain in cases of hydrocephalus – and to clear urinary tract blockages. Ultrasound is also used to guide the tiny forceps and scalpels used.

Intrauterine blood transfusions In some cases of Rhesus incompatibility (see p.202), in which a mother's blood is Rhesus (Rh) negative and her baby's Rh positive, the baby could become dangerously anaemic. If this happens, she'll need to be given one or more blood transfusions into one of the blood vessels in the umbilical cord to keep her going until she can be delivered safely. Fresh Rh-negative blood will be injected slowly, in amounts related to the baby's estimated weight and the seriousness of the anaemia.

Blood transfusions made to a baby in the womb have a good success rate, but in some severe cases, Rh incompatibility causes miscarriage or stillbirth, despite numerous transfusions. Until recently, if transfusions were unsuccessful there was nothing more that could be done. Research is underway, though, to find out whether injecting the baby with donated Rh-negative bone marrow will stimulate him to become Rh negative and so remove the incompatibility.

A more uncommon type of incompatibility between a mother and her baby results in the mother producing antibodies that destroy the baby's blood platelets. These platelets help blood to clot, and without them the baby could be in danger of suffering a haemorrhage and dying. This situation can be prevented by giving the baby transfusions of platelets and, in more severe cases, donor antibodies that counteract those of the mother.

Shunts for urinary tract problems Some unborn babies suffer a condition called hydronephrosis. In this, one of the baby's kidneys becomes swollen with urine because the ureter that drains it is narrow or blocked. If left untreated, this can lead to severe kidney damage; if it affects both kidneys, it can cause kidney failure. Hydronephrosis can sometimes be corrected by the insertion of shunts by fetal surgery.

Open fetal surgery

This is an even more extraordinary technique, used to correct some fetal defects that cannot be treated by ultrasound-guided surgery. It involves opening up a woman's womb and partially removing her baby so he can be operated on. Open fetal surgery has been used to repair diaphragmatic hernias – when a baby has a hole in his diaphragm that allows his intestines to protrude into his chest cavity and damage his lungs – and to remove certain types of tumour.

The operation Ultrasound-guided techniques are always carried out under local anaesthetic, but for open fetal surgery both mother and baby need to be given a general anaesthetic. When the anaesthetic has taken effect, the surgeon makes an incision in the mother's abdomen to expose her womb, and uses an ultrasound scan to find the exact position of the placenta. The amniotic fluid is then drawn off and kept warm. Next, an incision about 12cm (5in) long is made in the womb and amniotic membranes, taking care to keep well away from the placenta to avoid causing any damage. The baby is then eased gently out through this opening, just far enough for the surgeon to be able to repair the defect.

After the operation Once the surgeon has finished, the baby is carefully replaced in his mother's womb, along with the amniotic fluid. A small amount of antibiotic is added to the fluid to prevent infection. The incisions in the amniotic membranes and the womb are closed with absorbable stitches and surgical glue, and the incision in the abdomen is stitched together. The mother rests in bed for at least three days after the operation and she and her baby are intensively monitored. Although generally fit, most babies who undergo open fetal surgery are born before term, usually by Caesarean section.

Prospects for a baby

Fetal surgery is used to help babies who have defects that are easier to correct before they are born than afterwards, or who will die without it.

In general, the earlier in pregnancy fetal surgery is carried out, the better a baby's chances of survival. There are two main reasons for this. First, wounds heal relatively quickly in a developing baby. Second, organs that cannot grow until the defect is repaired have time to complete their normal development. For instance, if a baby's lungs cannot grow properly because of a diaphragmatic hernia, they'll need time to mature so that he'll be able to use them when he's born.

The exact timing of an operation depends on a number of factors – most importantly on when the defect can be diagnosed. Blood and antibody problems can usually be detected in the earliest weeks of pregnancy, and often, as in many cases of Rh incompatibility, they may be predicted. One baby who was given 25 transfusions of antibodies received the first at 11 weeks, when he was only about 5cm (2in) long. Most physical malformations cannot be diagnosed until the organ or organs they affect have grown enough for the defect to be apparent. As a result, surgery to correct defects of this type isn't usually carried out until after about week 18.

Miriam's casebook

Rhesus-negative mother

Elena's blood group is Rhesus (Rh) negative and her partner's, Chris, is Rh positive. Their daughter is Rh positive so Elena may have developed anti-Rh-positive antibodies. Their second baby has a 50:50 chance of being Rh positive. If this second baby is Rh positive, the baby's red blood cells may be damaged by the antibodies. To prevent damage, Elena will need special antenatal care.

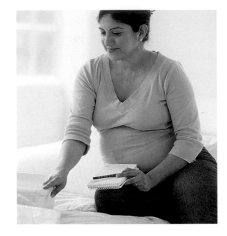

Mother and baby compatibility

I explained to Elena that about 85 per cent of people have the Rh factor in their red blood cells and they are Rh positive. The 15 per cent who lack the Rh factor are said to be Rh negative. A Rh-negative mother who's carrying a Rh-positive baby may develop antibodies to her baby's Rh-positive blood cells and injure them (see box opposite).

Elena's first pregnancy went without a hitch. This is usual with first pregnancies where the mother has Rh-negative blood and the baby Rh-positive blood (an incompatible pregnancy). However, when cells from this baby's blood mix with blood cells from the mother, for example during delivery, the mother's blood becomes sensitized. When the Rh factor from the baby's blood enters the mother's bloodstream, it acts as an antigen and stimulates the production of anti-Rh-positive antibodies. These attack and destroy the blood cells of her next Rh-positive (incompatible) baby. A newborn baby with Rh incompatability (see p.342) may suffer from various blood conditions ranging from mild jaundice to serious, possibly fatal, anaemia (see Haemolytic disease of the newborn, p.342). Fetuses who develop haemolytic disease can often be saved by intrauterine blood transfusion (see p.200).

Do all women become sensitized?

Not all Rh-negative women with Rh-positive babies become sensitized, as I explained to Elena, but there's no way of predicting which women will. All women who are Rh negative should be offered an Anti-D injection at 28 and 34 weeks of pregnancy and after delivery of a Rh-positive baby. Some units offer a double dose at 28 weeks only. Studies have yet to confirm which is the most effective.

Women who are Rh negative are also given an Anti-D injection after a late miscarriage, chorionic villus sampling, and amniocentesis or cordocentesis, especially if there's blood on the needle after it has been withdrawn from the uterus. Within 48 hours of delivering her first baby, Elena was injected with Anti-D (Rh immune-globulin) to help prevent the destructive antibodies from forming. If she'd miscarried, she would have also needed the injection, because her blood and her baby's would have mixed.

Birth expectations

I told Elena that if her antibody count remains low, she won't need further special care during her pregnancy. If the count rises moderately, her baby may be induced early to prevent serious consequences. In this case, home birth is out of the question. She'll need to deliver in hospital, probably by a Caesarean. In a very few cases the baby has to have a blood transfusion to replace his own blood cells, which have become damaged during pregnancy.

Elena's baby

Elena's baby is likely to be fit and healthy, thanks to the Anti-D injections. His cord blood will be tested for his group. If he is negative, no further Anti-D is needed. If he is positive, Anti-D will be given to Elena within 72 hours of delivery. The dose of Anti-D will be assessed by the amount of fetal cells in Elena's circulation.

If he is affected by Rh incompatibility, his bilirubin levels will rise quickly after birth because his liver can't get rid of it. A high level of bilirubin will make him look yellow. This can be treated by placing him under ultraviolet "bili" light, which converts bilirubin into a harmless substance. He may also need a transfusion – blood can be withdrawn from the baby via the umbilical vein and replaced with donor blood that's

compatible with his mother's blood. If severe haemolytic disease had been predicted before he was born, he may have been successfully treated by a transfusion while in the womb.

Rhesus disease in pregnancy

Rhesus disease only happens when a woman who has Rh-negative blood (symbolized by minus signs in the picture) is pregnant with a Rh-positive (symbolized by plus signs) baby. Most Rh-negative mothers carry their first babies without any problems – just as Elena did. If the woman then develops antibodies to Rh-positive blood (symbolized by triangles in the pictures below) any further babies that she has could be at risk.

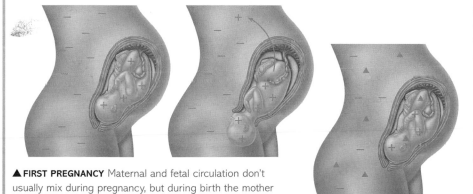

KEY
– mother's blood
+ baby's blood
▲ antibodies

▲ **FIRST PREGNANCY** Maternal and fetal circulation don't usually mix during pregnancy, but during birth the mother may be exposed to her baby's Rh-positive blood.

◀ **A FUTURE PREGNANCY** If the mother develops antibodies to her baby's red blood cells, they may cause problems in a future pregnancy.

Complaints in pregnancy

Very few women go through pregnancy without suffering a few complaints – most are uncomfortable rather than serious. Knowing what might happen is half the battle and also allows you to tell the difference between those that are just a nuisance and those that could be serious.

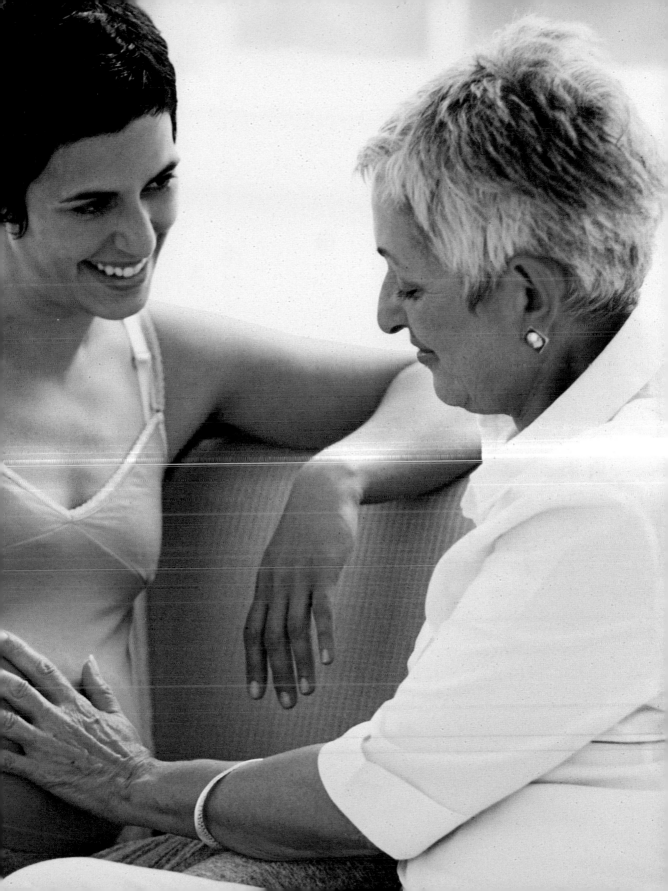

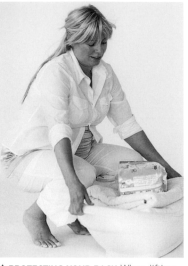

▲ **PROTECTING YOUR BACK** When lifting anything heavy, whether a pile of washing or a toddler, always use your thighs to do the work. Don't treat your back as a crane.

Common complaints

When you're pregnant you may find you're bothered by little ailments like backache, cramps, and constipation. These things are irritating but not serious, and most are caused by hormonal changes and the extra strain

Complaint	Why it happens
Backache is usually felt as general discomfort across the lower back, often with pain across the buttocks and down the legs. You can get it when you've been standing for too long with bad posture or after lifting something heavy, especially during the third trimester.	High progesterone levels soften the ligaments of the pelvic bones so they stretch to allow your baby to be born. But the ligaments of the spine also relax, putting extra strain on the joints of the back and hips.
You might also get intensely painful low backache when you rotate your spine and pelvis in opposite directions, such as when you turn over sideways in bed.	The baby is resting against your sacroiliac joint, which is some 7.5cm (3in) in from the top of your buttocks. Rotary movements of the spine and pelvis open and close the sacroiliac joint, causing pain.
Carpal tunnel syndrome feels like pins and needles, mainly in your thumb and first finger, with numbness and sometimes weakness. Occasionally your whole hand and forearm can be affected and this can happen from conception onwards.	Pressure on the nerve that passes from the arm to the hand along the front of the wrist. The pressure is caused by swelling of the carpal tunnel (a ring of fibres around the wrist under which the nerve passes) because of water retention.
Constipation is when you have dry, hard stools that are difficult to pass. This may happen from conception onwards.	Progesterone relaxes the muscles in the intestinal walls, so there are fewer contractions to push the food along. This means that much more water than usual is absorbed from the stool in the colon, which makes it hard and dry. Stools may be less frequent, too.
Cramps are a sudden pain in your thigh, calf, and/or foot, followed by a general ache. More common in the third trimester.	Cramps may be caused by low calcium levels in the blood, or they can be due to salt deficiency. Check with your doctor.

that pregnancy puts on your body. Most can be treated very simply, and are nothing to worry about. A few, though, can be serious, so it's important to be aware of what various symptoms can mean and be prepared to do something right away if you're worried. Always check with your midwife or doctor if you are concerned.

What can be done	Risk to baby
Massage may help (see p.152). Do exercises to strengthen your spine. Make sure your mattress is firm. Lift heavy weights correctly (see opposite). Try to improve your posture (see p.160), and don't wear high-heeled shoes. If the pain runs down the back of your leg towards your foot, check with your doctor in case it's a slipped disc.	None
Osteopathy can be helpful, even in severe cases. Backache usually eases in the fifth month when your baby tips forwards – although you may not be able to wait that long!	None
You will be given physiotherapy treatment. A splint on the wrist at night may help, as may holding your hand above your head and wiggling your fingers. Acupuncture may help too. Sleep with your arm on a pillow. Symptoms usually disappear soon after delivery.	None
Drink lots of water. Eat as much fibre in the form of fruit (especially figs and prunes), vegetables, and wholegrains as you can. Walk briskly for at least 20 minutes a day. Don't take laxatives without consulting your doctor. Natural laxatives are best as they increase the amount of water in the stool, making it soft.	None
Massage the area very firmly. Flex your foot up and push into the heel.	None

▲ RELIEVING FOOT CRAMPS Keeping your foot flexed up, carefully make circling movements with your lower leg.

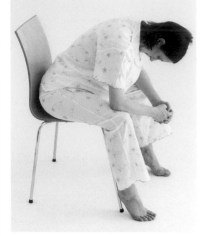

▲ **WHAT TO DO IF YOU FEEL FAINT** If you feel faint, sit down and bend your head towards your knees. When you feel better, get up slowly.

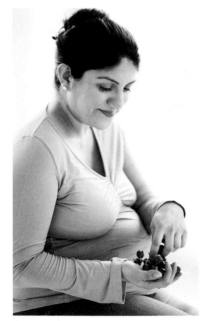

▲ **AVOIDING HEARTBURN** Eat smaller meals so your stomach doesn't get too full. Try snacking on nutritious foods such as fruit and nuts and eating little but often.

Complaint	Why it happens
Diarrhoea can happen at any time during your pregnancy. You'll have soft, watery stools and need to go to the toilet frequently.	Usually because you have an infection from bacteria or a virus.
Faintness is a feeling of dizziness or vertigo that comes on suddenly, making you unsteady on your feet. You may feel faint if you stand up too quickly, or you've been on your feet for too long, especially in hot weather.	A combination of a lack of blood supply to the brain, often caused by pooling of the blood in the legs and feet when standing, and the demands of the uterus for an increased blood supply.
Heartburn is a burning sensation just behind your breastbone and you may also bring up some stomach acid into your mouth. It can happen when you lie down, cough, strain when passing a stool, or lift something heavy.	Early in pregnancy, the muscular valve at the entrance to your stomach relaxes under the influence of progesterone. This allows stomach acid to flow up into your oesophagus, causing a burning feeling. Later in pregnancy, your baby can press up on your stomach, forcing the contents back into the oesophagus.
High blood pressure (hypertension) is an increase in blood pressure, which can be mild or severe. Although you may not experience any symptoms at all, headaches, visual disturbances, and vomiting are all warning signs. You may also have water retention (see p.212), with swelling of your feet, hands, and ankles. High blood pressure can happen at any time, but it's more likely near your due date. It's more common in women having their first baby, especially if they're over 35, and also in women having more than one baby. Your midwife will keep a close check on your blood pressure because a rise may be a warning of pre-eclampsia (sometimes called pre-eclamptic toxaemia), see p.224.	It's not clear why some women get high blood pressure in pregnancy. In some mothers, cells from the placenta produce chemicals called vasoconstrictors that may cause the blood vessels to constrict. This may raise the blood pressure and cause the kidneys to hold on to sodium, leading to water retention. Your blood pressure will return to normal once your baby has been born.

What can be done

Drink plenty of water – about 12–14 glasses a day – to replace the fluid you lose and make sure that your blood pressure remains normal. Check with your doctor, who will test your stools for infection and give you treatment if necessary.

Try not to stand for long periods. Always sit or lie down when you feel dizzy. Don't get up suddenly from sitting or get out of a hot bath too quickly. Keep cool in hot weather. If you feel dizzy, bend your head down towards your knees or lie down with your feet higher than your head.

Eat small meals so that your stomach is never too full. Sleep propped up with several pillows. Drink a glass of milk at bedtime to help to neutralize stomach acid. Your doctor may also suggest or prescribe antacids, and these are safe to take throughout your pregnancy.

If you suffered from high blood pressure before you were pregnant, tell your doctor. Keep an eye on your weight. Tell your doctor if you often have headaches and nausea.

Your doctor will test your blood pressure and urine, and look for any swelling (oedema – see Water retention, p.212) of your hands, face, and ankles at antenatal visits.

If your blood pressure goes up at any stage of your pregnancy, you'll almost certainly have to see your doctor more often and you may be asked to attend the antenatal day unit at the hospital for checking.

If the rise is severe, you'll need to go into hospital, where you can be monitored continuously. If your baby appears to be suffering, your labour may be induced or you may have a Caesarean section.

Risk to baby

If diarrhoea goes untreated for a long time, the dehydration and loss of calories it causes can put your baby at risk. If diarrhoea is profuse and protracted, you may need to go into hospital for intravenous feeding.

None, unless you fall very heavily on to your stomach.

None

Pregnancy-induced hypertension (see Pre-eclampsia, p.224) can slow your baby's growth rate, because blood flow to the uterus is reduced. Your baby may also be short of oxygen. Both these factors may lead to low birthweight. There is a severe form called eclampsia (see p.224), which can be life threatening, but thanks to good antenatal care this is now very rare in the West.

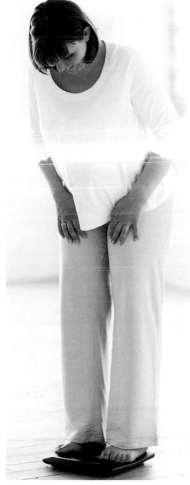

▲ **MONITOR YOUR WEIGHT** A sudden weight gain can be a symptom of pre-eclampsia, so tell your doctor if you notice any change.

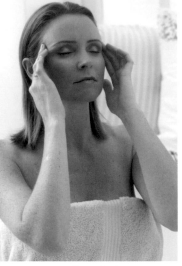

▲ **SELF MASSAGE** If you feel tense, massaging your face, especially your temples, and your neck is a good way to relax and can also help you get to sleep at night.

Complaint	Why it happens
Insomnia is the inability to sleep at night, making you tired and irritable during the day. It can happen at any time from conception onwards.	Your baby lives on a 24-hour clock, and his metabolism keeps going even when you want to sleep. This can affect your body's responses. Other causes of insomnia include night sweats and a desire to empty your bladder more often than usual, particularly during the third trimester.
Mood swings are rapid, uncharacteristic changes in mood, often with unexplained crying and anxiety attacks. They are common from conception onwards, but are especially likely to happen in the third trimester.	Changes in your hormone balance during pregnancy have a depressant effect on the nervous system, causing symptoms similar to those you may have before a period. Identity crises and the way you feel about the changes in your body may have a profound effect on you when you're pregnant, and mixed feelings about pregnancy and parenthood can cause sudden shifts in your moods.
Morning sickness is a feeling of sickness and nausea, sometimes with vomiting. Contrary to its name, it can happen at any time of the day, but generally when you haven't eaten for a long period, or after a night's sleep. Feelings of nausea are most common in the first trimester and then usually lessen.	The main cause is low blood sugar, but pregnancy hormones may irritate the stomach directly.
Piles are dilated rectal veins (see Varicose veins, p.212) that may protrude through the anus. They don't usually develop until the second trimester.	Your growing baby presses down on your rectum and can prevent blood flow to the heart. The blood therefore pools, causing the veins to dilate to accommodate the dammed-up blood.

What can be done	Risk to baby
A warm bath and a hot milky drink at bedtime may help, as may a relaxing massage (see p.152). Watch TV or read until you feel sleepy. Find a comfortable position, and try to stay cool. Doctors very rarely prescribe sleeping pills in pregnancy because they can cross the placenta and affect the baby (see also p.258).	None
These are natural feelings and moments of depression, anxiety, and confusion are common even in the easiest of pregnancies. Trying to analyze such feelings may only serve to prolong them. (See also Emotional changes, p.154.)	None
Food will help you avoid feeling nauseous, so eat little and often. Eat high carbohydrate foods such as wholemeal bread, potatoes, rice, and cereals, and avoid fried food and coffee, which trigger nausea. Keep glucose sweets in your car, desk, or handbag. To prevent sickness in the morning, put a glass of water and a plain biscuit by your bed at night, and have them as a snack 15 minutes before you get up. Cigarette smoke and other strong smells may also trigger nausea. Drink extra fluids such as fruit juice or skimmed milk – if you can keep them down.	In its severe form (called hyperemesis gravidarum), vomiting can deplete you of fluid and minerals, leading to low blood pressure. This may be harmful to your baby. Tell your doctor if you vomit more than three times a day for three days. In very severe cases, you may need to go to hospital for treatment to replace the fluids that you have lost.
Eat plenty of fibre to keep your bowels regular and your stools soft as this will help you avoid straining down. Don't lift weights, as this increases pressure in the abdominal area and in the rectal veins. Have coughs treated promptly for the same reasons. Aromatherapy may be able to relieve cough symptoms.	None

▲ A REASSURING CUDDLE A comforting hug from your partner can be just what you need when you're feeling anxious and upset.

Complaint	Why it happens
Rib pain can be felt as extreme soreness and tenderness of the ribs, usually on the right side, just below the breasts. The pain may be worse when you sit down and it tends to happen mainly during the third trimester.	It's caused by compression of the ribs as your womb rises in your abdomen. Also, your baby can bruise your lower ribs with his head, or by excessive punching and kicking.
Tender, painful breasts that feel heavy and uncomfortable, with a tingling sensation in the nipples, is often one of the first signs of pregnancy. Your breasts may feel tender throughout, but become more so towards term.	Hormones are getting your breasts ready for lactation. The milk ducts are growing and being stretched as they fill with milk.
Thrush is a yeast infection. Typically you'll have a thick, white, curdy discharge from your vagina, with dryness and intense itching around your vagina, vulva, perineum, and, sometimes, your anus. You may also have pain when passing urine. Thrush can happen at any time.	It's caused by an infection with the yeast Candida albicans, which is always in your bowel. Infection happens when the yeast grows uncontrolled by other bacteria, perhaps after a course of antibiotics. Thrush is more common in pregnancy, probably because increased vaginal blood flow can cause a leakage of sugar into body fluids. Excessive sugar intake often aggravates the condition.
Varicose veins are swollen veins just below the skin. Although most common in the legs or anus, they can also develop in the vulva.	The weight of your developing baby and growing uterus puts extra pressure on your veins. Also pregnancy hormones can relax the vein walls, making them more likely to expand to form varicose veins. See Piles, p.210.
Water retention happens when there's more fluid than usual in your body tissues. This causes swelling (oedema), especially of the feet, face, and hands. Your rings may become tight.	Standing all day, especially in hot weather, can cause fluid to pool in the ankles. High blood pressure (see p.208), which often happens in pregnancy, can force fluid from the bloodstream into the tissues, causing oedema. Pregnancy hormones can cause retention of sodium by the kidneys, which in turn causes the body to retain fluid.

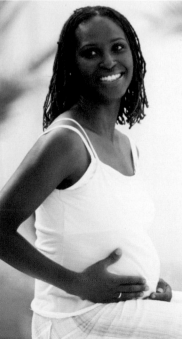

▲ **STAY COMFORTABLE** Don't be afraid to show off your bump in close-fitting clothes as long as they're stretchy and comfortable. Cotton is best.

What can be done	Risk to baby
Wear clothes that don't compress your ribs. Improve your posture. Prop yourself up on cushions when you lie down. The pain stops when the baby's head drops into the pelvic cavity before birth.	None
Wear a good supportive bra from early in pregnancy. If your breasts are large, wear a bra at night as well (see p.163). Wash your breasts gently once a day with a mild soap and pat dry. Put baby lotion or oil on your nipples if they're sore.	None
Tight pants and trousers can encourage infection. Choose cotton instead of man made fibres. The doctor will prescribe pessaries that you should place in your vagina at night, as directed. You'll also be prescribed a cream that you gently rub into the skin around your vaginal opening and anus, and on the thighs. This will stop the itching.	None
Don't stand for too long. Put your feet up. Wear pregnancy support tights. Gentle massage may help to prevent varicose veins, but do not massage the area if you develop them. Avoid leg-waxing treatments that may cause inflammation.	None
Don't stand for long periods. Put your feet up when you can. Avoid salty foods. Your doctor will check your hands, face, and ankles for any swelling at each antenatal visit. Diuretics are not recommended during pregnancy.	Potentially dangerous (see Pre-eclampsia, p.224).

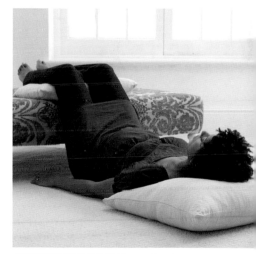

▲ **TAKE TIME TO RELAX** Remember to make time to put your feet up – this will help prevent water retention and varicose veins – but don't lie on your back for too long, you may feel dizzy.

Miriam's casebook

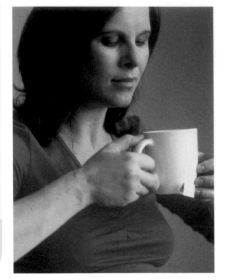

Mother with MS

When Kathy, now 29 and 14 weeks pregnant, developed multiple sclerosis at 23, a year after her marriage to Tom, both were devastated. They believed that Kathy's MS would make it harder for her to conceive, possibly even make her infertile. They worried that it wasn't good for a woman with MS to become pregnant because it could make the condition worse, with serious relapses and increased disability.

Getting new information

Five years after her diagnosis Kathy's walking was still steady, her eyesight was hardly affected, and she had no troublesome urinary symptoms or vertigo. She and Tom badly wanted a baby so they decided to see an obstetrician.

Kathy and Tom were given an encouraging picture by the obstetrician. He explained that MS doesn't affect a woman's fertility and has no effect on pregnancy, labour, or delivery. In a study of 36 pregnant women with MS, the only problems noted were two cases of mild vomiting. There's no increase in miscarriage, complications, malformations, or stillbirths.

A good prognosis

Kathy wondered whether pregnancy would make her MS worse. I reassured her that many research studies suggest that pregnancy is in fact a protection for women with MS. This is probably because the natural state of immuno-suppression that happens in pregnancy to prevent a woman from rejecting her baby also suppresses the inflammation that causes nerve and brain damage in MS. On the other hand, there's a slightly increased risk of a flare-up for three to six months after the birth. Between 40 and 60 per cent of women have a relapse during this time – 20 per cent of

these suffer from permanent side effects while 80 per cent go back to their pre-pregnant state of MS. Pregnancy does not appear to affect the long-term course of MS.

I reassured Kathy that the management of her labour and delivery would follow normal medical routine. She could be given analgesics – gas, injection, or epidural – and these would have no effect on her MS. A Caesarean would not affect her MS, nor would a forceps delivery.

Possible health risks

Tom was concerned that MS might be passed on to their child. I explained that in an area with a high prevalence of MS, one person in 1,000 would be likely to develop the disease. A study has shown that among children of people with MS, the figure could rise to one in 100. Dietary and genetic factors may be involved, although nothing has been proved. Most people feel that the risk of their child having MS is not great enough to stop them from trying to conceive.

Stopping medication

Kathy was worried that the drugs she's given for MS might harm her developing baby. I told her that in the first 12 weeks of pregnancy a woman is never given drugs, even if she does have MS, unless her life or the life of her baby is in danger. Drugs to stop painful muscle spasms would be discontinued before she conceived, as would long-term anti-inflammatory therapies. Drugs that help to control urinary frequency or incontinence would also be stopped. Steroids, which are only given if either the mother or the baby's life is in danger, are hardly ever needed during pregnancy.

When Kathy became pregnant, her obstetrician referred her to a neurologist who could give advice throughout her pregnancy and after the birth of the baby.

After the birth

Kathy wanted to know whether her MS would affect her ability to feed and care for her baby. There are no medical reasons for her not to breastfeed. It's extremely important for her to rest, though, so she'll need to have help with her baby and express milk so someone else can give night feeds. She was also worried that having a baby to look after might increase the sense of insecurity she already has because of her MS. Tom was able to calm Kathy's fears on that score.

Happily pregnant

Kathy and Tom thought about what they'd been told, and read the ARMS (Action for Research into Multiple Sclerosis) booklet, MS and Pregnancy (see Addresses, p.370). They decided to try for a baby, and Kathy is now 14 weeks pregnant. She's going to routine antenatal clinics and seeing her neurologist once a month. Kathy's doctors have told her that there's no need for special testing or monitoring. She's being given iron to avoid anaemia and her doctors are on the look-out for warning signs of a urinary tract infection, which would need prompt treatment. So far her pregnancy is going normally and her MS remains unchanged.

A mother with MS will need to rest regularly during the day. I suggested to Kathy that she should stop doing things if she gets breathless, learns to catnap in her spare time, takes two sleeps a day of at least 30 minutes each, and goes to bed early, say not later than 9.30pm.

The good news is that MS has no effect on a woman's fertility or on her ability to conceive, carry to term, and deliver a healthy baby. Bear in the mind the following:

■ consult your neurologist before becoming pregnant, so you can be advised on the best time to stop taking medication before conceiving

■ rest as much as you can during your pregnancy and learn to catnap as often as you need to recharge your batteries during the day

■ be prepared for the possibility of a flare-up in MS symptoms three to six months after delivery.

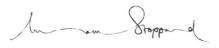

Kathy's baby

There's every expectation that Kathy's baby will develop normally and be born in a straightforward way without the need for any special medical intervention. I explained to Kathy that her baby cannot inherit MS by transmission across the placenta, and the risk of transmission through genes appears to be very small.

While in the uterus, Kathy's baby won't be at risk from the drugs given for MS because Kathy will be advised to stop taking medication. I advised Kathy to check with her doctor before starting drug treatment again following her baby's birth so her baby won't be at risk from any traces of drugs in her breast milk.

I explained to Kathy that breastfeeding would not present any difficulties and that Kathy would be wise to express milk so that someone else can help out by occasional bottlefeeding while Kathy rests to help keep her milk supply up. I suggested she practise breastfeeding a doll before the birth while lying on her bed or sofa with the doll resting on a pillow or cushion. That way Kathy can learn to conserve her energy as much as possible.

Emergencies in pregnancy

Emergencies tend to happen in the first and third trimesters. In the first, there may be miscarriage. In the third trimester, there may be complications such as pre-eclampsia, or problems with the placenta. Be reassured that most babies are delivered safely.

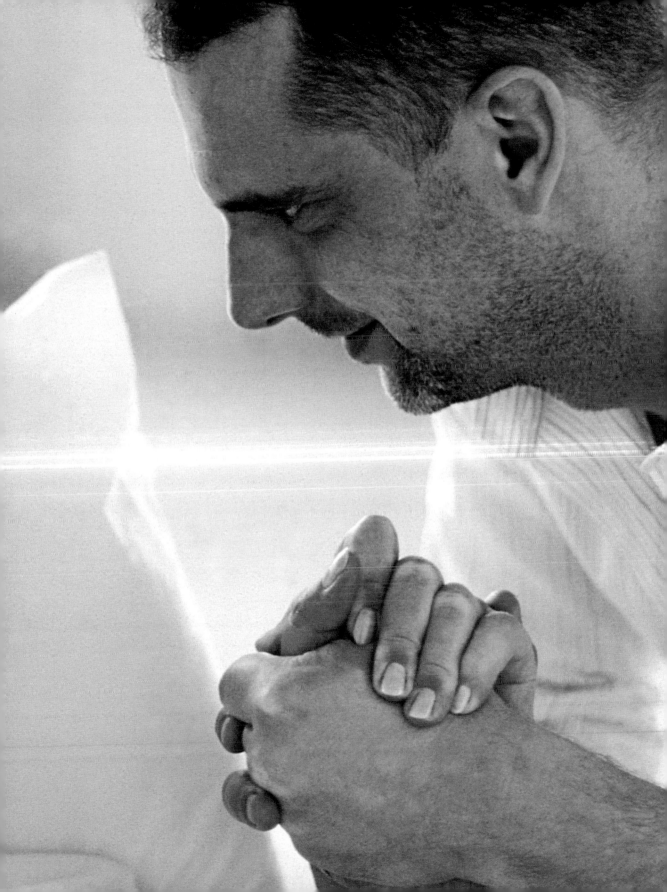

Vaginal bleeding

Don't disregard vaginal bleeding at any stage of pregnancy – it should always be taken seriously. Bleeding may be a sign of an abnormally placed placenta, placenta praevia (see p.222), or warn that a miscarriage is imminent. Both conditions need prompt medical treatment.

■ About one-quarter of all pregnant woman suffer some vaginal bleeding in the first trimester. More than half of these women go on to give birth to a healthy baby at term. If you have any bleeding, call your doctor or midwife, who will probably refer you to the Early Pregnancy Unit at your local hospital. These are walk-in clinics, where you can be scanned quickly to check for your baby's heartbeat. If it's confirmed, there's a very good chance (more than 90 per cent) that all will be well. Women with a history of repeated miscarriage may go to these units regularly to boost their confidence. Studies show that reassurance alone has a very positive effect.

■ If you start to bleed at any time during the second or third trimester, call your maternity unit and go there as soon as you can. There may be serious problems with your placenta, or you could be going into premature labour (see pp.298 and 299), but there arc other less serious causes. It's important to be seen right away just in case.

Medical emergencies

Most women carry their babies to term without any problems or emergencies. It's a good idea, though, to be aware of the danger signs just in case, so you know when to call for medical help.

Miscarriage

Spontaneous miscarriage is when a baby dies or is expelled from the womb before the 24th week. After the 24th week, this is called a stillbirth or premature delivery. About one-third of all pregnancies end in miscarriage in the first few weeks, but one-quarter of these happen before a woman even knows or suspects she is pregnant.

Miscarriages are more likely the older you are and the more pregnancies you've had. They are most common in the first trimester and the usual symptom is bleeding, which happens in 95 per cent of cases. If you notice bleeding at any time in your pregnancy, call your doctor.

Many early miscarriages are due to a seriously abnormal fetus failing to implant in the wall of the uterus, while 70 per cent are due to chromosomal abnormalities. In some, the baby itself never develops at all, just the amniotic sac and placenta. Causes linked to the mother include abnormalities in her uterus, such as large fibroids, and hormonal imbalances. Some miscarriages are also caused by bacterial and viral infections. Cervical incompetence (see p.223) accounts for only one per cent of spontaneous miscarriages. Factors linked to the father include abnormal sperm. Whatever the cause, at some point in the first three months the body starts to reject the pregnancy, and bleeding then pain occurs. Doctors divide spontaneous miscarriages into several categories:

Threatened miscarriage A mother suffers vaginal bleeding and sometimes pain; miscarriage is possible, but not inevitable. This happens in about ten per cent of all pregnancies and may be confused with the slight bleeding that can come at the time of the first "missed" period.

Inevitable miscarriage A woman has vaginal bleeding and pain because her uterus is contracting. Unfortunately if her cervix also dilates, she is bound to lose the pregnancy.

Complete miscarriage Heavy bleeding means the fetus and placenta are expelled from the uterus, and the uterus goes back to its previous size. Ultrasound examination can confirm this.

Missed miscarriage The fetus fails to develop, or dies, but the placenta keeps functioning. Eventually a miscarriage would result, but an ultrasound scan will confirm that there is no ongoing pregnancy. Different ways of treating this will be offered.

Incomplete miscarriage There's a miscarriage, but some of the products of conception, such as the amniotic sac or the placenta, remain in place.

Recurrent miscarriage A woman suffers a miscarriage on three or more occasions. This may happen at the same stage of pregnancy or at different stages and the reasons may be the same or differ each time.

Treatment If you're bleeding in the second or third trimester, call the hospital and go there as soon as you can (see column opposite). If you bleed in the first trimester, call your doctor and stop any physical activities such as strenuous exercise and sexual intercourse. If the bleeding and pain stop, you're likely to go on to deliver a healthy baby.

If a miscarriage seems inevitable, there's little that doctors can do to prevent it. You will have a scan to confirm that the pregnancy has failed and will then be offered either a natural approach in which you wait until the body expels all of the placenta, or a surgical option. If you're bleeding heavily, or have lost a lot of blood, you may need to have an emergency operation, an evacuation of retained products of conception (ERPC). This is similar to a dilatation and curettage (D and C) and is the procedure for clearing out the uterus. A general anaesthetic is usually given, along with painkillers. A blood transfusion may be necessary if the woman has lost more than 1 litre (1¾pts) of blood. There's no urgency in treating a missed miscarriage, but if, after a time, a spontaneous miscarriage hasn't taken place, a ERPC will be carried out.

If a baby dies later in pregnancy, prostaglandin pessaries or an oxytocin injection are given to stimulate delivery (see also p.312).

After suffering a miscarriage because of cervical incompetence (see p.223), some women can be treated by stitching the cervix shut at the beginning of the next pregnancy, though this is not always successful.

Other possible reasons for recurrent miscarriage are genetic or hormonal disorders or problems with blood clotting. Long-term infections, such as listeria, may sometimes cause repeated miscarriages, but these can be difficult to diagnose and treat.

Other contributing factors to miscarriage can be poor nutrition; chronic disease, such as renal disease; or tumours in the uterus (particularly fibroids).

Uterine septums

In all mammals, the uterus (womb) develops from two separate tubes in the embryo.

In some, for example cats and dogs, the tubes develop into two separate uteri. In monkeys, horses, and human beings, the tubes join to make a single uterus. If the tubes don't join completely this can leave a partition, or septum, in the uterus. If the baby is in an awkward position this may mean she needs to be delivered by Caesarean section.

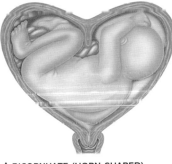

▲ **BICORNUATE (HORN-SHAPED) UTERUS** The baby is forced to lie across the uterus from the second trimester onwards.

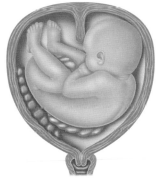

▲ **SUBSEPTATE UTERUS** The septum restricts the baby's movements, which can hinder birth.

Miriam's casebook

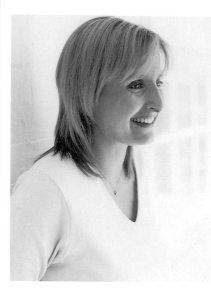

After a miscarriage

Liz and her partner, Alan, desperately wanted their first baby and were deeply upset by Liz's miscarriage at 11 weeks, nine months ago. Alan found it difficult to talk about their loss and buried himself in his work, while Liz struggled to cope with her feelings of bereavement. Liz is now eight weeks into her second pregnancy. Her pleasure at being pregnant is marred by fears that the same thing might happen again.

First reactions

When she miscarried nine months ago, Liz felt very alone as she battled with her feelings of guilt, despair, and anger. She felt that her doctor couldn't look her in the eye or talk openly about her lost baby. Her family and friends were sympathetic but on occasion their attempts to comfort her were rather clumsy. Some people said it was all for the best, because there must have been something wrong with the baby. Others reassured her that she could soon have another one. Her unborn baby was not real to them as it had been to Liz, and they did not understand her intense sense of loss.

Understandably, Liz began to wonder if her reactions were normal – perhaps she wasn't justified in grieving for a baby who'd never really existed? I reassured Liz that it is natural and healthy for a mother to mourn the loss of her child, even if the child has not been born. Her emotions as well as her body needed time to readjust. I also encouraged her to share her feelings with her partner, so that they could grieve together. At first Alan was reluctant to share his feelings with Liz, and she felt she had to force him to talk to her because he found it hard to put words to his emotions. She knew that it would be impossible to care for another baby until she had given herself time to come to terms with

losing this one, and this was something that they had to do together. I encouraged them to share their anxieties and frustration, talk through their feelings, and cry together. I explained how important it was for them to express their grief openly. I also suggested that it might help if they had a private memorial ceremony – perhaps something as simple as planting a tree in memory of their miscarried baby.

Concerns about the baby

After her miscarriage, Liz was taken to hospital and examined to make sure there were no fragments of the placenta left in her uterus, where they could cause bleeding. The doctors said they could find no particular cause for her miscarriage, which was reassuring. Often miscarriage occurs when no fetus has developed at all, or it has died very early on due to developmental abnormalities.

Liz began to blame herself – perhaps the miscarriage was her fault? I explained that one in three first pregnancies ends in miscarriage. There are thought to be two reasons for this. First, an immature uterus might need to mature by having a trial run before carrying a pregnancy to term. Second, defects in the sperm or egg can produce an abnormal fetus.

What research shows

Research on miscarriage in early pregnancy shows that a woman who's had one miscarriage is no more likely to miscarry again than other women. It is recommended that you wait for one normal menstrual period before trying to conceive again.

Some women do miscarry repeatedly, but even for them the chance of a successful pregnancy after three previous miscarriages is about 60 per cent. Women who've had several miscarriages are tested for uterine abnormalities, hormone imbalances, and disorders of the immunological system and blood clotting.

Why miscarriage occurs

The immune system is designed to repel foreign bodies because they can be harmful. Pregnancy normally overrides this, so that the woman's body protects the baby rather than rejecting it. But for unknown reasons, the override fails in some mothers – the immune system reasserts itself and the baby is miscarried.

Women suffering from polycystic ovary syndrome (PCOS) a condition usually characterized by multiple, tiny ovarian cysts – seem to have more miscarriages. This syndrome is caused by a hormone imbalance that causes the body to make too much testosterone and to overstimulate the ovaries so that immature eggs are produced. Women with PCOS and irregular or absent periods who are thinking of getting pregnant will be tested for hormone imbalances and checks on ovulation. They may be given fertility drugs such as clomiphene (see p.46), although this will not protect them against miscarriage.

Becoming pregnant again

Now that Liz is pregnant again, she's being extremely careful in every aspect of her life. Most importantly, she's given up blaming herself for the miscarriage and is taking a positive attitude towards her new pregnancy. I told Liz that although she can't be sure what the outcome will be, chances are all will go well this time and that she should try to enjoy her

Miriam's top tips

Talking over your feelings about losing your baby helps you both come to terms with your loss. It's only natural that the experience of a miscarriage may make you anxious about any future pregnancy.

■ Share your grief for the baby you have lost with your partner and close friends. Allow yourself time to mourn.

■ Before trying to conceive again, wait for one normal menstrual period.

■ Try to keep positive: eat well and get plenty of rest to allow your body to recuperate.

■ When you do become pregnant again, make the most of your antenatal check-ups to answer any questions you may have about your pregnancy.

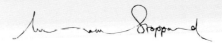

pregnancy. Alan is "sure it's going to be all right this time" but doesn't want to make plans for the future as he did before. Liz is fit and healthy and doesn't appear to have any condition that makes her likely to miscarry again. Because of her previous history, Liz will be given extra care during her pregnancy. The health of her baby will be closely watched for any signs of distress so that any problems can be averted. Her midwife or family doctor will be only too willing to answer any questions Liz may have.

Liz's baby has every chance of developing perfectly normally. In several ways, Liz's baby will actually benefit both before and after birth because of her mother's history of miscarriage: she will be well nourished because her mother is paying such careful attention to what she eats, and to relaxation and exercise routines. She will be comforted by the positive thoughts and feelings that Liz is directing towards her. When she's born, Liz's baby will be greeted with relief and delight by both parents because she's making up for a previous disappointment. She represents success.

Placenta in wrong position

If the placenta has implanted in the wrong position, it can obstruct a baby's birth.

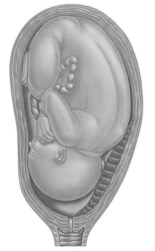

▲ **SIDE POSITION** In minor placenta praevia, the placenta implants on the side and extends to the cervix, but doesn't cover it.

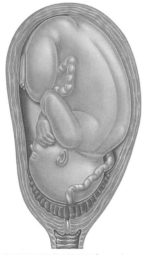

▲ **BLOCKING THE CERVIX** In major placenta praevia, the placenta implants centrally, completely covering the cervix – even when it's fully dilated.

Placental separation

The partial or complete separation of the placenta from the uterus can cause bleeding from the placental bed. Blood builds up in the spaces, and eventually escapes around the membranes and through the cervix into the vagina. This is known as placental abruption (abruptio placentae) and happens in about one in 200 pregnancies. The cause is unknown, but it tends to be more common in women who smoke or who use cocaine in pregnancy. Obstetricians divide placental separation into three types according to the severity.

In mild separation, your blood loss may be slight. You'll need bed rest, with ultrasound examination to monitor the situation. If it happens late in pregnancy, your labour may have to be induced.

In moderate separation, up to a quarter of the placenta separates and 0.5–1 litres (1–1¾pts) of blood is lost. You will need a blood transfusion and, if your pregnancy is at or nearing term, your baby will usually be delivered by Caesarean section.

Severe separation is an acute emergency, when at least two-thirds of the placenta shears off the uterine wall, and up to about 2 litres (4pts) of blood are lost. A rapid blood transfusion will be given, and sometimes an emergency Caesarean will be carried out to try to save the baby.

Placenta praevia

This happens when the placenta is implanted in the lower segment of the uterus instead of the upper part (see column, left) and it lies in front of the baby as he comes to descend the birth canal at the start of labour. The baby cannot pass down the canal without dislodging the placenta, so interrupting his own blood supply. Placenta praevia can be a cause of bleeding in the final two months of pregnancy. It's more common in women who've had several children, particularly if they've been born by Caesarean, but the cause is unknown.

The greater the proportion of the placenta lying in the lower uterine segment, the greater the likelihood of complications during delivery. Even though the growth of the placenta in both size and weight slows down after the 30th week of pregnancy, the lower segment of the uterus is increasing in length quite rapidly. There may be shearing stresses between the placenta and the uterine wall, leading to episodes of bleeding.

This potentially dangerous condition can be diagnosed well ahead of delivery using ultrasound (see p.180). Early symptoms include bleeding, with bright red blood, which may happen after sex. The doctor will advise a mother with these symptoms to go into hospital for ultrasound examination and bed rest, with blood transfusions if necessary. The baby will be delivered by Caesarean section (see p.308).

There may be a postpartum haemorrhage (severe bleeding) after the birth, but this is usually anticipated and drugs to prevent it will be given as soon as the baby is born. In a very few cases, haemorrhage will continue despite treatment and then a hysterectomy may be a possibility. For these reasons, placenta praevia should only be treated by obstetricians qualified to cope with these complications. The mother must be delivered in a well-equipped hospital, with a blood transfusion service on hand.

Placental insufficiency

During pregnancy the baby receives oxygen and nourishment and gets rid of carbon dioxide and waste products via the placenta and the umbilical blood vessels. A healthy placenta that can perform all these functions effectively is crucial for the baby's continuing health and wellbeing.

Assessment and treatment There's no reliable way of checking that your placenta is functioning properly. But doctors may suspect insufficiency if your uterus is growing too slowly, or if your baby's development is slower than normal.

Ultrasound is the most reliable way to measure your baby's growth. If it shows that your baby is not growing as expected, your doctor may need to do more scans, a non-stress test, and make a bio-physical profile that takes account of your baby's breathing and body movements, the tone and quantity of amniotic fluid. Placental insufficiency may mean that labour has to be induced or even that you have to have a Caesarean.

Incompetent cervix

Fortunately, this condition is rare. When you're pregnant, the cervix normally remains tightly shut and is sealed with a plug of mucus. This means that your baby is safely held in the womb until labour begins, when the cervix begins to dilate.

Occasionally, though, the cervix begins to open before it should, usually in the third or fourth month – termed cervical incompetence. This allows the amniotic sac containing the baby to sag through into the vagina and rupture, with a sudden loss of amniotic fluid followed by miscarriage. Unfortunately, an incompetent cervix is usually diagnosed only after a woman has suffered her first miscarriage. If cervical incompetence is thought to be the cause of previous miscarriage, a soft non-absorbable thread will be inserted around your cervix to tighten it (see right). After bed rest in hospital, you'll be able to go home, but you'll need plenty of rest during the remainder of your pregnancy. The thread will be cut at about 37 weeks of pregnancy and your baby will be delivered vaginally in the normal way.

Reasons for insufficiency

The placenta may be unable to support a baby sufficiently for a number of reasons:

■ the placenta may have developed abnormally

■ blood flow through the placenta may be restricted, or placental tissue lost because of a blood clot

■ the placenta may separate, or partly separate, from the uterine wall

■ the placenta may be too small

■ the pregnancy may go beyond the due date, so that the placenta becomes relatively inadequate for the baby (see p.260)

■ if a mother has diabetes (see also p.140), this can affect the placenta adversely.

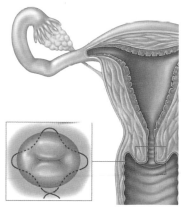

▲ SECURING THE CERVIX The cervix is kept closed by passing a thread right around it – rather like the strings of a purse. The thread is normally cut at about 37 weeks.

Postnatal infection

Postnatal infection, which used to be known as childbed fever, is now very rare indeed. Before antibiotics were available it was one of the main causes of death in new mothers.

Postnatal infection occurs at the site of the placenta, and is sometimes caused by remnants of the placenta remaining in the womb. The first symptoms are a high temperature, acute stomach pains, and bad-smelling lochia (vaginal discharge, see p.354).

If you should develop any of these symptoms, tell your doctor at once. Any remaining placenta will be removed and you'll be given antibiotics to treat the infection.

Pre-eclampsia

This is a potentially serious condition, also called pre-eclamptic toxaemia (PET). It affects as many as one in 10 women, especially first-time mothers and those carrying more than one baby. It's unique to pregnancy and starts in the placenta, so the baby may grow more slowly than normal. We don't know quite why it happens, but it tends to run in families.

Symptoms Pre-eclampsia itself doesn't really have any symptoms, but your midwife or doctor may suspect its presence if you have significantly raised blood pressure and protein in your urine. Both of these symptoms should be picked up at an antenatal check, which is why it's very important to have your blood pressure taken at each antenatal visit. You may also have oedema – swelling of the ankles and wrists – although you can have this without pre-eclampsia. Pre-eclampsia never happens before the 20th week, but your blood pressure may start to rise steadily after this. Delivery of the baby and placenta ends the problem.

Treatment You'll be admitted to hospital or asked to go to a special day unit, so that arrangements for the birth of your baby can be made before you suffer any serious complications. Your blood pressure, kidney and liver function, and blood clotting, will all be monitored closely as they may be affected by the condition. Very rarely, pre-eclampsia can develop into eclampsia. This is one of the most dangerous complications of pregnancy, causing coma and convulsions. It's nearly always preceded by pre-eclampsia, which acts as an early warning signal, and can be prevented by delivery of your baby.

Eclampsia

The word eclampsia derives from the Greek words meaning "like a flash of lightning" – the condition seems to strike from out of the blue with fits and, eventually, coma. Eclampsia is a potentially life-threatening condition for both mother and baby and used to be quite common. Fortunately, it's now extremely rare in the Western world because doctors can diagnose the condition in its earliest phase (pre-eclampsia, see above).

Symptoms Eclampsia is an emergency because the blood vessels in the uterus go into spasm, cutting down the blood flow to the baby so that the level of oxygen in her blood becomes dangerously low.

The mother's brain oxygen is also lowered, causing heightened brain sensitivity, which shows as seizures. Tissues become waterlogged because of fluid retention and haemorrhages can happen in tissues such as the liver. The earliest signs of the condition are drowsiness, headache, and dimness of vision, as well as rising blood pressure, some protein in the urine (see p.177), and oedema (see p.212).

Treatment If eclampsia does develop, doctors try to increase the blood flow to the mother's brain, sedating the brain and reducing high blood pressure. Her baby is delivered, usually by Caesarean section. As soon as the baby is born, the condition begins to subside, although the mother may be at risk of having fits for up to five days after the birth.

Ectopic pregnancy

In an ectopic pregnancy, the fertilized egg implants somewhere other than in the cavity of the womb, usually in a Fallopian tube. The rapidly growing embryo causes the tube to distend, and the invading placenta weakens its walls, causing bleeding. Eventually the tube bursts under the strain.

Before a Fallopian tube bursts, there are usually certain symptoms around the sixth week of pregnancy that signal all is not well. If you should notice any of these, it's important to report them to your doctor immediately. Doctors define two forms of ectopic pregnancy.

Unruptured After a positive pregnancy test, warning signs of an ectopic pregnancy may be pain in the abdomen, usually only on one side, sometimes accompanied by vaginal bleeding, fainting, and pain in the shoulder (on the same side as any pain in the abdomen). Sometimes an ectopic pregnancy is detected by an ultrasound scan after a small amount of bleeding from the vagina early in the pregnancy. Although there's some leakage, there is no rupture as yet, and it may not be detected until eight to ten weeks' gestation.

This kind of ectopic pregnancy can sometimes be treated by injecting a drug into the embryo, causing it to die and then be reabsorbed, which can save the Fallopian tube. Otherwise the part of the tube with the pregnancy in it can be removed by laparoscopy (see pp.45 and 51).

Ruptured This happens when the affected tube bursts, leading to severe pain and shock, with extreme paleness, weak but rapid pulse, and falling blood pressure. A woman suffering this form of ectopic pregnancy will need emergency surgery. The pregnancy will be removed along with that part of the Fallopian tube.

Outlook Almost 60 per cent of women who've had an ectopic pregnancy become pregnant again; 30 per cent avoid further pregnancy voluntarily; the rest are infertile. If you've had a previous ectopic pregnancy, you will need special care during your current pregnancy.

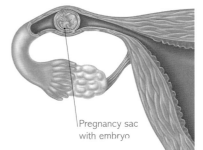

Pregnancy sac
with embryo

▲ **TUBAL IMPLANTATION** About one in every 300 pregnancies is ectopic. In 99 per cent of ectopic pregnancies the blastocyst (see p.32) implants in the Fallopian tube. Very rarely, the blastocyst may implant in the abdominal cavity, the cervix, or on one of a woman's ovaries.

Miriam's casebook

A mother with pre-eclampsia

During Amie's first pregnancy three years ago she had very mild pre-eclampsia in the last trimester. Amie had a normal delivery and a healthy baby, but she's worried pre-eclampsia will come back during her second pregnancy, with more complications. Amie's mother had high blood pressure during pregnancy, a symptom of pre-eclampsia, so Amie knows she has a higher risk of developing the condition.

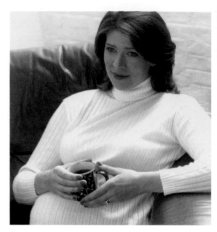

Understanding pre-eclampsia

This condition, which is unique to pregnant women, has the following symptoms: a rise in blood pressure, swollen ankles, feet, and hands, and protein in the urine. Although nothing can be done to prevent pre-eclampsia, good antenatal care can make sure that the condition does not get worse.

Pre-eclampsia is most common in first pregnancies, so I would hope that in a way Amie's been exposed to the highest risk already. Second, her pre-eclampsia was very mild. Her symptoms were slight oedema – swelling of the hands, fingers, feet, and face – and a marginally raised blood pressure that needed no treatment. She didn't have the other important sign of pre-eclampsia, the appearance of protein in the urine. Best of all, the pre-eclampsia came on only four weeks before the birth. Statistics show that the later pre-eclampsia starts in pregnancy, the lower the risk of it happening in a second pregnancy. In the end, Amie had a normal vaginal delivery and her baby was healthy.

What causes pre-eclampsia?

Pre-eclampsia is an illness that happens only in pregnancy, potentially affecting mother and baby, and is most common towards the end of pregnancy. We don't really know what

causes pre-eclampsia, although it seems to run in families – the daughters of women who have had pre-eclampsia are slightly more likely to get it themselves. Pre-eclampsia isn't caused or prevented by what you eat; by how you feel about your pregnancy; by whether or not you exercise; by how hard you work; or by how much rest you take.

Amie ate healthily and had heard that a high-protein diet might protect her against pre-eclampsia, but I had to tell her that there's nothing to support this theory. Some people say that calcium and fish oil supplements may help, but the evidence isn't strong enough for me to recommend that she add any supplements to her diet.

How the placenta is affected

What's known for certain is that pre-eclampsia starts in the placenta. Towards the end of pregnancy the placenta gets as large as a dinner plate, about 5cm (2in) thick, and needs a large and efficient blood supply from the mother to keep her baby growing healthily. In pre-eclampsia the placenta seems to run short of an adequate blood supply, and this has potentially serious consequences for mother and baby.

Key symptoms of pre-eclampsia are a rise in blood pressure and swelling of the fingers, hands, feet, and face.

An antenatal urine test may also show that protein has leaked into the urine from kidneys that can't function as effectively as before and the blood-clotting mechanism may also be affected. It's likely that if pre-eclampsia did come back in her second pregnancy it would be milder than before. Nonetheless I advised Amie to take a close interest in the results of her antenatal tests.

I told Amie to make sure she has excellent antenatal care throughout her pregnancy. Because she's had the condition before, she may be asked to come for more frequent antenatal visits than usual, especially if any signs of pre-eclampsia are detected.

Understanding tests and treatment

While there are no screening tests that can predict Amie's risk of developing pre-eclampsia, there are some baseline tests that she could have done in the first half of her pregnancy. These can be repeated at regular intervals to give early warning of the onset of pre-eclampsia. So apart from the normal checks on blood pressure, urine, and her weight, she may be offered tests for kidney and liver function; ultrasound scans to track her baby's growth; and Doppler scans to measure the efficiency of blood flow to the placenta.

I reassured Amie that at the first sign of pre-eclampsia, in even its mildest form, she would be taken into hospital so that both she and her baby could be monitored. If necessary, her baby could be delivered before complications set in. Pre-eclampsia is progressive and doesn't get better, so once admitted Amie shouldn't expect to be allowed home until after her baby's been born.

Doctors may prescribe drugs to bring down a mother's blood pressure if it's found to be too high. Although these drugs don't affect the underlying disease, they can reduce the risk of some of the complications that are linked with it.

It's also possible that Amie may be given small daily doses of aspirin during her pregnancy, which could prevent or delay the onset of pre-eclampsia. The dose of aspirin works directly on the clotting blood cells, known as platelets, which are involved in pre-eclampsia.

Miriam's top tips

Naturally, Amie wants to be as well prepared as possible should there be any signs of pre-eclampsia during this pregnancy. My advice is to:

■ keep an extra-careful watch for symptoms such as swollen ankles, hands, fingers, or face. Regular urine tests will alert carers to any traces of protein

■ be vigilant about keeping antenatal appointments to ensure close monitoring throughout pregnancy.

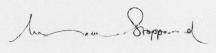

Ensuring a safe delivery

If pre-eclampsia is getting worse, if the baby shows signs of distress, or if the mother's condition is deteriorating, there's only one treatment: urgent delivery of the baby – sometimes by Caesarean section if the situation demands. Last time Amie had a normal delivery and the chances are she'll have the same this time. I reassured Amie that even if she did have a Caesarean, this wouldn't affect any subsequent deliveries. Women who've had one Caesarean section can try for a normal delivery next time. I suggested to Amie that if she did need a Caesarean, she could have regional rather than general anaesthesia, so she and her partner, Ed, could still take an active part in the birth of their child.

Seeking expert advice

All obstetricians are able to care for women at risk from or with pre-eclampsia. Research shows that the most important factor in a happy outcome to a pre-eclampsia birth is the involvement of doctors and midwives who are familiar with the condition and who can take action at once if there are any warning signs.

I advised Amie to get in touch with Action on Pre-Eclampsia (APEC), 84–88 Pinner Road, Harrow, HA1 4HZ.

A sensual pregnancy

The very high levels of female hormones in your body when you're pregnant mean that you may find you enjoy all aspects of sex, from massage to lovemaking, far more than ever before. You may also experience some sexual problems, but most can be resolved easily as long as you and your partner are open with one another.

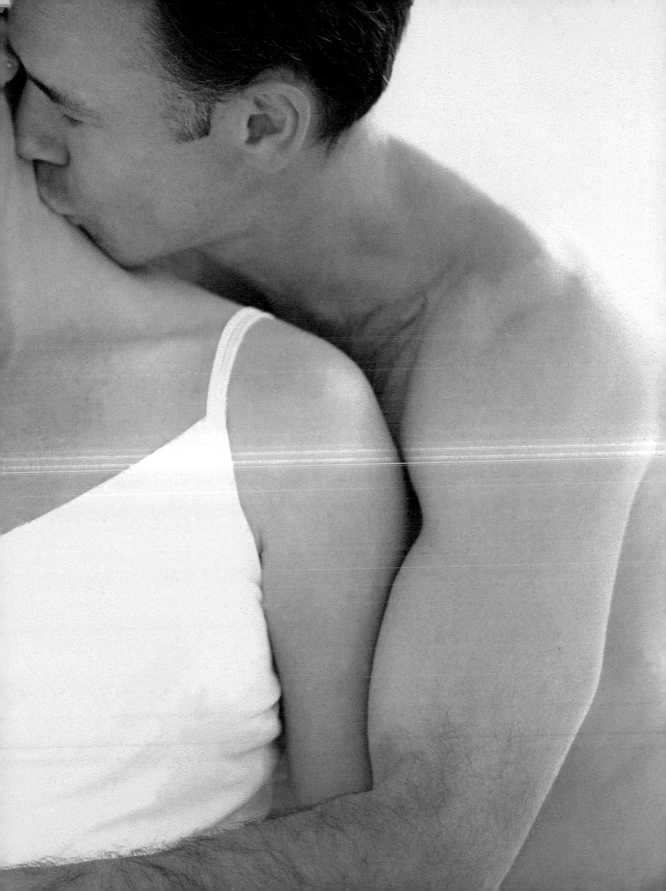

Your hormones

You may go through all kinds of physical, emotional, and psychological changes during your pregnancy, which can affect how you feel about sex. These changes are mostly due to the vastly increased levels of hormones circulating in your body.

The most important hormones involved in maintaining your pregnancy are progesterone and oestrogen. In the early days of a pregnancy these are produced by the corpus luteum in the ovary. Once the embryo has implanted in the uterine lining, it and the developing placenta take over as the primary sources of progesterone and oestrogen.

The increase in the amounts of progesterone and oestrogen circulating in the body is swift and dramatic. The level of progesterone rises to ten times the amount before conception and you produce as much oestrogen in one day as a non-pregnant woman in three years. In fact, during the course of a single pregnancy, a woman produces as much oestrogen as a non-pregnant woman could over 150 years.

Progesterone and oestrogen bring a sense of wellbeing, giving you shining hair, supple and glowing skin, and an aura of tranquillity and contentment.

Your relationship

It's perfectly safe to enjoy lovemaking during your pregnancy, unless there are medical reasons why you should abstain for a while. Every pregnant woman has the potential to enjoy sex – and some enjoy it more than they've ever done before.

How much you want and enjoy sex can vary during pregnancy, not only from one woman to another, but also in the same woman at different times throughout the 40 weeks. Most women feel less interested in lovemaking during the first trimester (especially if suffering from tiredness and nausea). Desire generally increases in the second trimester and declines again in the third.

When you do have sex, you may find it far more exciting and satisfying than it was before you conceived. In fact, some women have their first orgasm or multiple orgasms while pregnant.

This enhanced sexuality is mainly due to the very high levels of female hormones and pregnancy hormones circulating throughout the body during pregnancy (see column, left). These cause changes to your breasts and sexual organs, making them more sensitive and responsive than usual. Also, being pregnant is such an affirmation of being female that you may find yourself feeling much more feminine and sensual.

Sexual excitement during pregnancy

One effect of the high oestrogen levels during pregnancy is an increase in blood flow, especially in the pelvic area. Because of this, the vagina and its folds, the labia, become slightly stretched and swollen. This stretching and swelling, which normally happen only when you're sexually excited, make the sensory nerve endings hypersensitive, and you become aroused much more rapidly than usual.

One of the first things that happens when you get pregnant is your breasts start to get bigger – one of the classic signs of pregnancy is sensitive, enlarged breasts and tingling, even painful, nipples. The increased sensitivity of the breasts makes them a focus of sensory arousal, and you may feel the most exquisite pleasure when your partner kisses and caresses your nipples and breasts. This sexual foreplay can also arouse the clitoris and the vagina, which will swell very readily.

The increased blood flow makes your vaginal secretions quite profuse, so you'll find you're ready for penetration earlier than usual. Penetration is particularly easy because of the plentiful vaginal fluid, and you may climax quite quickly if your clitoris is stimulated at the same time. You may find the intensity of your orgasms reaches new heights and the time taken to "come down" from an orgasm is much longer. The labia minora and the lower end of the vagina can remain swollen for anything up to two hours after orgasm, particularly in the last trimester.

As well as stimulating the whole of the genital tract, the pregnancy hormones stimulate the production of a hormone within the brain called melanocyte-stimulating hormone (or MSH). This causes areas where the skin pigmentation is deeper anyway to get darker – as in the darkening of the nipple area. Darkening of the nipples can act as a sexual signal to a man, making his partner's breasts very attractive to him.

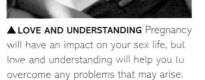

▲ **LOVE AND UNDERSTANDING** Pregnancy will have an impact on your sex life, but love and understanding will help you to overcome any problems that may arise.

When to make love

You can make love whenever you want to, provided that you don't try to get too athletic and that there are no medical reasons for you to avoid sex (see p.236). Good sex in pregnancy is not only very enjoyable, but also helps to prepare you for childbirth by keeping your pelvic muscles strong and supple. It helps strengthen your bonds with your partner, too, which will help you cope much better with the stresses of parenthood.

There's no physical reason why a woman having a normal pregnancy shouldn't continue enjoying making love with her partner. If both partners are happy, sex can continue right up to when you begin labour. In a low-risk pregnancy, the uterine spasms that you have with orgasms are perfectly safe, and in late pregnancy they help prepare the uterus for the rigours of labour.

It's not true that sex can cause an infection during pregnancy and may harm the baby. Infection is virtually impossible because the cervix is plugged with a tough mucus that prevents bacteria getting into the uterus. Also, the baby is completely enclosed inside the amniotic sac, which resists rupture even when under great pressure and cushions him against all external forces (including the weight of a partner during intercourse). That said, extremely athletic sex is not a good idea, because it may cause soreness and abrasions and a pregnant woman should be free of these unnecessary discomforts.

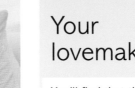

Your lovemaking

You'll find that the missionary position becomes awkward and uncomfortable as your pregnancy goes on, but there are other sexual positions you can use to enhance your enjoyment – without in any way diminishing that of your partner.

Side-by-side positions are often pleasurable, as is vaginal sex from behind, because in these positions your abdomen is not under any pressure from the weight of your partner. Sitting positions can be very enjoyable in the later months of pregnancy, allowing you to adjust your position but still see your partner's face and feel very close to him.

If you are feeling sexy, but you don't really want intercourse, you and your partner could explore other forms of sensual and sexual pleasuring, such as erotically stroking and kissing each other, massage (see p.232), mutual masturbation, and oral sex.

As your pregnancy advances you may find you have to change your sexual habits. Try to understand any changes in your own and your partner's sexual desires. Be open and ready to talk to each other about your needs, but don't let your sex life become the dominant feature of your overall relationship. Concentrate on loving rather than lovemaking, and rediscover the intimacy and joy of simply being with the one you love.

Good for you

Use sensual massage as a source of pleasure in itself, or as part of your foreplay.

Sensual massage is a lovely way of keeping up a close physical relationship with your partner during your pregnancy, especially if intercourse isn't possible for medical reasons, or if you find it uncomfortable or undesirable. If you make the massage as sexy as possible, and masturbate each other while you do it, both of you will probably be able to reach orgasm without penetration. If you're still having intercourse, use sensual massage as a loving, prolonged, and highly effective method of foreplay.

Sensual massage

A loving massage can be relaxing and highly erotic for you and your partner, and reinforces the feelings of love and tenderness you have for each other, particularly if making love is difficult for some reason. Begin with loving hugs, cuddles, and stroking, then take it in turns to massage each other all over, from head to toe. Use slow, sensuous hand movements and plenty of massage oil.

A shared pleasure

Massage is a way of discovering what gives you sensual pleasure, so let yourself be open to the experience and see what happens. You may both be pleasantly surprised at how sexy it feels to have certain parts of your bodies that you'd never thought of as erotic caressed by your partner.

Preparing for massage Choose a time when you're not likely to be disturbed (switch on the answering machine and put your mobile on to voicemail). Spend a little time getting your bedroom ready, making sure it's warm and comfortable. If your bed is too soft for giving a massage,

Back and leg massage

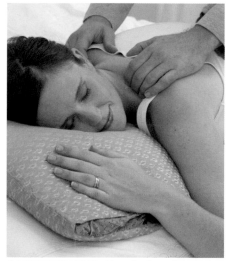

▲ **BACK MASSAGE** Working slowly and sensuously, gently massage her back. Start with her neck and shoulders and work down to her lower back.

▶ **LEG STROKES** Put both hands on her ankles, fingers pointing in opposite directions. Slide your hands up to her thighs and back down again, going gently over the backs of her knees.

▶ **LEG MASSAGE** Hold her legs with both hands, thumbs uppermost. Pressing firmly, slide your hands up to the back of the knee. Work down again without pressure.

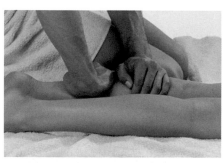

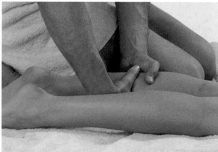

put a mattress, duvet, or a pile of folded blankets on the floor and cover them with a large, clean towel or sheet. Dim the lighting, light some scented candles if you like them, and play some gentle music to create a soothing, relaxing atmosphere.

Lubricating the skin It's best to use a proper massage oil or lotion – you'll find that hand cream or ordinary body lotion is absorbed into the skin too quickly, and baby oil leaves an oily film on the skin. Warm the oil before you use it (the simplest way is to put the bottle in a bowl of warm water) and check that your hands are warm and your fingernails are short and smooth. When you're giving the massage, pour some oil into your hands and smooth it on to your partner's skin. Never just pour the massage oil directly on to your partner; it doesn't feel good as well as being wasteful and messy.

Touching intimately Lightly coat your fingertips with massage oil and delicately trace the outlines of each other's lips, cheeks, jaws, ears, and neck. Then, using plenty of oil, work your fingers and the palm of your hands sensuously over breasts, chest, sides, and abdomen, and across the shoulders and down the arms. Stroke firmly up the inside of each thigh in turn, using the lightest of finger pressure on the return stroke. Always handle her breasts carefully as they will be tender.

Good for your baby

Your baby may also respond with pleasure as your body is stroked and caressed, and she'll share some of the benefits you gain from massage.

■ From about the fifth month onward, your baby may feel stroking movements through your abdomen, which she'll find very comforting and soothing.

■ Learning to massage your own and your partner's body during pregnancy will help you to soothe your baby through touch after her birth.

■ Continue to massage your baby after she's born: babies find massage soothing too.

SENSUAL MASSAGE

233

Foot massage

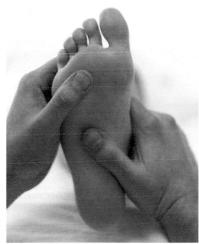

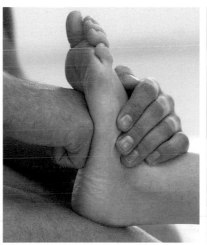

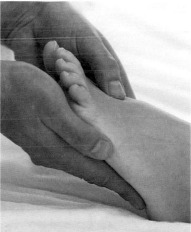

1 CIRCLE WITH YOUR THUMBS Using both your thumbs, gently circle over the whole area of the sole. Apply as much pressure as feels comfortable for your partner.

2 PRESS WITH YOUR FIST Holding the foot with your left hand, press your right fist into the sole of the foot. Using small movements, gently circle over the whole area.

3 DOWN THE GROOVES Support the foot with one hand. Using the thumb of your other hand, press down the grooves between the tendons at the top of the foot. Work from ankle to toes.

Partner's dos and don'ts

If you're happy to make just a few changes to your lovemaking, you can improve the experience for your partner.

Do:

■ be tender, romantic, patient, and understanding

■ use different kinds of stroking, such as using a firm hand over her abdomen if the baby kicks

■ keep your weight off her stomach and breasts when you make love

■ use lots of pillows for greater comfort and to get the right angles around the curves of her body

■ take your time when you're making love, and don't be afraid to experiment.

Don't:

■ force her to make love if she doesn't feel like it

■ expect her to have simultaneous orgasms – or even one orgasm.

Making love

Keep on making love as late into pregnancy as you wish, as long as there are no medical reasons for abstaining (see p.236). Your baby is safe in your uterus. He's not harmed by normal sexual activity (see column, left), and probably enjoys sex as much as you do as your hormones reach him via the placenta (see p.192).

Lovemaking positions

In the early months, use any lovemaking position you like, but as your abdomen gets bigger you may find some positions uncomfortable. After about 24 weeks it's best to avoid lying on your back for any length of time so don't use the missionary position, with your partner on top – there are lots of other exciting options.

Woman on top You may find these the most comfortable positions from the second trimester onwards. As your abdomen grows, you can lift yourself further off his stomach by supporting yourself on your bent legs. This also prevents too much pressure on your abdomen and breasts. In these positions, too, it's easier for you to control the depth of penetration and the speed and rhythm of lovemaking.

These positions allow a great deal of intimacy. You and your partner have your hands free to caress and stroke each other and he can easily reach your breasts with his mouth.

Kneeling and side by side Kneeling positions allow your partner freedom of movement and let him vary the amount of penetration. Side-by-side positions are comfortable and permit plenty of kissing and caressing. The "spoons" position, so called because the partners nestle together like a pair of spoons, is also good to try if you feel any soreness when you start making love again after you've given birth, especially if you've had an episiotomy.

Sitting These positions are good in the middle and late months. They don't allow much movement, but are comfortable for you both and ease pressure on the abdomen. Also, the depth of penetration can be controlled. Your partner sits on a chair or the edge of the bed and you sit on his lap, either facing him, facing to one side, or facing away. Your partner can use his hands to caress your body and stimulate your clitoris. His range of movement is limited, so you control the sexual tempo.

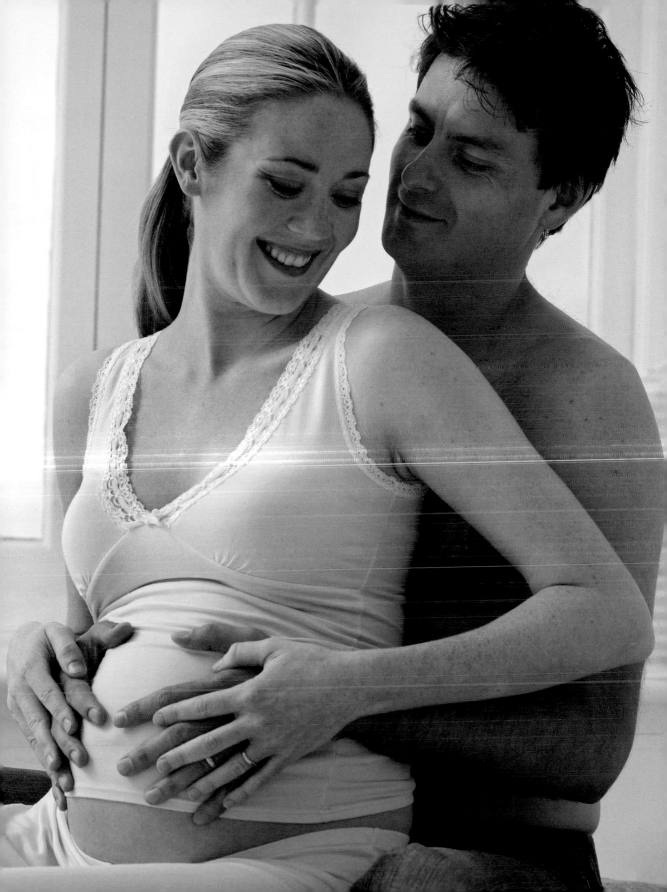

When sex may be dangerous

If yours is a high-risk pregnancy, you may need to avoid sex at certain times or even completely.

Your doctor will warn you if there's any risk of sexual activity being a danger to your pregnancy, and advise you on what (and when) is safe. Make sure that your doctor explains the problem fully so you're completely clear about what you can and cannot safely do.

The most common reasons and times for restricting intercourse during pregnancy are:

■ whenever there's any sign of bleeding. The bleeding may well be quite harmless, but you should check with your doctor immediately

■ if placenta praevia is suspected or confirmed (see p.222)

■ in the last trimester if you have a multiple pregnancy

■ in the last 12 weeks if you have a history of premature labour or if you're showing signs that you might go into premature labour

■ if your waters have broken.

Sexual problems

When you're pregnant, there are many physical and emotional factors that can lessen your enjoyment of lovemaking. Fortunately there are very few that actually prevent you from having sex, and these are relatively rare.

For many women, the most common reason for taking less pleasure in sex is the feeling that your body is becoming less and less attractive to your partner as your pregnancy goes on. Some women become shy and defensive about their appearance, believing that their femininity has gone, and start to feel embarrassed about being seen naked. In fact, the opposite is probably true and most men find their pregnant partners very attractive. Talk to your partner about your fears – he'll probably be astonished that you feel unsure about your appearance.

Loss of libido

While you may find your sex drive increases during pregnancy, it must be said that some women don't feel like making love very often during the first trimester. Morning sickness, which can make you feel thoroughly wretched and unattractive in every way, is one reason for this. Tiredness is another enemy of the libido, and because pregnancy can be exhausting, you may sometimes feel you just don't have enough energy to enjoy sex with your partner. Both morning sickness and tiredness are common problems in the first trimester, although they usually lessen, or disappear, during the second trimester.

Once free of the discomforts of morning sickness and exhaustion, most women find that their interest and pleasure in sex increase in the second trimester. Towards the last weeks of pregnancy, though, libido may wane again as tiredness increases. Sadly, many women feel like beached whales at this time and don't enjoy their rounded beauty. Some may feel shy about stripping bare and making love.

Hormone levels can swing quite violently during pregnancy and you'll probably find yourself emotionally volatile, switching from feeling very contented to sadness and tearfulness, and then to great elation. This is perfectly normal but, of course, it can be difficult for your partner to understand and can disrupt your sexual relationship.

If you do have problems, try to be open with your partner and be honest about your feelings. If you don't want to make love because you feel physically ill or excessively tired, tell your partner the truth. That way he won't feel rejected.

Discomfort

The hormone-controlled changes in your breasts and genitals make them more sensitive and responsive to touch. This increased sensitivity can heighten your sexuality, but can also sometimes cause discomfort. This is especially true of the breasts in early pregnancy, and you may find that they're very tender for the first couple of months. Explain this to your partner and ask him to avoid touching them during love play.

The engorgement of your genitals may also cause some slight discomfort, particularly later in pregnancy, as they remain swollen and aching after orgasm. This can create a feeling of unrelieved fullness, which may make sex less satisfying. Some women find they can overcome this lack of satisfaction by masturbation, especially if they usually tend to have better orgasms through masturbation (by themselves or by their partners) than they do via intercourse.

A common source of discomfort comes when the baby gets bigger and it's difficult for you to make love in the missionary position. Instead, try other lovemaking positions (see p.234).

When to stop

Stop having sex if you're bleeding at any time, and check with your doctor as soon as possible to find out why this might be happening. The bleeding is probably not serious, and may simply be because of changes in the cervix that make it soft and easily damaged by deep penetration, but you'll need medical advice. If the bleeding is caused by the sensitivity of the cervix, it's best to avoid deep penetration when you make love.

It's not a good idea to have sex if the mucus plug that seals the cervix has become dislodged (a show, see p.271). And you should also abstain after your waters have broken. Both are signs that labour is about to begin, although you can have a show seven to ten days before contractions start. Both usually happen near term, although they can be earlier and could be a sign that you're going into premature labour (see p.298).

Anxieties

In any relationship, it's difficult to enjoy relaxed, happy lovemaking if either or both of you are feeling anxious, tense, or nervous. During pregnancy there are lots of things to feel anxious about, including fears about the safety of having sex, and the difficulty some couples or individuals have in adjusting to the idea of imminent parenthood.

Worries about the safety of sex during pregnancy are usually unfounded. As for anxieties about your relationship, the best thing to do is talk frankly and fully with your partner about how you feel. If you can't resolve your problems, seek professional advice and counselling.

Sex without intercourse

When you don't want, or can't have, intercourse, there are other ways of enjoying sexual pleasure.

Extended foreplay Sensual massage and passionate kissing and caressing can stop short of or lead to orgasm, as you want.

Mutual masturbation You and your partner can give each other sexual pleasure, and bring each other to orgasm, without having intercourse. To make the experience more sensual and also to avoid harming the delicate skin of your genitals, have your partner smear his hands and fingers with a suitable lubricant such as saliva.

Oral sex Fellatio and cunnilingus, as well as or instead of mutual masturbation, are perfectly safe when you're pregnant. The vaginal secretions generally have a much stronger odour during pregnancy than at other times, though, and some men find this off-putting.

Getting ready for your baby

From the 36th week, nesting begins
in earnest. You'll find there's plenty to do –
getting your baby's room ready, choosing
equipment and baby clothes, and finalizing
your choice of names. You'll also want to
make preparations for the birth and to
decide what kind of child care you'll need
if you're going back to work.

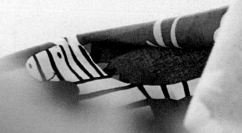

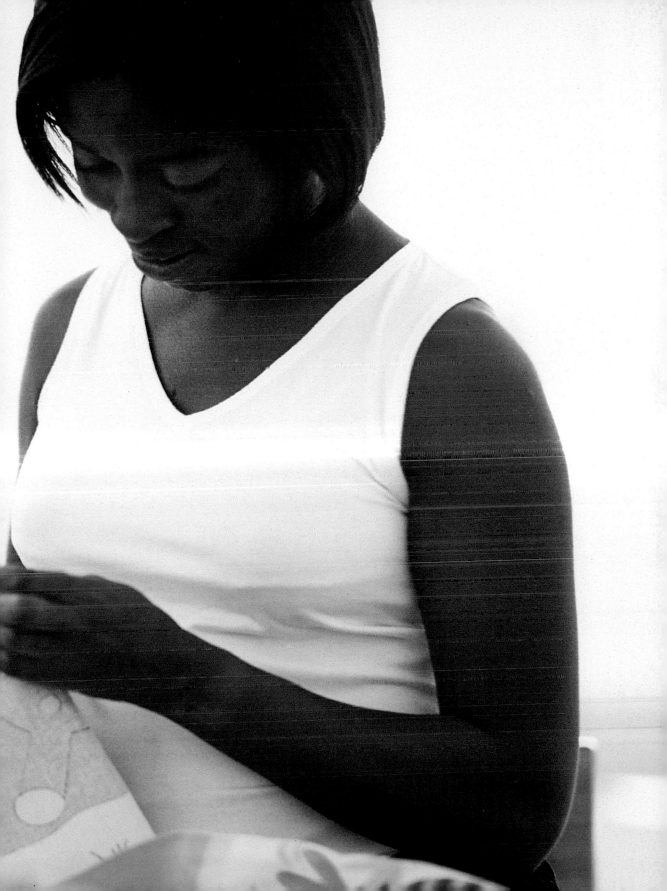

Pointers for parents

When arranging your baby's room, remember to think of your own needs – make sure you can reach equipment easily and safely.

■ Put up shelves so that you're able to see everything at a glance and find things quickly.

■ Keep creams and wipes on shelves close to the changing mat but out of your baby's reach.

■ Check there aren't any things in the way between the changing table, bath, your chair, and her cot.

■ Make sure there are no cords running across the floor. Set any lamps close to the wall socket.

■ Put a comfortable, low chair in your baby's room for night feeds – make sure it's easy to get out of and gives you good back support.

Preparing for your baby

Getting everything ready for your new baby can be great fun and you'll feel very excited once her room is prepared and you have a stock of tiny baby clothes. So you don't get overtired, start doing things a little at a time. Get your partner involved too – the preparations will help you both to bond with your unborn child.

Your baby's room

It's a good idea to prepare the room before the birth – once you have your baby, most of your time and energy will be taken up by her care. Make safety and comfort for both of you your main priorities.

Sleeping

You'll probably want to have your baby sleeping close to you in your own room for the first few weeks of her life. But it's a good idea also to have somewhere that's a special space for your baby – this may be either a whole room, or an area in another child's room. Make sure you have enough space for sleeping, feeding, bathing, nappy changing, and dressing. A baby's room doesn't have to be expensively decorated and if you keep it simple there'll be fewer changes to make as she grows up. You can usually find most of the essentials secondhand, or you can sometimes adapt existing furniture to your needs (see below). Whether your baby has her own room or shares yours at first, she needs to be kept warm. Try to keep a constant temperature of around 16–20°C (60–70°F) and if possible, install a thermostatically controlled heater.

Furniture and storage

A chest of drawers with a sturdy frame and legs is ideal both for storing your baby's clothes and to use as a table for changing nappies. It should be high enough (about hip-height) to allow you or your partner to use without bending too much. Make sure the surface can be cleaned easily and, if it's wooden, check that there are no cracks or splinters. Choose a chest with at least three spacious drawers. Keep nappy-changing equipment in the top drawer so it's close to hand or on wall shelf units nearby – these can be used later for books and toys. Put a plastic-covered changing mat with raised sides on top of the chest and have a small pedal-bin, lined with a plastic bag, nearby for dirty nappies. Keep a straight-backed chair in the room so that you or your partner can feed your baby in comfort. If possible, place a small, sturdy table nearby so you have somewhere to put drinks, bottles, and so on.

Lighting

You're bound to want to check your baby while she's sleeping at night so it helps to have lighting that you can put on without disturbing her sleep. Fit a dimmer switch to the overhead lighting system and adjust it so you can put on the light without waking your baby. You could also use a night light or shaded lamp, but be very careful to avoid any trailing wires.

Floors and walls

The floor in your baby's room needs to be non-slippery, warm, and easy to clean. Don't use small rugs or mats as you may trip or slip on them. Linoleum and vinyl floor coverings are hardwearing and easily washed, and wood or cork tiles are warm and practical. Paint the walls with a non-toxic, washable emulsion paint, or use wallpaper that can be wiped clean.

Windows and curtains

Keep your baby's room well aired, but make sure the windows are draughtproof, and above your baby's reach. Put up well-lined curtains, or blinds plus curtains, to block out light when your baby is sleeping during the day. Always choose non-flammable materials.

Safety precautions

- Fit a safety lock on each window in your baby's room, as well as bars if the window is close to the floor.

- Use flameproof fabric for bedding, upholstery, and curtains.

- Place childproof covers over all power point sockets.

- Screen electric bar and gas fires with a fire guard secured to the wall.

- Coat walls and furniture in non-toxic, lead-free paint or varnish.

- Put childproof safety catches on all cupboards and drawers, especially in the kitchen. You can also get locks for the fridge, freezer, and oven.

- Install smoke alarms and check them regularly.

- Check that all electrical flexes are well out of your baby's reach.

- Use non-slip mats in the bath and on the bathroom floor.

What's good for baby

A brightly coloured environment with lots of sounds is very stimulating for a young baby.

A musical mobile placed low over her cot will give your baby lots of pleasure. Hang plastic-coated photographs or a specially designed baby mirror in the cot – she'll love to look at faces close up. Give her rattles and toys that make a noise when thrown, batted, or shaken. Moulded soft toys are good for sucking. Check that soft toys are safe, and that items such as eyes and noses are firmly attached and cannot come off.

▼ **COT MOBILE** A mobile over her cot gives your baby something interesting to watch when she wakes up and keeps her entertained.

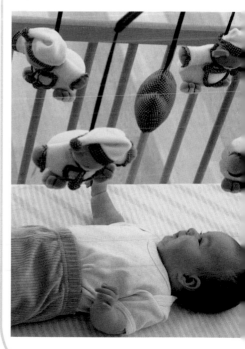

Meeting your needs

You don't need much equipment at first – just something in which to transport your baby, somewhere for him to sleep, and something to bathe him in.

Make sure that your pushchair or buggy has handles that are at a comfortable height so you don't strain your back. Good brakes are essential: you must be able to apply them without letting go of the handle.

Your baby will quickly outgrow a baby basket, so it may be cheaper to start with a cot, some convert into beds. Make sure the height can be adjusted so you don't have to bend low to lift your baby.

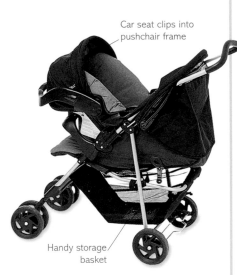

Car seat clips into pushchair frame

Handy storage basket

▲ **ADAPTABLE TRANSPORT** The latest models can be used from birth to around three years and combine pushchair with a removable car seat.

Choosing equipment

Babies grow quickly and some items of equipment may be more expensive than they're worth for the short time they're in use. Try to choose equipment that has a long life – a cot that becomes a bed for a toddler, for example. Baby equipment is rarely worn out, simply outgrown, and there's no need to buy everything new – ask friends and family or check for secondhand items on the Internet.

Travel

You'll need something to carry your baby around in as soon as he arrives. Before you buy anything, think very carefully about how much space you have for storage, and the kind of lifestyle you lead. A simple baby sling is perfect for the first few months.

Pushchairs The newest models can be used from birth until your child is about three. Most have a seat that reclines in several different positions so a young baby can lie flat or an older baby or toddler can sit up and watch the world go by. Some also include a car seat, shopping basket, canopy, and so on.

Car seats By law, your baby must be safely restrained in a car, so make sure you have an appropriate safety seat before taking him home from the hospital and check that it's securely anchored. The seat must meet UK safety regulations. Never buy a car seat secondhand because it might be damaged.

Portable baby chair Your baby will enjoy sitting in one of these so he can see what's happening around him and a bouncing chair will be fun when

▶ **BABY SLING** Your baby will enjoy the warmth of your body and the sound of your heartbeat when carried next to your chest.

he kicks his feet. These are easy to carry around, but check that the base is wide and sturdy so that he can't tip himself over. Always strap him in securely, and never put it on a raised surface like a table.

Sleeping and bathing

At first your baby will fit snugly into a baby basket, carry cot, or even a drawer! The important thing is that his bed is the right size and is comfortable. Choose a thin, close-fitting, waterproof mattress and cotton sheets. He must not have a pillow. It's important to keep your baby's room draught-free and at an even temperature. Warm, light cotton cellular blankets are probably best for bedding. Remember that if your sleeping baby seems to be chilly, don't just add an extra covering as this will trap cold air inside, making him colder. Pick him up and cuddle him until he's warm, then add an extra blanket to his bedding.

His cot If your newborn starts off in a baby basket, he'll need a cot as soon as he's too big for it. You can buy a new or secondhand cot. Get a large cot, it may seem enormous at first, but it will last him longer. Make sure it's sturdy and has non-toxic paint or varnish. The bars should be no further than 6cm (2½in) apart so your baby can't push his head through. The sides of the cot should be high enough to stop him from climbing over, and have safety catches at each end of the drop side to stop it being released by accident. Choose a close-fitting, waterproof mattress, with no gaps between the edges of the mattress and the cot frame. Don't use cot bumpers as the baby can get too hot, and an adventurous baby may even use it as a step to help him climb out of his cot.

Changing and bathing

All you really need is a plastic changing mat that can be used on the floor, a sturdy table, or a chest of drawers. But if you do want a special changing unit, choose one with plenty of storage.

You can bathe your baby in a sink, but if you want a baby bath on a stand, check that the stand is stable and at the right height.

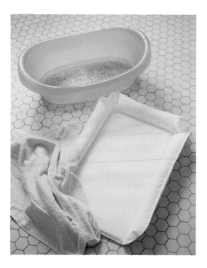

▶ **BATHTIME** Choose sturdy (but lightweight), practical equipment for bathtime.

Meeting your baby's needs

Safety is the most important thing when choosing equipment for your baby, as any number of items can take care of his basic needs.

■ Choose blankets and quilts without any fringes or loose ends that your baby could choke on.

■ Use closely woven blankets that don't trap fingers and toes.

■ If you use a baby sling, choose one with a neck support and wide straps that will support your baby's weight as he grows.

■ Check that cots, prams, and pushchairs don't have any sharp edges or sharp screws.

■ When choosing a pushchair make sure there's adequate protection for your baby's head.

■ Check there's nothing on the pushchair that will trap his little fingers or toes.

■ Choose covers with bright colours and patterns to stimulate your baby.

Don't wait until the last minute to buy your baby's clothes; shop while you still feel comfortable enough to enjoy it.

■ Don't try to get everything all in one go, and ask your partner or a friend to help you carry any heavy shopping bags.

■ Your baby doesn't care what colour and style her clothes are, so choose garments that are easily machine washed in colours that won't run.

■ Don't buy too many clothes for the first months in advance as you don't know how fast your baby's going to grow or what the weather will be like. But don't skimp on the number of essential items. You always need more than you think.

■ Choose medium-priced items from reliable stores. Cheap baby clothes often fall apart at the seams, the fabric becomes rough and irritating, and they may have to be thrown out after only a few washes.

Your baby's clothes

Most of us over-prepare for a new baby, especially if it's our first. Don't forget babies grow extremely fast, and tiny garments will soon be outgrown. On the whole, it's better to buy bigger, rather than smaller, as clothes that are too close-fitting may make your baby hot and rub her skin. The golden rule is to keep all clothing simple and comfortable, causing fewer problems for both of you.

Choosing clothes and accessories

Baby clothes are getting better all the time in terms of fabric, design, and washability, so get a feel for what's available before you make a final choice. You'll see lots of things you don't need and would never use, so don't waste your money on unnecessary items. Ask a friend with a baby what she found useful – perhaps she can pass on some clothes to you.

You'll need several changes of sheets, stretchsuits, vests, and shawls so that you can have a few in the wash without running out. Choose patterned sheets and clothing, rather than solid pastels so that every little stain doesn't show. Natural fibres are best as they allow sweat to evaporate. Choose vests with wide necks, as babies hate having tight things pulled over their heads. Don't buy any clothing with buttons or zippers that are close to the neck. Also, think about what's convenient for you. Even if you prefer terry nappies, keep a supply of disposable nappies on hand for times when you need to make a quick change.

Essential baby items

■ 1 hat – the type will depend on the season
■ 6 cotton vests with wide or envelope neck
■ 2 plain cardigans, jackets, or loose jumpers
■ 2 pairs cotton socks or slip-on fabric bootees
■ 2 shawls
■ 6 stretch suits
■ gloves or scratch mittens
■ 2 soft new towels

■ 1 packet cotton wool
■ baby lotion
■ blunt-edged scissors
■ nappy rash cream
■ 1 box newborn-size disposable nappies or 2 dozen reusable nappies and liners (or packs of disposable liners)
If using reusables you'll also need:
■ 2 nappy buckets
■ 6 pairs plastic pants and 12 safe nappy pins or plastic snap fasteners

Choosing clothes for your baby Buying clothes for your new baby can seem like a daunting task as there is so much to choose from. The most important thing is to be practical in your choice so bear in mind the points below when you shop.

▼**STRETCHSUITS** These are ideal for keeping baby warm all over. Fastenings in the crotch and inside leg will make nappy changing easy.

▼**NIGHTWEAR** Babies move in their sleep. Choose nightwear that allows your baby to move freely and does not entangle her limbs.

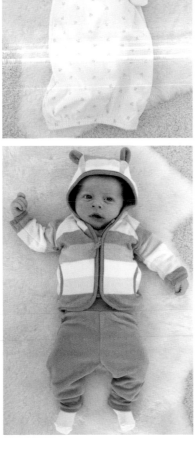

Your baby's needs

Comfort and safety, rather than style, are the main priorities when choosing your baby's clothing.

■ Look for soft, machine-washable fabrics. Cotton is ideal. Synthetic fabrics don't always absorb sweat, and wool can irritate the skin of some newborn babies.

■ In warm weather two layers are usually ample. In winter add more layers, but do not wrap her up too much with tight clothes.

■ A baby's gestures are jerky and expansive, so make sure garments are loose, and easily stretched.

◀**OUTDOOR WEAR** When choosing clothing for outdoors, warmth is the most important thing. Don't be distracted by colour or fashion. Your baby's head and feet are vulnerable to the cold, so make sure they're covered.

◀**VESTS (FAR LEFT)** Envelope neck vests are ideal as they slip over your baby's head easily. They should be made of soft cotton or thermal material.

Mother's experience

Unless there are good reasons not to, it's best to breastfeed your baby if you possibly can.

Breastfeeding Your baby is getting the ideal food; breastmilk is always available and doesn't require any special equipment or preparation. Many women really enjoy breastfeeding, and it's also better for your body: for instance, it helps your uterus to return quickly to its normal size.

There are a few drawbacks, which can be easily overcome. The quantity and quality of your milk depend on your overall health, so eat well and look after yourself. Feeding can lead to sore nipples or breast infections (see p.356), which need prompt treatment. It can also be tiring so make sure you get lots of rest.

Bottlefeeding Infant formulas are very nourishing, but they are still only second-best to breastmilk. Bottlefeeding costs more and you need to purchase equipment.

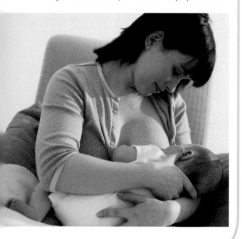

Breast or bottle?

Breastfeeding is better for your baby than bottlefeeding. But if for some reason you can't breastfeed your baby, don't worry – modern milk formulas are good and he will be adequately nourished.

The best possible preparation for breastfeeding your baby is to make sure you and your partner are aware of all the benefits it has (see below). Check that you know what's involved, and that you're physically and mentally ready for it. Physical preparations are simple and straightforward: all you need to do is keep yourself well nourished, avoid hazards that could affect your milk supply, and make sure you look after your breasts properly. Your midwife, doctor, obstetrician, childbirth teacher, or health visitor should be able to answer any questions you have.

Breastfeeding

Breastmilk is the perfect food for a baby. It contains all the essential nutrients (fat, protein, carbohydrate, vitamins, and iron) he needs; it's never too rich or too watery; it's clean, readily available, and always at the right temperature. Like the colostrum that's made by your breasts before your milk comes in (see Producing milk, p.326), it contains antibodies that help protect your baby from infections such as gastro-enteritis.

Breastfeeding is a fulfilling and enjoyable experience that will enhance the loving relationship between you and your baby. What's more, despite occasional snags such as sore nipples or engorged breasts, it's good for you too. The extra calories you use in producing breastmilk help to use up the fat reserves you gained during pregnancy, so you get back to your pre-pregnant weight more easily. When you breastfeed, the hormone oxytocin that makes your milk glands contract when your baby suckles (see p.326) also causes contractions in your uterus, which helps it to return to its normal size more quickly.

There's also some evidence that women who have breastfed are less prone to breast cancer and to osteoporosis (brittle bones). From a purely practical point of view, breastfeeding is quick, easy, and convenient. It's free and you don't need to carry round any special equipment.

Breastfeeding does have some drawbacks, though. Until your milk supply is sufficiently well established for you to collect and store some for later feeding by bottle (see p.327), you're the only person who can feed your baby. If you prefer privacy when breastfeeding, you may find it difficult when away from home.

Breastfeeding can lead to sore or cracked nipples and other breast problems (see p.356); illness, tiredness, worry, and menstruation can reduce your milk supply; if you're taking any medication or drugs while breastfeeding, these can pass into your milk and possibly cause harm to your baby; and some foods that you eat, such as oranges, may upset your baby's stomach.

Most of the problems and difficulties that you may have in getting your baby to breastfeed tend to lessen after the first couple of weeks. So if you find feeding trying at first, persevere. Stick with it for a while, get advice if you need it and once the initial difficulties have passed, you'll probably find it easy, immensely rewarding, and enjoyable.

Bottlefeeding

Although modern infant formula provides adequate nourishment for your baby (as you can see from the chart below), it doesn't contain the protective antibodies found in colostrum and breastmilk. Other disadvantages are that it's harder to digest than breastmilk (but because of this, your baby will need feeding less frequently); it gives more formed bowel movements with a stronger smell than those of a breastfed baby; formula may lay the foundation for a milk allergy later on; preparing it is time-consuming; and you may find it harder to lose weight because you're not using up calories in producing milk. If you decide on bottlefeeding (see pp.332 and 334), you'll need to buy supplies of formula, bottles, and teats, as well as sterilizing equipment, before your baby is born. When you go out you'll need to take feeding equipment with you.

Comparing breastmilk and formulas

NUTRIENT (PER 100 MILLILITRES)	HUMAN MILK	COW'S MILK FORMULA	SOYA-BASED FORMULA
Energy (kcal)	68	66	65
Fat (g)	3.8	3.7	3.6
Protein (g)	1.25	1.45	1.8
Carbohydrate (g)	7.2	7.22	6.9
Vitamin A (mg)	60	80	60
Vitamin D (mg)	0.025	1.0	1.0
Vitamin C (mg)	3.7	6.8	5.5
Iron (mg)	0.07	0.58	0.67

Baby's experience

Your baby will greatly enjoy being breastfed and breastmilk is specifically designed to give him the best start in life.

Breastmilk is nutritionally superior to formula, easy to digest, and, like colostrum, protects against many common infections, particularly those of the gastro-intestinal and respiratory tracts. Even if you only breastfeed your baby for the first few weeks, the antibodies in your colostrum and milk will do him a great deal of good, and the close contact between you will strengthen your relationship.

Formula If you're unable to breastfeed, your baby will, of course, thrive on formula. Whenever you bottlefeed, give your baby lots of skin and eye contact, and talk or sing to him to help to intensify the bonding between you.

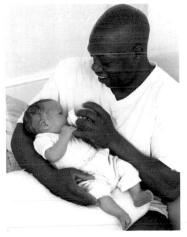

▲ **CLOSE CONTACT** As you bottlefeed your baby, keep your attention focused on him. Maintain eye contact, and smile and talk to him.

Points to think about

Here are a few things to bear in mind when you're choosing a first name for your newborn baby.

- Will the name be suitable for your child at all stages of life?

- Is it obvious how the name is spelled and pronounced?

- Does the name sound right when put together with the middle name(s) you like and your surname?

- Do the initials of the full name make a word when put together?

- Are you happy with any associations with the name – famous people or people you know, for example?

- Is there any reason why your child might be teased because of the name you've chosen?

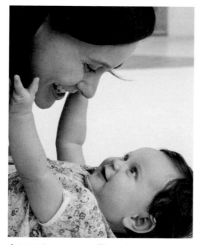

▲ COMMUNICATION Choosing your baby's name as early as possible helps you talk to her too. She will learn to recognize her name very quickly.

Choosing a name

Naming your baby can be surprisingly difficult. There are so many things to think about – will the name you've chosen go with the family name? Is it likely to go out of fashion? You may be influenced by many different associations and considerations, but the main thing to remember is that the name you choose is for your baby, and hopefully it will please her throughout her life.

Fashion

This does influence lots of parents, either consciously or unconsciously. A name can suddenly become very popular – often because of a particular celebrity – and then fall out of fashion equally suddenly, so dating the children bearing it. It's very difficult to predict which will be the "in" names in any given year, although some are always popular and many parents define what is fashionable or unfashionable by their own social set. The annual publication *The Top Ten of Everything* lists the most popular names for boys and girls in any given year, and the National Statistics Office (www.statistics.gov.uk) has the top 100 names for both sexes over the past five years.

Some people like old, familiar names and shrink from new, invented, or imported names; others prefer to choose something that is meaningful to them and the time in which they live.

Associations

Parents often choose names because of their association, rather than their particular meaning. Meaning tends to play a much smaller role in the Western world than it does in some other parts of the world.

Personal associations can have a positive or negative influence. Some people like to name a child after a friend or a family member – a much-loved grandparent, for example. You won't want to use names you associate with someone you don't like. Godparents are sometimes honoured, and public associations might include royalty, celebrities, pop singers, and film and television stars. Place names, too, have begun to be used if they have particular meaning for parents (Brooklyn, Phoenix), but take care when combining these with surnames (Brooklyn Bridge) to avoid your child being teased. Characters in books and films can also inspire parents and some parents like to name their children after characters in popular television series such as soap operas.

For many people, a name can conjure up a particular image or character and they may expect children to fit or suit a name. As this can influence the way a child is treated, and consequently how the child responds, children may well grow into the names they're given. Other names, such as Patience or Faith, can reflect the parents' desire for the child (usually female in the Western world) to possess particular virtues, and were first introduced by the Puritans (see column, right).

Some first names are inspired by where a baby is conceived or something that happens around the time of the birth. These can include time of birth – Noël or Natalie for a Christmas baby; month names such as May, June; Dawn or Eve for the actual time of birth.

Family traditions

Names that have been passed down through a family from generation to generation were at one time the automatic choice for many parents, especially for a first-born. If the traditional name was masculine, it was sometimes feminized for a girl (Thomas, Thomasina), especially if there was no male heir. These customs have lapsed in recent times, leading to many traditional family names being dropped, although they are sometimes used as a child's middle name.

Some families, particularly among the aristocracy in Scotland, and in the American South, used the mother's maiden name as the first-born son's given name. This appears to be dying out, although the maiden name is still given as a middle name. Because of this custom, surnames such as Russell, Howard, Cameron have become normal as first names, particularly for boys. Couples who are not married or in which the woman prefers to keep her maiden name sometimes like to give the mother's surname as the child's middle name.

Many parents choose names for their children that work together, although few go as far as the Victorians (see column, right). Some parents like all their children's names to start with the same initial, although this can cause confusion with letters and official documents.

Nationality

Many parents choose names that reflect where they come from, even though they no longer live there. This can lead to problems of spelling and pronunciation, so the spelling may be simplified – from Gaelic to English, for example (Síle – Sheila; Aodán – Aidan). In other cases, first names that are perceived as being "national" may not be used in their country of origin. Colleen, for example, comes from the Celtic word caitlín, meaning "girl" or "wench", and is popular for girls of Irish origin in America and Australia, even though it's not used as a name in Ireland.

Naming fashions

There are trends in name-giving just as there are in other things. Many of today's first names have been used for centuries.

Norman After their British conquest in 1066, the Normans introduced a fixed name system. Norman names included Alan, Henry, Hugh, Ralph, Richard, Oliver, William, Alice, Emma, Rosamund, and Yvonne.

Biblical In the 16th century there were many names used primarily by Catholics. These included Mary, and saints' names such as Sebastian, Benedict, and Agnes. The Protestants turned to the Bible for inspiration, and Adam, Benjamin, David, Joshua, Michael, Samuel, Abigail, Hannah, Rachel, Ruth, and Sarah became popular. The Puritans in the 17th century produced the "virtue" names – Faith, Charity, Grace, Hope, Patience, and Prudence.

Victorian At the end of the 19th century, there was a vogue for using gemstones or flowers as first names for girls. Thus Pearl, Ruby, Lily, Ivy, and Rose became popular.

Contemporary The 20th century saw the rise of exotic spellings, such as Nikki and Debra, as well as descriptive names like River and Rainbow. Popular choices in the early 21st century include Olivia, Grace, Sophie, and Chloe for girls, and Jack, Thomas, Oliver, and Joshua for boys.

Naming twins

There's a tradition of giving twins names that are related. The names may reflect an association; begin with the same initial (Paul, Patricia); sound alike (Suzanna, Hannah); or have a similar rhythm (Benjamin, Jonathan).

But there are lots of reasons why your twins won't thank you if their names are too closely associated for comfort.

First, and most important, people will be much more likely to get them confused if there's a strong link between their names. Names are used as labels and twins, perhaps more than other children, need individual labels that belong solely to them.

Secondly, official forms, examination papers, and letters can easily become confused, especially if initials are shared.

Thirdly, if the names are closely linked by association, twins are likely to come in for a lot of name teasing or punning.

Meanings

The meaning or origin of a name tends to be less important than its associations for most modern Western parents. Many Western first names have had a more convoluted history than those of other cultures. This is because these names, along with other traditions and customs, have been transferred from one society to another, often by invasion followed by integration, migration, or contact between different cultures. For this reason, many names have become divorced from their original meanings, but some Western parents do still choose names primarily because of what they mean.

Form of a name

The way our names are pronounced and spelled, and the shortened forms we prefer, are very important to most of us. It's irritating if your name is constantly misspelled or mispronounced, and it can be very annoying if someone uses a short version you don't like, or the formal version that wasn't actually bestowed.

Diminutives The pet forms of names (Megan, Kate, Jamie) are often used, and sometimes given, in preference to the full versions (Margaret, Katherine, James). Even if you intend always using the diminutive, it's worth considering giving your child the formal name since there may be times when it's more appropriate. On the other hand, if you intend always to use the full version of a name (Patricia, Edward), it's as well to consider how you feel about any pet forms (Pat, Patty, Patsy, Trish, Tricia; Ed, Eddie, Ted, Ned) as your child's name will almost certainly be shortened by friends as she grows up.

Sound You may like a name because of its sound – it could be that the name is naturally harmonious or perhaps it sounds good alongside your surname. Most parents take particular care to select a happy partnership, with surnames balanced by given names. Indeed, some parents bestow names in the order they feel sounds best (Elizabeth Anne, Arthur James), but call their child by the middle name (Anne, James).

Spelling and pronunciation It's worth giving your child a name that everyone can spell and pronounce easily to avoid confusion and irritation for your child in later life. In the last 50 years or so, there has been an increasing tendency to choose exotic spellings of ordinary first names (Jayne, Kathryn, Jonothon). Some names have more than one pronunciation (Helena), while others are confusing (Phoebe), and still others have more than one spelling (Clare, Clair, Claire).

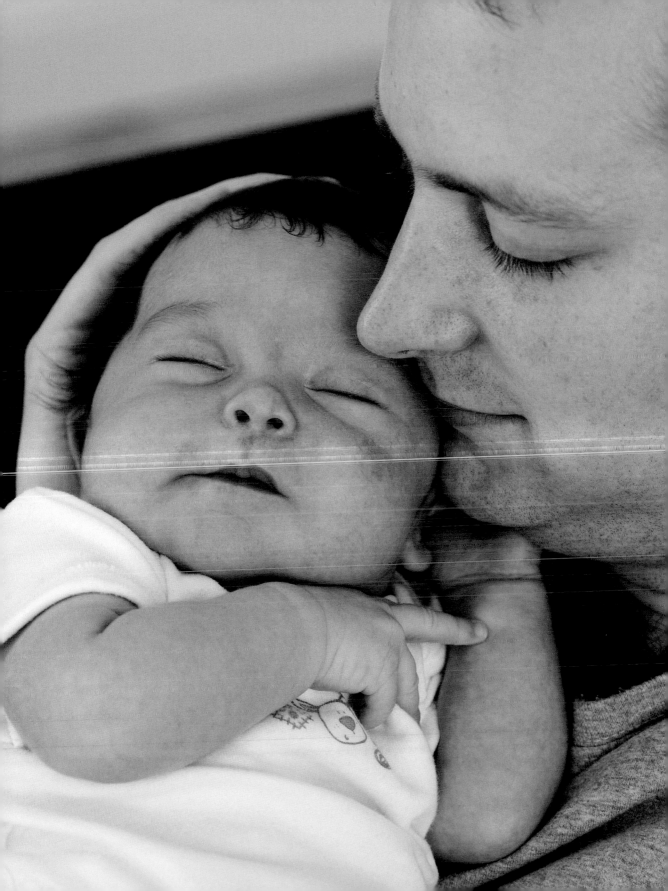

Preparing siblings for a new baby

Any child who's enjoyed the undivided attention of both parents for any length of time will suffer what child psychologists call "dethronement" when a new baby arrives. Nearly all toddlers suffer a deep sense of loss of parental love when a new sibling arrives. It's not surprising that their psychological disturbance shows in changes in their behaviour after the new arrival.

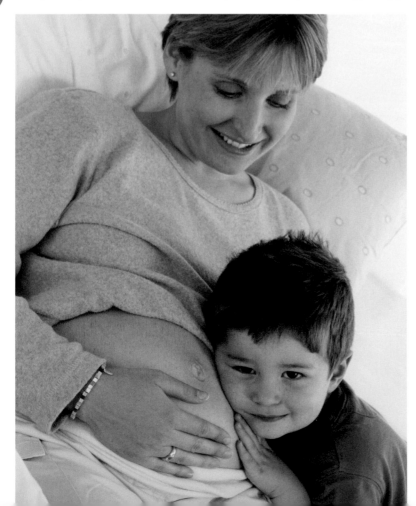

▼ **KEEP HIM INVOLVED** Talking to your child about the arrival of your new baby will help him feel involved and avoid feelings of neglect.

Helping a young child To a young child, the arrival of a new baby topples him from pride of place, from being first in his mother's considerations, from being the apple of her eye, and the focus of her love, nurture, and attention. He may feel that he's taking second place with mum and dad and has less attention than before. A child feels this displacement very dramatically and of course responds as only a small child knows how by using all the tactics at his disposal to regain his parents' love and attention.

The result can be "regression", which means the toddler goes back to earlier, happier times when he couldn't feed himself perhaps, or when he wet and soiled his nappies, or before he'd learned to talk. This may look to adults like some sort of rebellion, but a toddler can't help it, so the worst you can do is punish him for it. In fact, the opposite is essential – he needs extra-special time alone with you, with loving care, plenty of rewards, praise, and physical affection with games, kisses, and cuddles and lots of jokes and laughter.

Armed with this knowledge of how your toddler is likely to react to the arrival of a brother or sister, you can ease him through this painful time with some careful preparation and planning.

Involving your older child in the pregnancy Be honest with your child from the start. Tell him that a new baby is on the way and he's going to have a new brother or sister. You might even ask him what his favourite names are. Make a list, put them up in the kitchen, and talk about them from time to time.

Encourage your child to put his hand on your tummy as it gets bigger to feel the baby kicking. You could also tell him that your baby loves the sound of his voice and that he should talk to her through your tummy. Ask him to sing her songs and nursery rhymes through your tummy.

Incidentally, this isn't all hot air. Your developing baby does remember the voices of those around her and will bond with them after birth. She'll respond instantly on hearing her brother's or sister's voice once she's born, if she's heard it constantly during your pregnancy.

Helping your child to understand what's happening Show him what's happening in your tummy month by month using the pictures in this book (see pp.72–89). Copy them on large sheets of paper so that it's all very clear. Point out how the baby is developing and put up the drawings round the wall at a height where your toddler can see them easily. Perhaps you could then make up stories about each stage of the new baby's development, saying things like, "Now your new baby's heart is beating." "Now your new baby can move his hands and legs and we can feel him kicking." "Now your new baby can suck her thumb." "Now your new baby is getting ready to be born", and so on.

Try to encourage your child to take ownership of his new sibling by using the word "your", as in "your baby", "your new sister". If you do, very soon he'll develop a sense of ownership, and of a desire to take care of his new brother or sister. If you and your partner always talk about "our new baby" he may feel excluded and frozen out.

It'll help your toddler to feel included if you involve him in the preparations for the new baby – helping to make up the cot and setting out equipment, for example. You might even suggest that he could try getting into the baby bath first, saying something like "Wouldn't you like to see what the bath feels like before your sister uses it?"

All toddlers like to help and love to imitate your actions. So, give your toddler small jobs to do and be very appreciative of all his efforts. You can show him all the new baby's tiny clothes and encourage him to feel special by saying how much he's grown since he needed them.

After the birth

Try to arrange for your child to see you and the baby as soon as possible after the delivery.

When your toddler visits, have eyes only for him. Ideally, your new baby should be asleep in the bedside cot. Make a fuss of your toddler until he asks about the new baby. Only then show him his sister, but not for long, and not paying too much attention to her. Make his visit short so that you can attend to your baby once he's gone.

Bringing the baby home Try to help your toddler to feel secure and bond with the new baby.

■ When you greet him, make sure someone else holds the baby so that you are free to cuddle him.

■ For the first few minutes give him all your attention.

■ Give your child a present from the new baby, something he's really been looking forward to.

■ In the first weeks set aside some time when the two of you can be together without any interruptions.

■ Involve your child in the new baby's bath times, changing, and feeding times. Describe everything that your new baby is doing so that he can get to know her and relate to her.

■ A newborn baby has a well-developed grasp reflex. Put one of your child's fingers into her hand – she'll grasp on to it very tightly and he'll interpret this as love from his newborn sister.

Dad as carer

In many households, dad is the main helper when his partner arrives home with their new baby. Some men immediately involve themselves in caring for their partner and child, but others need to be encouraged.

What you need from your partner more than anything else at this time is understanding, sympathy, and a readiness to go along with you and the baby. It's best to have a serious discussion about this before your baby is born.

You may find it best to divide the work between you. For instance, your partner could take over the cleaning, shopping, and laundry, leaving you free to concentrate on looking after yourself and the baby. Or you might prefer to share all the household and child care work.

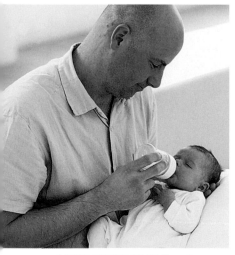

▲ HELP AT MEAL TIMES If you're breastfeeding, express milk into a bottle (see p.327) so that your partner can enjoy feeding the baby.

Arranging for help

In the last weeks of pregnancy, it's a good idea for you and your partner to talk about how you are going to organize things at home once your baby is born. If your partner is taking time off and able to play a full part, you'll be able to cope without too much difficulty; if not, you'll need someone else to give you some help and support, especially for the first few weeks.

The first few days of motherhood will be harder than you think. Labour and birth are physically and emotionally draining; you'll feel you've very few reserves left, and you'll be very tired. You'll realize, once at home with your baby, that one job or activity succeeds another almost without a moment's pause, and in the middle of all this you're still learning about being a mother. Even if you've read every baby book going, you'll find that your baby conforms to no typical schedule or plan, and that you have to work out your life around your baby's routine. Trying to impose a routine on your baby only causes you more work; it's best to take your lead from him. As far as sleep is concerned, you need to get it when you can – new babies don't know night from day and need the same attention during the night as they do in the day.

Sources of help

So that you don't become overtired, and even depressed and weepy, you'll need some help to tide you over at least the first few days, and preferably the first week or two. Don't be too proud to ask for or accept help – if you don't say what you need, you may soon come to regret it. Having help does not make you an inadequate mother. The best possible solution is to have someone living in your house, so that your day can be split into shifts. That way you can at least make sure that you get enough rest and time to pay attention to what you're eating.

Family and friends Your mother and your mother-in-law are probably the people you trust most in the world when it comes to child care They've had children and are experienced at looking after babies, and they'll give you lots of helpful support and advice. If possible, ask one of them, or another close relative who has the flexibility and time, to come and live in your house around the time you go into labour. That way your helper can establish herself in your home with your partner and other children if you have them, and be ready to receive you when you come home with the baby.

Such a helper is invaluable. You'll feel confident that the household is ticking over quite normally. She can take over all the organizing and see to meals, laundry, shopping, and so on. This also takes some of the responsibility from your partner so you can both devote more time to your baby. And if your helper has had children of her own, she'll probably have lots of valuable information and advice for you.

Nannies Nannies can either live with you or come on a daily basis. If you decide that you'd like a nanny, it's best to arrange for her to be settled in with your family before your baby is born so you can get to know each other. Having a newborn baby in the house is quite a traumatic event, and it's important to have a helper who'll fit in with your routines and lifestyle. It's also vital for you to feel confident about her abilities and happy with her relationship with your baby. You can find a nanny through personal recommendation, advertising, or through a really reliable nanny agency. I recommend contacting the Recruitment and Employment Confederation for advice (see Addresses, p.370).

However you recruit your nanny, you'll need to see her at least twice before you hire her. Make sure you get two good references, and follow up these references with a telephone call to tease out any "between the lines" information. The first time you meet, suggest you relax over tea or lunch together or maybe go shopping. Follow this up with a formal interview. Both you and your partner should be involved in the process, because you'll probably see different aspects of her character.

Draw up a contract of employment with a proper job description in which you cover all the tasks you expect her to undertake, and include the approaches and attitudes you expect. Your nanny should be prepared to bend her usual practices in order to fit in with yours. Remember that you are her employer and as such you are responsible for her welfare. She has the same employment rights as an employee in any other line of work.

Au pairs These are young women (or occasionally young men) from other countries who help you with your baby in exchange for room, board, and a small wage. They are much cheaper than nannies but bear in mind that most have no special child-care training and may speak little English. An au pair is supposed to live with you as part of the family; she is not an employee. It's not a good idea (and not fair on your au pair) to leave her in sole charge of a baby under one year of age for any length of time. In fact in the UK, au pairs are not supposed to work more than five hours a day. They must be given time off to go to language classes if they wish.

Live-in helpers

If you want live-in help for a short time, you could hire a maternity nurse for a few weeks. She'll join your household just before or after your baby is born and she will help you with all the baby care.

As well as providing welcome help with your baby, maternity nurses are invaluable teachers. They'll show you how to see to your baby's daily care: how to change nappies, and how to breast- or bottlefeed him, for example, how to know when he's had enough, and how to take the baby carefully off your breast to avoid soreness and cracked nipples.

But it's up to you and your maternity nurse to work out what kind of regime you would like. You may decide, for instance, that you'd like to have a night's sleep without interruption so the nurse will be on duty all the way through the night. You'd then take over at, say, 7am, so that she can get some rest. Maternity nurses are expensive, but will get you off to a good start if there's no one else around to help.

Another option is a doula (see Useful addresses, p.370). A doula is an experienced woman who offers help and support during and after the birth of your baby. Some doulas are willing to live in for a few weeks after the birth. A doula is trained and experienced in childbirth and baby care, but she is not medically qualified.

Miriam's casebook

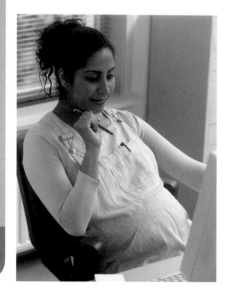

A working pregnancy

Vicky, a junior partner in a firm of accountants, passed her accountancy exams while she was expecting her first child, now six years old. She knows that she can combine work and mothering, having worked since shortly after the birth of her son. Her challenge now is to combine pregnancy with her working life, be a mother to a schoolboy, and keep up a good relationship with her partner.

Combining motherhood and work

Vicky decided to continue with a very demanding job while she had her second child. To do this, she had to fit the pieces of her life together like a jigsaw puzzle.

She told her colleagues that she was pregnant right away and arranged to talk to them about her maternity leave. I advised her to eat well so she had all the energy and nutrition she needed to keep working while her pregnancy progressed and her baby developed.

I explained that as no two pregnancies are alike, Vicky could not know how she would feel this time around. I advised her not to commit herself to staying at work beyond the 32nd week, but suggested that perhaps she could make an informal arrangement to do so if she felt well enough when the time came.

Planning maternity leave

When to return after maternity leave is a more complicated decision. Vicky's menstrual cycle may take only three months to get back to normal, but her muscles and various organs would probably need more time. The process takes a year altogether. I explained to Vicky that she would need to make special feeding plans if she went back to work before

her baby was six months old. As she didn't want to give her baby formula milk, she'd have to express her breast milk and freeze it (see p.327) and would need to allow time to build up a stock of milk initially, then a further six weeks for her baby to get used to breastfeeding and taking breast milk from a bottle.

I suggested that Vicky could arrange a provisional date for her return to work, and check with her doctor as she neared her return date. When choosing a carer, I suggested that she checked out all the available options well in advance – crèches, daytime nannies, childminders, au pairs – to find a carer who was just right.

Making time

I advised Vicky that she would need to plan to have some time alone with her new baby every day, and her son, Jack, who would also need lots of attention and reassurance at this stage. I explained to Vicky that the best way to give him this was to make sure he has his own special time with her, so that he doesn't feel shut out. She would also need to factor in time alone with her partner, Peter, so that their relationship didn't suffer. Above all, I advised Vicky to ringfence some time to herself – one free hour a week when nobody made any demands upon her. Many mothers feel guilty about taking time out for themselves but it's really important if you're going to be relaxed and happy.

Settling into a routine

We agreed that Vicky would feel less overwhelmed if she had a routine to work to, and that the rest of her family would also feel happier if their days were structured. For example, Vicky could spend time with her baby when she gets back from work. She could encourage Peter and Jack to bring her a cup of tea, make sure she's comfortable, then leave her with her baby while they went off to play and chat together. Her special time with her son could be his bedtime, when she could read him a story and listen to him talk about his day. She and Peter could then have an evening meal together and chat, before the baby's late-evening feed.

Adjusting to changes

I suggested to Vicky that six weeks before she returned to work, she should start weaning her baby off the breast for her daytime feeds, replacing one feed with bottled breast milk. Her baby would also need time to get used to the new carer. In fact, her baby developed close bonds with her carer, who'll be an important person in her life. But this won't affect her relationship with her parents.

When Vicky returned to work, her baby adapted to a new routine. She accepted bottles of expressed milk quite easily as she had been introduced to bottlefeeding before she was five weeks old. Initially she had refused to accept milk from a bottle so Vicky experimented with bottles with different types of teat until she found one her baby liked.

Expressing and storing breast milk

I explained to Vicky that she'd need to keep up a good supply of breast milk by feeding her baby or by expressing it regularly. Leaving milk in the breast discourages further milk production and supplies soon dwindle. Vicky was sure that she would have enough milk for her to be able to express some just after feeds so that she can gradually stockpile milk

Miriam's top tips

Vicky needs to make her own well-being and her baby's the top priority in all her plans. The keys are managing her time well and being sensitive to her own needs. My advice is to:

■ make arrangements about when to leave work and when to return, and set up childcare well in advance to smooth the transition

■ build a support network with other local working families so you can help each other out.

■ make time in a busy schedule to relax and take stock.

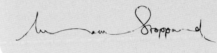

for future use. When back at work, Vicky found that her breasts became full twice a day, so she made time to express using a breast pump. She expressed her milk in the comfortable ladies' room and stored it in a refrigerator in her office until she went home. She sterilized all containers and kept her milk in the refrigerator no more than 48 hours – it can be stored for up to six months in the freezer.

Coming home to the family

At home, her carer was responsible for defrosting each day's supply of breast milk. This should usually be done in the refrigerator, although if you need to defrost breast milk quickly, you can place the container under running lukewarm tap water. Leftover milk must be thrown away and never kept or refrozen for later use.

Now, when Vicky gets home from work her breasts are full of milk and her baby is ready for a feed. I did warn Vicky that her baby will be quick to figure out that although mummy is away during the day, she is there all night, and may become a wakeful baby, as two of my own sons did. I advised Vicky that she would need to establish a routine that helps her baby sleep through the night so that she, too, could get a decent night's sleep.

Getting enough sleep

A good night's sleep is one of your top priorities in the late stages of pregnancy.

If you can, have eight hours of sleep a night, but you may find you suffer from irritating insomnia. Although your metabolism slows down at night your baby's doesn't, and he may be active and kicking through the night hours. If you can't sleep, there are a number of things you can try:

■ have a warm (not hot) bath before going to bed to relax you and make you sleepy and calm

■ a hot milky bedtime drink helps you drop off; also, read a calming book, listen to music or the radio, or watch television

■ deep breathing and relaxation exercises are excellent treatments for insomnia, so find a bedtime routine that suits you

■ instead of worrying about your lack of sleep, get up in the middle of the night and do something – perhaps a job that you've been putting off for some time – or go into your baby's room, look at things, touch them, rearrange them, and feel happy at the thought of your baby

■ if you have worries that stop you sleeping, visualize each one as being written on a piece of paper. Then mentally screw it up and throw it away.

The late stages of pregnancy

Very little goes wrong in the last few weeks of pregnancy. From week 32 onwards, your doctor and midwife will be mainly keeping an eye on the continued growth of your baby and your own health. You'll need to have check-ups more often than before, probably every three weeks from week 32 to week 36, and then fortnightly up to week 40.

One of the problems of later pregnancy is that it's harder and harder to get comfortable. As your abdomen grows larger, sitting or lying in your usual positions can become difficult. If you lie flat on your back, the weight of your growing baby will press down on your major blood vessels and nerves that lie against the spine and cause numbness and tingling pain, even dizziness and shortness of breath. Experiment with your sleeping position in bed and find ways to make yourself as comfortable as possible. It may help to use some cushions or soft pillows (see below).

Tense and relax technique

Good relaxation techniques combine the release of tension in the mind and body with deep, regular breathing. You'll find it helps to practise these techniques so that towards the end of pregnancy they've become second nature. A good way to relax your whole body completely is to use the

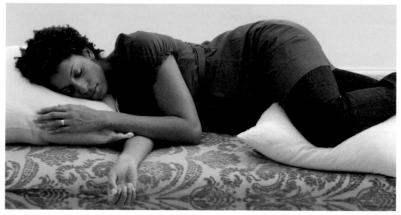

▲ **RESTING ON YOUR SIDE** In late pregnancy it's often most comfortable to lie on your side, with your uppermost leg propped up with lots of cushions or pillows.

tense and relax technique. This is a pleasant way to relax during pregnancy, and will also serve as a good preparation for labour, when it's a great help to be able to relax most of the muscles in your body, so that your uterus contracts without the rest of your body tensing.

What you do is tense and relax different parts of your body one after the other. Your partner can help by touching you where he can see you are tensing up: you respond to his touch by relaxing. Practise this technique twice a day for 15–20 minutes if you can, before meals or an hour or more after eating. You'll find it really helps you feel better.

Find a comfortable position, either lying on your back or propped up with cushions on a chair. Close your eyes and then try to clear your mind of any stressful thoughts, anxieties, or worries by breathing in and out slowly and regularly and concentrating all your attention on your breathing actions. Let pleasant, relaxing thoughts flow through your head, and if anything worrying or nagging tries to surface, prevent it from doing so by saying "no" under your breath, then go back to concentrating completely on your deep breathing.

When your mind is totally relaxed and your breathing deep and regular, begin the tense and relax routine. Think about your right hand: tense it for a moment, palm facing upward, relax it and tell it to feel heavy and warm. Work up through the right side of your body, tensing and relaxing your forearm, upper arm, and shoulder. Then repeat the process on the upper left side of your body. Next, roll your knees outward, and then in turn tense and relax your buttocks, thighs, calves, and feet. Press your lower back gently into the floor or cushions, then release and relax.

Finish off by relaxing your head and neck. Relax your face, eyes, and forehead, and smooth away any frowns.

▶ **RELAXING IN A CHAIR**
Sit up straight as this helps strengthen your back muscles. Keep your knees at right angles (raise your feet if necessary) and put a cushion at the small of your back.

Your baby's position

As a baby reaches full maturity at about 37 weeks, he usually becomes heavier and tips head down. But some babies remain breech (see p.307) until term.

If a baby is in the breech position at term he may be delivered by Caesarean section (see p.308). If your baby is breech in the last weeks of pregnancy, though, don't worry – he'll probably turn himself before labour actually begins:

■ 30 per cent of babies are breech at 30 weeks. More than half of these babies will turn spontaneously during the next two weeks

■ 14 per cent of babies are still breech at 32 weeks. There's a 60 per cent chance that a baby who is bottom down will turn of his own accord before labour starts

■ fewer than five per cent of babies are still breech at 37 weeks. One-quarter of these will turn on their own, although this is less likely if the legs are extended or there isn't much room in the uterus for some reason – for example, if you're having more than one baby or a large baby.

When your baby's overdue

If you go past your EDD your midwife will keep a very close check on your baby by a number of different methods.

Fetal movement recording The most accurate sign that all is well with your baby is if you can feel regular movements. Since all mothers, and babies, are different, the amount of movement that's normal differs from one pregnancy to another. You are the best judge of whether your unborn baby is acting normally, and you may be asked to monitor his activity using a kick chart (see p.195).

Electronic fetal monitoring This may be used to check your baby's heartbeat by providing a continuous sound or paper recording (see p.275). If the heartbeat is satisfactory, you're unlikely to need other tests or your labour induced.

Ultrasound You'll probably be given an ultrasound scan to assess the volume of amniotic fluid. If this is becoming dangerously low, your doctors will probably advise you to have your labour induced.

Are you overdue?

Only about five per cent of all babies arrive on the actual date that they're expected. The expected date of delivery (EDD) (see p.63) is only a statistical average, and studies have shown that as many as 40 per cent of babies are born more than a week after their EDD. Of the 40 per cent of babies who are "overdue", 25 per cent of babies are born in the 42nd week.

Being overdue

The exact date of conception in any particular pregnancy is extremely difficult to pinpoint , which makes it difficult to decide whether a baby is actually overdue or not. Even if you have a regular menstrual cycle of 28 days (the standard on which the EDD chart is based), the date of ovulation is known only approximately (see p.63).

As well as this uncertainty about the exact date of ovulation, every baby is different and so it's unrealistic to expect them all to mature in precisely the same number of days. Since labour is initiated by your baby producing certain hormones as he reaches full maturity, it makes sense that the actual date of delivery can vary fairly widely – even in "textbook" pregnancies. Early ultrasound scans are helpful in confirming, or sometimes even changing, your due date. The earlier the scan is performed the more accurate it is.

Doctors do become worried, though, if a pregnancy continues much beyond two weeks after the estimated date of delivery. This is because post-maturity and possible problems with the placenta (placental insufficiency) pose some risks to the health of your unborn baby (see Post-maturity, Risks, opposite). The longer your baby goes on growing inside your womb, the larger he is likely to become, which, in turn, will increase the chances of a difficult labour. There's also the risk that the placenta will not be able to continue to support your baby over an extended period (see Your baby's placenta, opposite).

Doctors will also ask you about your family history – have you or your mother had longer than average pregnancies (lasting 43 or 44 weeks for example)? If this is the case, your doctor will probably be more willing to let you go more than two weeks overdue without suggesting that you're induced – although you'll be closely monitored in case any problems do develop. In practice, most women are quite desperate to have their babies by this stage of pregnancy.

Post-maturity

An overdue baby may be in danger of being post-mature. A post-mature baby will have lost fat from all over his body, particularly from his tummy. His skin will look red and wrinkled as if it doesn't fit him, and it may have begun to peel. Very few babies are actually post-mature because post-maturity depends not only on the baby's condition, but also on his placenta (see below). It is difficult to predict which babies will be at risk.

Risks A post-mature baby tends to be bigger than average which can make your labour longer and more difficult. Also the bones in his skull tend to be harder, which means that his descent through the birth canal is likely to be more traumatic both for him and for you. In addition, there's an increased risk of stillbirth: the risk of stillbirth doubles by the 43rd week of pregnancy and triples by the 44th week.

Your baby's placenta

At term, the placenta – the organ that links the blood supplies of the mother and baby – looks rather like a piece of raw liver. It is about the size of a dinner plate, and measures about 2.5cm (1in) thick. The maternal side is divided into wedge shaped chunks called cotyledons.

The placenta has substantial reserves, readily adjusts to injury repairs damages due to ischaemia (lack of oxygen), and does not undergo ageing. The widely held view that the placenta ages progressively during your pregnancy is due to a misinterpretation of the appearance of different parts of the placenta over the duration of the pregnancy.

There are, though, changes in the character of the villi (small projections) around the placenta during the pregnancy, and by 36 weeks there may be deposits of calcium within the walls of the small blood vessels, and a protein deposit may appear on the surface of many of the villi. Both of these changes can limit the flow of nutrients and waste across the placenta to your baby, but this is balanced by the fact that the fetal blood vessels and villi are close together, which makes the exchange of nutrients easier.

Risks If labour does not begin as expected (this varies from pregnancy to pregnancy, but is usually considered to be two weeks either side of the EDD), the placenta may then start to become relatively inefficient. This does happen slowly and at 42 weeks the placenta should still be supplying your baby with enough nutrients for his needs. There can be problems when, occasionally, the placenta fails to nourish and support your baby adequately. This is known as placental insufficiency and in these circumstances you may be advised to have your labour induced.

Late engagement

When engagement is late in a first pregnancy, doctors may suspect pelvic disproportion. This means that if your baby is very big it might be hard for him to pass through your pelvis.

To check whether your baby's head will actually engage in, and pass through, your pelvis, your doctor will perform a simple test.

Step 1
You'll be asked to lie on your back. In this position, your doctor will be able to feel your baby's head resting just at the pelvic brim.

Step 2
You'll then be asked to prop yourself up on your elbows. If your baby's head slips easily into your pelvis, it shows that you've no problem with pelvic disproportion.

Managing your labour

Labour is the culmination of your pregnancy. Very few labours are pain-free, but you can choose the method of pain relief that suits you best. The help and support of your partner can be invaluable in making your labour a smoother, more comfortable experience.

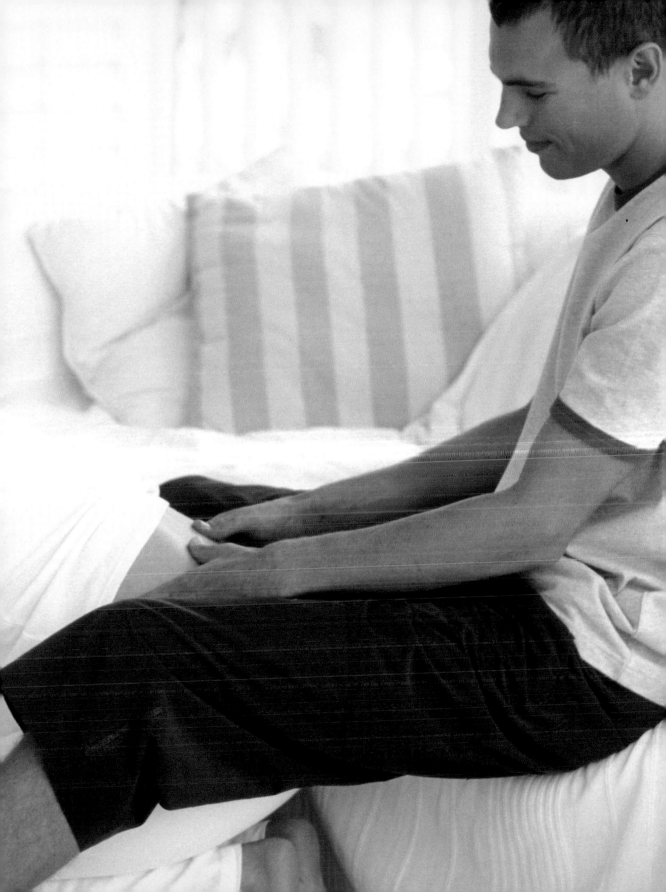

Your checklist

Most preparations can be made well in advance, but you'll still have a few things that you need to take care of at the last minute.

When you go into labour (see p.270), you should:

- call your midwife

- make contact with your partner or birth coach

- get in touch with whoever's going to care for your other children, if it's not your partner

- check that the room is ready

- check that your labour aids are conveniently to hand

- make yourself a hot, sweet drink.

▼ **ADVANCE PREPARATIONS** Get as much as possible ready well in advance so you don't have a last-minute rush.

Preparing for a home birth

If you're planning to have a home birth, your midwife will tell you all about what preparations you need to make. Do as much as you can about four weeks before your due date so that you don't have to rush around getting everything organized at the last minute, and you are at least partly prepared if your baby comes early.

Advance preparations

Decide which room you're going to use for the birth and arrange everything so that it's convenient and comfortable for you and your midwife. Put the bed at right angles to the wall, with plenty of space on each side so your midwife can reach you easily. A week or two before your due date, she'll bring round a home birth pack of medical equipment. The contents will be sterile, so don't open the pack.

Protection Whether you want to deliver your baby on to the floor or your bed, the bed itself and the floor area below and immediately around you will need to be protected during the birth. Make sure you have some old clean sheets, big towels, and a large piece of plastic sheeting to hand so that it can be put down quickly when the time comes.

What your midwife will need
It's useful to put a small side table or a tea trolley next to the bed so your midwife has somewhere to put her instruments and other equipment, although a couple of tea trays will do. She'll also need a bright, adjustable reading lamp so she can direct light on to your perineum. Have a torch (with spare batteries and bulb) ready too, just in case there's a power cut.

Stock up on food, drink, and other essentials in the few days

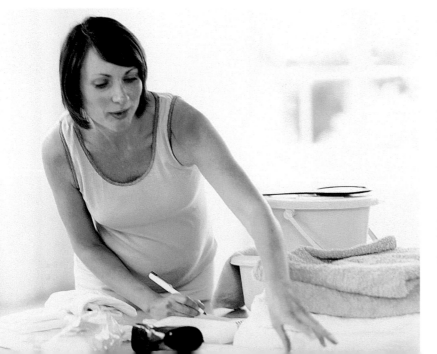

before your baby's due. When shopping, remember that you'll need food for your midwife and for any visitors you may have as well as for yourself, your partner, and your other children (if you have any).

When labour starts

When your contractions are coming every 15 minutes, are about one minute long, and don't die away when you move around, telephone your midwife according to your arrangements. First labours often take a while to get going so, although your midwife will want to know that things have started happening, she's likely to suggest that you try to relax and get some rest until you're in full labour – it's important to conserve your energy. All independent midwives can be contacted by mobile phone, so it's easy to keep in touch.

Final preparations Make sure everything else that you and the midwife will need, for the birth and immediately afterwards, is ready – including your comfort aids (see p.268), bowls for washing, a bedpan (or a clean bucket), clean towels, and large plastic bags for the soiled sheets, sanitary pads, and used dressings. Then put out a clean nightdress or large nightshirt for yourself, make sure you have clothes and nappies ready for your baby, and prepare her cot.

Your midwife Her equipment will include a sphygmomanometer to take blood pressure; Pinnard stethoscope or sonicaid (see column, p.178); Entonox (gas and air) cylinder; urine-testing sticks; local anaesthetic and syringes; scissors; suture material; mucus extractor; resuscitation equipment; intravenous equipment, in case of bleeding; syntometrine. If you want to make sure there are pain-relieving drugs available, she'll give you a prescription in advance.

Going to hospital unexpectedly With the help of a skilled midwife or doctor, a home birth is completely safe for both you and your baby. But, as is also the case with hospital births, there can be complications, and if there's a serious problem you might have to go into hospital instead of having your baby at home. If that should happen, your midwife or doctor will go with you.

It can be bitterly disappointing if you can't give birth at home after all your plans, but if you and your partner accept that this might happen and talk about it in advance, it'll be easier to cope with if it you do have to transfer to hospital. It's better to tell yourself that you're going to start your labour at home and see how it goes before deciding where your baby will actually be born.

Factors against a home birth

Normally, it's as safe to give birth at home as it is in a hospital, but there are circumstances when a hospital birth is your only option.

Factors that will rule out a home birth include:

■ if you have a condition such as diabetes before your pregnancy, or you develop it during pregnancy

■ when you've had complications in previous pregnancies

■ when your pelvis is too small for your baby's head to pass through

■ when your baby is in the breech position

■ when you develop a medical problem that puts you, your baby, or both of you at risk, such as: high blood pressure; anaemia; excess amniotic fluid; active herpes; placenta praevia; abruptio placentae; pre-eclampsia; or eclampsia

■ when you have a multiple pregnancy

■ when your baby is premature

■ when your pregnancy goes well beyond your EDD (see p.260).

Your checklist

When your contractions begin, keep calm and don't rush: labour can last 12–14 hours for a first child and about seven hours for subsequent children.

When labour starts you need to:

■ notify the hospital

■ contact your partner or your birth coach to arrange your journey to the hospital. You should only call an ambulance in an emergency, for example, if you're bleeding heavily

■ advise whoever's going to look after your other children, if it's not your partner, that you are in labour

■ check that your hospital bag, your baby's bag, and your bag of labour aids are packed

■ sit down and wait calmly for your transport to arrive

■ make yourself a hot, sweet drink.

▶ **GETTING READY** Make sure that you have everything ready for your labour well in advance. Keep your bag packed and near the door.

Going to hospital

If you get everything ready in advance and pack the things you'll need to take with you to hospital, you won't have to worry about being caught unprepared.

What to take

The items you'll need with you in hospital fall into three groups: clothes and other personal things for you; the comfort aids you'll need for labour (see p.268); and clothes and nappies for your baby.

For you You'll need two or three maternity bras and front-opening cotton nightdresses, a supply of breast pads, a dressing gown and slippers, pants, and a supply of super-absorbent, stick-on sanitary towels (these may be supplied by the hospital). Pack an overnight bag with your hairbrush and shampoo, toothbrush and toothpaste, a couple of towels and facecloths, a small mirror, some make-up, face cream, hand cream, and tissues. If you've made a birth plan (see p.122), take it with you, along with your maternity notes.

For your baby Hospitals don't provide baby clothes or nappies so take your own. Take a blanket in which to wrap your baby when you leave the hospital, and a car seat if you are coming home by car.

Is it time?

When your due date is near, your body will begin to give you signals that it's preparing for the birth. You may have some symptoms of pre-labour (see p.270) and, in some cases, labour. Although you don't have to rush to hospital when you have any of the following, you do need to be ready for them and make your final preparations. The show normally comes first, and either the waters breaking or contractions will follow, although sometimes contractions come first. For more information see p.270.

The show The plug of blood-tinged mucus that has been sealing your cervix prior to birth becomes dislodged during the early first stage of labour, if not before. It can happen days or even weeks before labour.

The waters break Pressure caused by contractions or your baby's head pressing on the membranes of your amniotic sac may cause it to rupture before labour starts. The amniotic fluid will then escape.

Regular contractions Whether or not you've been aware of any contractions before, you start to experience them as severe cramp-like pains that come at regular intervals and last longer and longer. The interval between contractions gets shorter.

When to go

If, over an hour, you notice your contractions are coming every five to 15 minutes, are about one minute long, and don't die away when you move around, or when you feel you can't cope without pain relief, call your labour ward or midwife, depending on what you've arranged. At this time, your first level of breathing (see column p.282) will probably no longer be enough, and you'll be getting ready to use other breathing patterns as pre-labour eases into the first stage. There's still plenty of time to check that you have everything you need and to get to the hospital.

There's absolutely no need to rush into hospital because the first stage usually lasts at least eight hours for a first baby and can be 12–14 hours. But if you live a long way from the hospital or you're particularly worried about getting there in time, go as soon as you feel that you have to.

Transport You'll probably travel to the hospital by car, by taxi, or, in an emergency, by ambulance. Never try to drive yourself. If you call an ambulance or taxi, be sure to give your full address and, if necessary, a clear description of how to get to your house so there's no delay. If you are planning to go by car, make sure that the car has been serviced recently and that there's plenty of fuel in the tank from about week 38.

Your journey to hospital

If you're travelling to hospital by car or taxi, do what you can to make your journey safe and comfortable.

In the weeks leading up to the birth, make sure that both you and whoever's going to drive you to the hospital know the route really well. Find out how long the journey is likely to take at different times of the day, and work out alternative routes in case there's exceptionally heavy traffic or other delays on the day. Find out if you need to take any money for the car park and make sure you have the right change ready. It's also a good idea to check the different entrances to the hospital and find out how to get to the labour ward from each of them — especially at night.

The car The bigger the car you travel in, the more comfortable you're likely to be. You'll probably feel safer and more comfortable in the back seat.

Sudden birth If your baby starts to arrive while you're still on your way to the hospital, stay as calm as you can. If you're close to the hospital, you have a good chance of getting there before your baby is actually born, but if you're farther away, stop the car at the nearest telephone, call for an ambulance, and then get ready for an emergency delivery (see also p.304).

Drinks and food

It's important to save your energy during the first stage, in case you have a long and tiring labour.

Many hospitals suggest that you don't eat anything during labour in case there's an unexpected emergency and you need a general anaesthetic. Take glucose sweets to suck, and high-energy isotonic sports drinks to help you keep up your energy levels. Your partner will also need food so he should make himself a snack to take – perhaps sandwiches and fruit and a flask of coffee.

Take something for you to have later as well – you'll probably be ravenous after the birth and you'll want something to eat right away.

You'll also need plenty to drink – a bottle or vacuum flask of diluted unsweetened fruit juice or cold water is ideal.

Comfort aids for labour

When you're gathering together all the things you'll need for the birth, think about any items that will make your labour a more comfortable experience. It's best to get your comfort aids ready in advance. That way you won't forget anything in the excitement when labour starts, and you won't be caught unprepared if your labour starts sooner than you expect.

Items you'll find helpful

Your midwife or hospital attendants will suggest things you might find helpful during labour. If you're having a home birth, keep all your comfort aids together in the room where you're going to give birth. If you're having a hospital birth, pack them in a bag, and put it next to your case. Make sure your birth assistant knows where they are, and doesn't forget them at the last minute.

Keeping warm During the later stages of labour, and particularly immediately after the birth, some women begin to shake quite visibly with cold. Have some warm clothes and leg warmers or thick socks ready in case this happens to you.

Keeping cool If you want something wet and cool in your mouth but you don't want a drink, try sucking an ice cube or crushed ice. Most hospitals will now provide ice. Alternatively, moisten your lips and mouth by sucking on a small natural sponge that's been dipped in cold water. If you feel hot and sweaty, ask your partner to bathe your face with a cool face cloth and create a refreshing breeze with a hand-held fan.

General comfort If your hair is long or falls in your face, tie it back with hair grips, slides, or a hairband so that it doesn't irritate you. Your lips are likely to become dry because of breathing through your mouth, so include a lipsalve or chapstick to stop them cracking.

If you feel nauseous and actually vomit, you'll feel much better if you can clean your teeth, so don't forget to take your toothbrush and some toothpaste. A box of tissues may come in handy, as may some scented wipes in single packs that can be opened when needed and used to

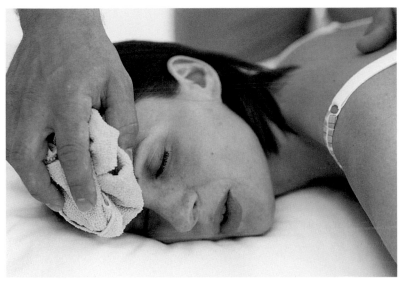

▲ **COOLING DOWN** If you start to feel very hot and sweaty during labour, a gentle wipe with a cool flannel can be very soothing.

Your birth partner

Your birth partner will need to take along his own comfort aids to help him through the labour. Here are some suggestions:

■ a pack of wipes for freshening face and hands

■ snacks and drinks

■ change of clothing

■ camera, or video camera if that's allowed

■ telephone numbers of family and friends, and coins or phone card – generally, you can't use mobile phones in hospital.

cleanse your face, neck, and hands. For freshening up you may want to splash on some eau de cologne.

Distractions Many women find that massage soothes the discomfort of labour (see p.202). Your partner can provide counterpressure with his hands, a spinal roll, or even a tennis ball or rolling pin! Use a small amount of talcum powder or vegetable-based massage oil to stop your skin from being dragged or pinched. A hot water bottle or a hot pad placed in the small of your back can act as a compress to soothe backache. In the early stages before labour really gets going, you might feel that nothing much happens for long periods. You might find it helpful to distract yourself with books and magazines or even some playing cards and board games.

Your checklist

Use the following as a checklist when packing your bag of comfort aids for a home or hospital birth.

■ Food and drink
■ Spinal roll or tennis ball
■ Massage oil or talcum powder
■ Hot water bottle
■ Books, magazines, cards, games
■ Some favourite music
■ Small natural sponge

■ Face cloth and hand-held fan
■ Warm clothes and thick socks
■ Hair clips, slides, or hairband
■ Lipsalve or chapstick
■ Toothbrush and toothpaste
■ Box of tissues or wet wipes
■ Eau de cologne

Your mood changes

As you wait for signs that your baby is ready to be born, you may feel a number of emotions.

Contentment As your body changes in preparation for labour, you may find that you respond to the ripening of your womb in a sensual way. Particularly if this is your first baby, you may like to enjoy these last days on your own indulging your whims, sharing moments of intimacy with your partner, or spending the time just daydreaming.

Elation You may feel a great sense of joy when your body alerts you to the moment that you've been waiting for with such excitement. Don't try to quench this feeling; share it with the people around you as it may help to release any pangs of nervous tension.

Anxiety The signs of pre-labour can make you feel apprehensive. You may worry about the pain of labour and its effect on your baby and you may wonder if you'll be able to cope. You may feel nervous about your waters breaking in an embarrassing situation.

Impatience If your expected date of delivery comes and goes, don't be depressed. Remember it's only an approximate date and that most babies arrive sooner or later than expected. This is particularly likely if you were born sooner or later than expected.

Pre-labour and labour

Medically, labour is divided into three stages. In the first stage, your cervix opens fully to allow your baby to pass through; in the second stage, your baby descends through the vagina; in the third stage, the placenta is delivered. All these stages are discussed in detail over the following pages. As well as these stages, most women experience pre-labour.

Pre-labour

Before real labour begins, hormones from your uterus and your baby prepare your body for birth in a number of ways. During the last few weeks, you'll probably notice signs of your coming labour. But just as each woman's experience of labour and birth is unique, so these pre-labour symptoms affect everyone in different ways. They do provide useful signals to warn you that labour is imminent.

Engagement To position himself for the journey through the birth canal, your baby will move lower down so that his presenting part, usually his head, settles into your bony pelvis (see opposite). This is known as engagement and you'll experience it as a feeling of lightening.

If this is your first pregnancy, your baby will probably engage two to three weeks before the labour starts. If you've had previous babies, your baby's head may stay higher until just before labour starts, because your uterine muscles have stretched and so exert less pressure on your baby.

You'll know when your baby has engaged because there's less pressure on your diaphragm and breathing becomes easier. On the other hand, you'll probably find you have to pass urine more often, as your baby will now be pressing down on your bladder.

Braxton Hicks contractions Your uterus practises for the strong contractions needed in labour with weak, irregular contractions, named after the doctor who first described them. Most women feel these during the last few months. If you place your hand on your abdomen, you may feel a hardening and tightening of your uterus, which lasts for approximately 25 seconds. Unlike real labour contractions, these are usually painless, although some women find them uncomfortable. If you do feel any discomfort, sit down quietly until the feeling eases. You may find you get more and stronger Braxton Hicks contractions as real labour approaches. This is your body's way of preparing the cervix to dilate and increasing the circulation of blood to the placenta.

When you feel a run of Braxton Hicks, practise the relaxation techniques you're going to use during labour; the tightening and relaxing of your uterus will give you a good idea of how a contraction feels as it waxes, and then wanes. Some mothers misinterpret Braxton Hicks for real labour pains and go to hospital, only to be told they can go home again (see A false labour? p.272).

Nesting instinct You may suddenly feel like making final preparations for the arrival of your baby. If you want to rush around cleaning or decorating the house, or cooking large meals, try to restrain yourself. Save this extra energy for coping with labour and delivery.

The show A sign that labour is coming soon is the appearance of the show – a thick sticky discharge that occurs when the plug of mucus that seals your cervix in pregnancy, providing protection against infection, becomes dislodged. Although this often doesn't appear until labour is underway, the cervix may widen enough for the mucus plug to be dislodged up to 12 days before labour begins. The show may be slightly brown, pink, or blood-tinged from the capillaries that attached it to the cervix. The show signals dilation of the cervix.

Premenstrual feelings You may notice some physical and emotional changes similar to those you have before a menstrual period. You may also feel crampy, with some pressure in your rectum, and feel the need to empty your bowels and pass urine more often than usual.

Your baby's descent

Your midwife will check your baby's progress down your birth canal by an internal examination. She measures the baby's position in "stations", or lines, calculated in centimetres from −5 to +5 in relation to the level of your ischial spines (specific anatomical points on your pelvis) and the top of your baby's head, see right.

What your baby's doing

While no one actually knows for certain why labour starts, there's increasing evidence to suggest that your baby plays a major role.

Hormones The start of labour is triggered by hormones – the levels of some pregnancy hormones drop, others rise. New hormones are secreted, one of which is produced by your baby.

Engagement Throughout your pregnancy, your baby will be floating in his amniotic sac above your pelvic brim. As his birth approaches, his head, or his bottom if he is in a breech position, will descend lower down into your pelvis and become engaged.

Kicking less You may notice that your baby becomes quieter than in previous months. From time to time you may feel a slight flurry of movement, but if his actions seem to stop completely, get in touch with your doctor or midwife.

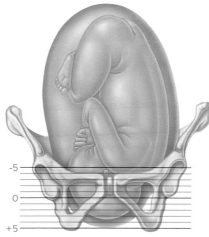

-5

0

+5

◀ **YOUR BABY'S PROGRESS** When the top of your baby's head first enters your pelvis it's at station −5. When it is level with your ischial spines it is then at station 0 (engaged). The other stations describe the position of the baby's head as it passes via the birth canal to the vaginal opening – station +5.

A false labour?

In a first pregnancy it's not always easy to tell false from real labour. As a general rule, if you're in doubt, you're not in real labour.

Although false labour is only a rehearsal, don't be too disappointed – it means that real labour isn't too far off. There are some very simple differences between the contractions of false and real labour.

Regularity False contractions never really settle down and become truly regular.

Frequency False contractions are sporadic. They may vary from 10 minutes to 20 minutes to 15 minutes, with no steady pattern.

Effect of movement False contractions usually weaken or stop altogether if you get up and move around, whereas real contractions increase.

Strength False contractions do not get progressively stronger. They may even weaken from time to time and disappear altogether.

Some women, especially if they are working and get overtired or overexcited, slip in and out of false labour for a few days before real labour begins.

Tell your doctor or midwife about the contractions if you're concerned. If you can't contact them, check with your hospital and go to hospital if you want to. If you stay at home keep on the move and stay upright to help labour.

The first stage

In medical terms, the first stage starts when your contractions bring about the opening (dilation) and thinning (effacement) of the cervix, and ends when these are complete. At this point, your midwife will confirm that you are fully dilated.

What happens in labour

It's difficult to be sure about the onset of labour as it differs from woman to woman. Certain classic signs – intense contractions, dilatation and thinning of the cervix, and rupturing of the membranes – are taken to mean that labour is underway.

Contractions When true labour starts, the nature of your contractions changes. They become more rhythmical, more painful, and they come at regular intervals. These contractions are not within your control and, once they have begun, won't stop until your baby is born.

You can time your contractions from the start of one contraction to the start of the next. In early labour, contractions are usually 30–60 seconds long and come at intervals of five to 20 minutes. This can vary as some women may not notice their contractions until they are closer together, say every five minutes. During the active phase, contractions usually last 60–90 seconds, at intervals of two to four minutes.

As your uterine muscles tighten, you may feel something like menstrual cramps, spreading around your lower abdomen like a tight band. This is because the uterine muscle becomes short of oxygen as its blood vessels are compressed. The uterus is a huge muscle and needs a lot of energy during contractions.

Every woman feels contraction pains differently, but in early labour they may be similar to menstrual cramps or a mild backache. Some women experience severe backache (see p.296). Very often a contraction feels like a wave of discomfort right across your abdomen that reaches a peak for a few seconds and then diminishes. At the same time, you can feel a hardening and tightening of the uterine muscle, which is held at the peak of its intensity for a few seconds before the muscle begins to relax.

Women assume that contractions will get steadily longer, more frequent, and stronger. This is not so; don't be disturbed if your contractions seem to vary. It's as normal for a strong contraction to be followed by a weaker one that doesn't last quite as long as it is for contractions to follow one another relentlessly.

Your cervix dilates and thins The cervix is usually a thick-walled canal about 2cm (¾in) long, and firmly closed. In the last few weeks, pregnancy hormones may soften your cervix, but the intense contractions of first-stage labour are needed to dilate and thin it. Dilation is measured in centimetres from 0–10cm (up to 4in). Your cervix will only dilate about 4cm (1½in) during the latent phase, then progress to 8cm (3in) in the active phase (see column, right). The pain increases as it becomes fully dilated during transition. Eventually, the whole cervix opens up and is made one with the body of the uterus, creating a continuous channel that your baby can pass through.

Your waters break The membranes of the amniotic sac may rupture painlessly at any time during labour, although this usually happens towards the end of the first stage. Fluid may leak or gush out; the flow depends on the size and site of the break and whether or not the baby's head is plugging the hole. Usually, if the membranes rupture spontaneously near term, labour follows within a short time, although occasionally it's delayed.

How long does labour last?

Labour times vary greatly, but an average labour lasts 12–14 hours for first-time mums, and about seven hours for subsequent labours. If labour lasts longer than 14 hours the first time, or nine hours in subsequent labours, your doctor will want to find out why and may intervene. The first stage of labour can be further divided into three separate phases. The latent phase is the longest, lasting about eight hours for first babies, and you'll feel contractions coming with increasing frequency and length, but they won't be too distressing. The next, active phase, will be shorter, lasting about three to five hours, but this is when your contractions become more painful, and you may want some pain relief (see p.280). The final, transitional phase, is the shortest and most intense of all, usually lasting just under an hour, and comes right before the delivery.

Transition Your contractions will now last about 60–90 seconds, with intervals of only 30–90 seconds. As the contractions become more forceful, you may find it hard to relax and this is the time you may feel the most discomfort. You may also feel a very strong urge to push, but should not do so unless you're fully dilated.

The intense pain may make you feel extremely irritable, even bad-tempered, with your birth partner. You may also feel that you can't go on any more, but you'll find hidden resources of energy to help you cope. Remind yourself that your baby's birth is now just minutes away.

What happens to your cervix

During the first stage the cervix, which is normally tough, must be stretched thin and needs to open wide before your baby's head is able to pass through.

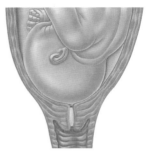

▲ **LATENT PHASE** Your cervix remains about 2cm (¾in) long until contractions start thinning it out (effacing).

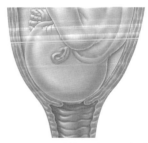

▲ **ACTIVE PHASE** When the cervical canal is thinned out, further contractions will widen (dilate) your cervix.

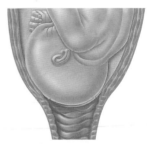

▲ **TRANSITIONAL PHASE** The last part of your cervix at the front has opened to 10cm (4in). You are now fully dilated.

Going to hospital

When you arrive at the hospital, your midwife will prepare you for the birth and give you a few routine checks.

■ Your midwife will look at your notes and ask you some questions about how your labour's going – whether your waters have broken and how often you're having contractions.

■ Then she'll examine you: she'll palpate your abdomen to feel what position your baby's in; she'll listen to your baby's heartbeat, take your blood pressure, pulse, and temperature; and give you an internal examination to see how far your cervix has dilated.

■ You'll be asked to give a urine sample to test for the presence of protein and sugar.

■ You'll be asked when you last moved your bowels. You won't be given an enema or a suppository unless you ask.

■ Then you'll have a shower or bath and settle in to your delivery room. If you've any questions or there's anything you want to tell the hospital staff about your preferences, now is the time.

Hospital procedures

Hospitals can be intimidating but are much less so when you get to know them, so it's a good idea to have a look at the labour and delivery rooms, meet the staff who'll be looking after you, and get some idea about ward routine before your due date.

Admission to hospital You'll have outlined in your birth plan (see p.122) how you'd like your labour to proceed, and once you've met your midwife or doctor, this is the time to make sure they have a copy of your plan so that you can look over it with them, and talk to them about it. They'll also make some checks and ask you a few questions about your labour (see column, left, and p.116).

If there's anything you're not happy with, if equipment, lights, and needles frighten you, for example, or if you're upset by a staff member, do something about it right away. Don't wait, letting your fears and anxieties fester and grow. Your partner or birth coach can voice your feelings if you aren't feeling strong enough to be assertive.

Examinations Your baby's heart will be checked regularly by a sonicaid, or an electronic fetal monitor (see below). Your midwife will probably give you an internal check every four hours during the first stage to see how far your cervix has dilated but there's no hard and fast rule.

Each time you have an internal check, ask how things are going. It's very comforting to know how far your cervix has dilated between examinations. If you're asked a question while you're having a contraction, concentrate on your relaxation techniques and answer the question when the contraction is over.

Pain relief Once you've been admitted, an anaesthetist will visit you if you've asked for an epidural (see p.281), and the procedure will be set up. This usually takes ten to 20 minutes. If a top-up is needed, this can usually be given by your midwife. If you've decided not to have any medical pain relief, you will be left with your birth coach and a midwife who'll stay with you throughout your labour.

Electronic fetal monitoring

This high-tech replacement for the ear trumpet is used to track your baby's heartbeat. In all high-risk pregnancies, electronic fetal monitoring (EFM) or a cardiotocograph (CTG) will be used throughout labour for your own and especially your baby's safety. You'll have monitoring if you are being induced or your labour is being accelerated for any reason, or if you're having epidural anaesthesia. The main function of the monitoring is to give early warning if your baby is in any distress.

What it is There are two kinds of electronic monitors, external and internal. A hand-held external monitor is used for routine short periods of monitoring. Sometimes it's necessary to monitor the baby's heartbeat over a longer period of time. For this a special belt with sensors that record the baby's heartbeat and your uterine contractions is strapped around your abdomen, the readings are then printed out on a graph.

The internal monitor is slightly more accurate. You'll have a belt strapped around your body and a tiny electrode will be clipped on to your baby's scalp once your cervix is 2–3cm (1–1¼in) dilated. The baby's heartbeat is printed out on a paper trace.

How it works During a contraction, the blood flow to your placenta is reduced for a few seconds, and your baby's heart rate may dip. The heart rate should return to what it was before when the contraction passes. If it doesn't or the return is delayed, your baby may be distressed and your medical team may need to take action to protect his wellbeing.

If the medical staff are worried that your baby is not getting enough oxygen, they may want to take a tiny sample of his blood – a fetal blood sample (FBS). Analysis of this blood gives your doctor and midwife a good idea of how your baby is coping with labour.

How monitoring helps doctors EFM provides medical staff with a second-by-second report on your baby's condition. It alerts the doctors if your baby is in distress so that they can intervene before anything untoward has happened. If your doctors decide that you and your baby would be better off with monitoring, try not to resent it. Look on it as something that gives reassurance that your baby is doing fine.

Disadvantages The use of monitoring means that there'll be more electronic equipment in the delivery room, making the atmosphere very clinical. You may also feel that the midwifery staff might concentrate more on the machine than on you. As they are aware of any tiny changes that may take place, they're more likely to intervene rather than letting labour take its natural course.

However, many mothers do find it comforting to know that the doctors and midwives will know right away if there are any problems with the baby during labour.

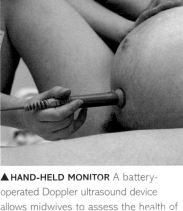

▲ **HAND-HELD MONITOR** A battery-operated Doppler ultrasound device allows midwives to assess the health of the fetus's heartbeat throughout labour. Alternatively, a belt may be strapped around your abdomen for a short while, which is connected to a machine that gives a printout of the heartbeat.

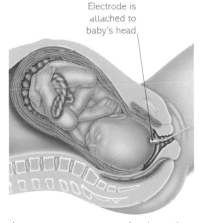

Electrode is attached to baby's head

▲ **INTERNAL MONITORING** An electrode is attached to the baby's presenting part, usually his head, by piercing the skin. This provides an electrical contact that picks up his heartbeat. Some babies' heads will be bruised or have a rash where the electrode was attached to them. Many mothers do find this device reassuring as they can watch their baby's heartbeat throughout labour.

Partner's role in labour

The more secure and relaxed a mother feels during labour, the better she'll be able to cope. Her partner is the natural person to give this loving support. Otherwise, a friend who's had children makes a good birth coach.

▼ **SUPPORTING YOUR PARTNER** If your partner leans back against you, you can support her weight and cuddle her at the same time.

Understanding your role

It's normal to feel nervous about the idea of supporting at a birth, so the best thing to do is prepare yourself. Find out as much as you can so you're able to help the mother meet the physical and emotional demands of labour. At antenatal classes there'll be demonstrations to describe labour's onset and the effect of contractions, and you'll be taught techniques to help her relax.

If it's going to be a hospital birth, visit the hospital's labour and delivery rooms and introduce yourself to the staff. If the birth is to be at home, make sure you know the route to hospital in case of an emergency, and find out all you'll need to do; trust will create a calmer atmosphere.

How to help during labour

You may have a very active role throughout the labour and birth, but sometimes your presence is all the mother needs. Make sure you're very familiar with her birth plan and the alternative version (see p.122) and that you know all her wishes.

Use your intuition Judge the situation by observing your partner's moods. She may want to stay quiet, going through contractions alone without being touched. Or she may need lots of encouragement, or distractions.

Provide emotional support Remain as close and intimate as you can, using loving words, and keep your movements slow, quiet, and steady. Be positive: praise her and don't criticize. If she wants to hear your voice, constantly tell her how well she's doing (how far dilated) and how she can relax herself. Tell her what the midwife is doing and what will soon happen. Also, help her to see how much she's achieved already – it's easy for her to be overwhelmed by how far she thinks she has to go. Massage and stroke her slowly, but if she just wants to hold your hand, you can encourage her by the expression on your face and lots of eye contact. Sometimes just the look of love in her partner's eyes can help a woman bear the pain of contractions.

Combat tiredness Before labour, encourage her to rest as much as possible. If her labour is long and tiring, try to help her relax between contractions and save her energy for the second stage. If she's not feeling nauseous, provide her with any drinks or nourishment she wants (see also p.268).

Help her cope with pain It's hard to see someone you care about in pain, but try not to show your anxiety as it could make her feel more worried. On the other hand, don't dismiss her suffering. Acknowledge it positively, telling her each contraction is bringing the baby's birth nearer, and make different suggestions for relief. Help her not to be embarrassed about saying what hurts – encourage her to be as uninhibited as possible. A woman in labour should never be ashamed of needing pain relief.

It she feels particularly anxious during a contraction, it might calm her fears to talk about how she felt before the next one starts. Don't take it personally if she's critical or aggressive towards you – this often happens when the pain is very intense.

Help with breathing You'll probably have practised your partner's preferred method in antenatal classes, but let her follow her own rhythm. If she seems to lose control, stay close by and slowly guide her through the pattern until she's able to carry on alone. Be ready to adapt – very few people follow exactly what they practised at antenatal classes.

Make her comfortable You can be a great help here. Suggest different positions (see p.278) and support her with cushions or blankets, or let her lean against you while you cuddle, and rock together. Look out for signs of tension in her neck, shoulders, or forehead, and gently stroke these areas. Massage may give some relief from pain, and if she's using visualization techniques, gently talk her through them. She'll probably find having her face and hands wiped very soothing, and give her ice cubes to suck. If she feels cold, help her put on socks, or leg warmers. As labour progresses she may want to talk less, but you can keep in touch by touching or caressing, or by using eye contact.

How your partner can help

A birth partner can do a lot to help you during labour, not only providing reassurance and comfort, but also dealing with staff. Try to remember that although the hospital uniforms and equipment may appear daunting, the medical team is there to support you.

Your birth partner can:

■ answer questions for you (if allowed to by the staff), which saves you having your concentration disturbed

■ support you in the positions you choose for pain relief and/or to give birth

■ stroke and massage you if you find it comforting

■ change the atmosphere (dim the lights, change the music) for you

■ ask people to leave if there are too many in your personal space during a home birth, and ask any students present at a hospital delivery to leave if they are inhibiting you

■ be the one you can really rely on to deal with the medical staff and to stand by your decisions on pain relief – whether to accept it or not, and if so, when and how much. If you do decide to ask for relief, he should encourage you to have a breathing space of 15 minutes before it's administered, as things can change quickly, and you may find you don't need it.

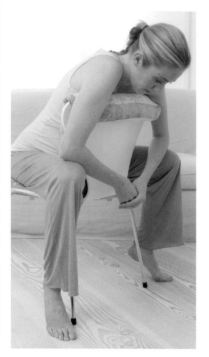

First stage positions

There are many different positions that you can take up to ease your discomfort. Some women prefer to stand and move around during labour, as this helps to strengthen contractions, which in turn accelerates labour. If you do stand, try leaning forwards against your partner or a wall. This will take the weight of your baby off your spine and make your contractions more efficient. As your contractions get stronger, you may prefer to sit or kneel, using cushions or chairs for support.

◄ **SITTING** If you find it more comfortable to sit down, try leaning forwards with your legs wide apart. You can sit facing the chair back, resting on a pillow or cushion. Or you may prefer to support yourself by leaning against your birth assistant, who can also rub your back.

▶ **KNEELING** As your contractions strengthen, you may find it less tiring to go down on to your hands and knees. This helps to ease any backache. Keep your legs wide apart, and rock your pelvis. Between your contractions, lean forward on to your folded arms or sit back on your heels.

Rock your pelvis backward and forward during contractions to relieve backache

Make sure your back is straight and don't allow it to arch

▶ DURING TRANSITION If your cervix isn't fully dilated towards the end of the first stage, just before giving birth, use gravity to slow down your baby while your cervix continues to open. Lean on to a pile of cushions with your legs wide apart, or kneel with your head down and your bottom raised.

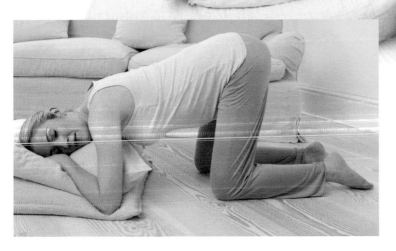

◀ RELIEVING BACKACHE Kneeling on the floor with your bottom raised and your head down helps to take the pressure off your lower back and relieve backache. Put your head on a couple of pillows or cushions.

▼ LYING DOWN There may be times during labour when you just want to lie down. Try lying on your side, and place cushions under your head and upper thigh. Keep your legs wide apart.

Relax your shoulders, and concentrate on your breathing with your eyes closed

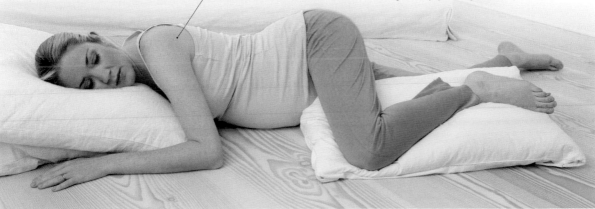

How drugs affect you

Drugs give you relief from pain but they can affect your experience of childbirth in other ways. Make sure you opt for the type that will help to improve, rather than detract from, the pleasure of your baby's birth.

Drowsiness This is a common side effect of gas and oxygen, and narcotics. Some women enjoy the feeling of drifting, but sometimes the sleepiness can make mothers feel they lack control. After using narcotics such as pethidine, a few women become so lightheaded that they're unaware of what's happening around them, and give birth without even realizing it's happening.

Dizziness Pethidine and other narcotics can sometimes bring on a feeling of confusion, or disorientation, and some mothers have even had hallucinations.

Nausea The sensation of nausea is usually quite slight with gas and oxygen, but is common after using pethidine and other narcotics. A few mothers may experience vomiting attacks.

Your state of mind can have a major influence on how much pain you feel during labour. If you feel very tense your uterus may be affected, slowing down labour and adversely affecting your baby (see column, opposite), so if having some pain-relieving drugs makes you feel less anxious, there's no point in depriving yourself.

Pain relief

For many women, excitement about their baby's birth may be overshadowed by worry about pain during labour. Build up your confidence by preparing for the intensity of contractions, by understanding your own limits of pain tolerance, and by learning about methods of pain relief. Try to think of the pain in a positive way – each contraction brings the birth of your baby nearer.

Coping with pain

The kind of pain you'll experience during contractions varies. Very often, it feels like a thick band being squeezed around your abdomen as the uterine muscles harden and tighten for a few seconds before relaxing. Some women describe it as being like severe menstrual cramp, others feel backache, but there may be a mixture of sensations as the contraction peaks, culminating in a wave of discomfort, which then subsides.

Individual response You may prefer not to use drugs during labour because they can dim your awareness of what's happening and deprive you of the sensation of giving birth. It's difficult, though, to know your own pain threshold, particularly if this is your first baby. Some women are surprised by the overpowering intensity of their contractions; for others the pain may be made worse by fear and anxiety.

Pain relief in childbirth can be complete, as in epidural anaesthesia, or it can reduce pain to bearable levels as with gas and air and narcotics. Many women choose to have no drugs in the early part of the first stage, then have a low dose of gas and air towards transition. Don't blame yourself if you want some pain relief with drugs. Your labour isn't a test, and the use of drugs may even be essential for you to deliver your baby.

If you haven't made up your mind about the use of painkillers, you may want to do without drugs for as long as possible. If so, a useful tip is to wait 15 minutes after you feel you want pain relief before actually having it. During that time your labour may progress well, and it gives you and your birth partner time to discuss whether or not you can get by with encouragement, or whether you really do feel the pain is increasing to the point where you need some relief.

If you want to participate fully in your baby's birth without dimming your consciousness of the feelings involved, there are alternatives to drugs for pain relief. Also, your body can provide its own brand of painkiller and relaxant, endorphins. The more natural your labour, the more quickly your own endorphins will be produced and your pain threshold increased.

A clear choice Find out as much as you can about the types of pain relief available. Talk to your doctor, midwife, and hospital staff, and outline your choices in your birth plan (see p.122). Have an alternative version ready in case any complications arise. Don't hesitate to question the use of drugs, or ask your midwife's advice.

Pain-relieving drugs

Some types of pain relief will only be available in large or teaching hospitals; others are available in all hospitals. Your midwife will also have certain types for use in a home delivery.

Regional anaesthetics These remove feeling from part of your body by blocking the transmission of pain from nerve fibres. There are several different sorts. Most widely used is the epidural block (see below). This prevents pain spreading from your uterus by acting as a "nerve block" in your spine. A well-managed epidural removes all sensation from your waist to your knees, but you remain alert. Doctors may recommend an epidural if you have a difficult labour, pre-eclampsia, or severe asthma, or if you have a forceps delivery.

If you choose an epidural for pain relief, you'll be given a local anaesthetic in your back to numb the area for the injection. The anaesthetist then inserts a fine, hollow needle into the epidural space and a thin tube known as a catheter is threaded down inside the hollow needle. The needle is removed, leaving the catheter in position. Anaesthetic is syringed down the catheter, which is then sealed, although it can be topped up if necessary.

Most mothers who have a Caesarean now have a spinal instead of a general anaesthetic so they're awake during the birth. A spinal anaesthetic is similar to an epidural but is a single injection and no catheter is left in place.

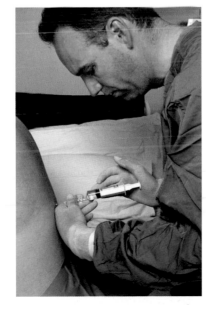

How drugs affect your baby

Once they're in your bloodstream, most drugs will cross the placenta to affect your baby. There'll be a higher concentration of the drugs in your baby's blood than in your own.

Drowsiness Pethidine can make your baby drowsy after the birth, which may affect his ability to suckle and to respond to you after he's born.

Breathing difficulties Narcotics can depress your baby's respiration. If you take pethidine late in your labour it will remain in your baby's bloodstream for longer.

Drugs used in epidural anaesthesia cannot enter your baby's blood. A baby born after anaesthesia stands a very good chance of being alert and of breathing well.

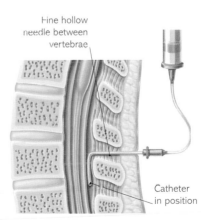

Fine hollow needle between vertebrae

Catheter in position

◀ **EPIDURAL ANAESTHETIC** You'll have an injection of local anaesthetic in your back, to numb it (see left). A fine, hollow needle is inserted between the vertebrae (see above), through which a catheter (tube) is threaded. The anaesthetic is delivered via the tube.

Ways you can breathe

Relaxing your body and focusing on your breathing will help to soothe your tension and anxiety and let you ride out your contractions. Practise breathing patterns beforehand with your partner or birth coach so they can help you during labour.

Slow breathing In the early stages, calmly and deliberately breathe out through your mouth as the contraction begins. Then slowly breathe in through your nose. Keep up the same steady pattern throughout the contraction, which may last about 45–60 seconds.

Light breathing As your contractions become more intense and frequent, you may find it easier to breathe above them. Take light, short breaths that seem to involve only the upper part of your body and not your abdomen where the contraction takes place.

You'll probably find that you'll use different breathing techniques at different stages of your labour.

Inhalation analgesics This is a gas that consists of nitrous oxide and oxygen (entonox), commonly called "gas and air". You administer it yourself using a face mask or a mouthpiece. You inhale deeply as the contraction starts, and carry on until it peaks, or you've had enough. You then put the mask aside and breathe normally. Gas works by numbing the pain centre in the brain, and can make you feel as though you're floating. You may be shown the inhalation technique in an antenatal class.

Narcotics The most commonly used narcotics are pethidine and meptazinol (Meptit). Both are morphine-like drugs and are given by injection in your thigh or buttock in varying dosages during the first stage. They dull the pain by acting on the nerve cells in your brain and spine. If you choose to take a narcotic, ask for a small dose (50–75mg) to see how you're affected – you can always have more, but once injected it can't be taken away. Narcotics usually take about 20 minutes to work.

Relief without drugs

Make sure you know as much as you can about your chosen pain-relief method, and you've shown your birth coach the technique, before you go into labour. If you need any special equipment, check it's available at home or in hospital. One method on its own may not be enough – you may need a combination for more complete relief.

Positions Walking around, leaning against your partner or the wall, and rocking your pelvis will probably feel much more comfortable than lying on your back. There are some positions that may feel more comfortable than others, as these will relieve the pressure on your back (see p.278).

Massage This is a wonderful way of relieving discomfort, whether you're lying, standing, or squatting, and greatly reassuring. It's particularly good if you have backache in labour, as about 90 per cent of women do (see column, right), or if you suffer from a backache labour (see p.296). Your partner will need to practise the technique beforehand.

Sounds You may find it helps to diffuse the pain and anxiety of labour to make different sounds. Sighing, moaning, groaning, and grunting are all ways of releasing tension. Don't feel inhibited about the noise you make, or worry about disturbing others – just go ahead and make as much noise as you want. Many women find that listening to music is helpful. Light, uplifting music may help you rise above your contraction. When your contractions intensify, more dramatic music, building to a crescendo, may help you cope.

Water Lying in warm water can be very relaxing and soothing. When in water you're virtually weightless and this brings relief between contractions. More and more mothers are using birthing pools under supervision (see p.107) and many hospitals have this facility. You can also hire a pool for use at home. If you want to use a birthing pool, check early in pregnancy so that you can be sure one will be available.

Visualizing Creating images in your mind can be a very effective way of calming fear and reducing pain. As your contraction begins, imagine something that you find particularly soothing, for example warm, bright sunshine. Contractions in the first stage are opening your cervix and you may find it helpful to imagine the bud of your favourite flower opening very slowly, petal by petal. Many women find thinking about ocean waves comforting, matching the flow of the waves with their own contractions.

Hypnobirthing If you choose hypnosis for pain relief during labour you'll need to be prepared by a trained hypnotherapist during five or so 30-minute visits throughout pregnancy. Hypnosis is a natural and safe state of profound relaxation. You remain fully present and aware during the birth. Research shows that hypnosis can lessen the pain of labour, shorten its length, and reduce the incidence of postnatal depression.

Acupuncture Only choose this method if you've already found that it can relieve pain in other situations. You'll also need an acupuncturist who's familiar with labour and delivery. Acupuncture may not completely relieve pain, but it will certainly reduce it, and it helps to stop nausea.

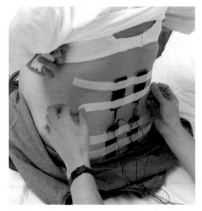

▲ **POSITIONING A TENS MACHINE** Sticky-pad electrodes are fixed in position on either side of your spine with adhesive tape. TENS is not addictive and doesn't have any side effects.

TENS (transcutaneous electrical nerve stimulation)

In this technique, pain impulses conducted by nerves are blocked by an electric current, which also stimulates the production of the body's endorphins. A battery-powered stimulator is connected by wires to electrodes placed on either side of your spine. You'll be given a handset that regulates the stimulation, allowing you to control the amount of pain relief that you receive. If you'd like to try out a TENS machine ask your midwife.

Relieving backache

Many women suffer from backache during labour, sometimes because of the baby's head pressing against the sacrum. Your partner can help to relieve any discomfort by gently massaging your lower back during labour.

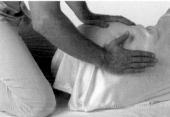

▲ **RUBBING THE SACRUM** Using the heel of your hand, rub all around your partner's sacrum and lower back.

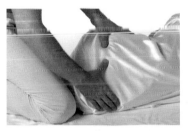

▲ **CIRCULAR PRESSURE** Press your thumbs over the sacrum and move them gently in a circle. Rest your hands on your partner's hips for support.

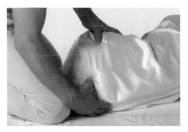

▲ **DEEP PRESSURE** Press your thumbs into the middle of each buttock. Encourage your partner to focus on her breathing to help her relax.

Breathing in the second stage

You'll be shown breathing exercises in antenatal classes. I can't stress enough how important good breathing techniques are during the second stage of labour. They help you feel in control of your own body and this is very empowering.

As you begin the second stage of labour, you may want to accelerate your breathing. This is the most shallow form of breathing you use in labour. Instead of using your chest and throat, focus on breathing only through your mouth. Breathe lightly in and out through your lips, starting slowly and gradually speeding up. Be careful not to breathe out too deeply or you'll start to hyperventilate. If you start to feel at all dizzy, place your hands lightly over your nose and mouth while you're breathing.

▶ **INTO THE SECOND STAGE** At the end of the first stage of labour your cervix will be fully dilated. The first sign that this has happened can be that you'll feel a tremendous urge to push, but always ask your midwife to check that your cervix is fully dilated. Once you know you're dilated you can push with force. Stay as upright as you can so that gravity can help make your contractions more efficient. Your partner and midwife can help support you. Your mood will change and you'll feel energized and positive as you work hard towards the birth – now only a short time away.

The second stage: delivery

Delivery is the main event: it's what you've been waiting and preparing for over the last nine months. Your expectations are realistic – a manageable labour, not necessarily painless but happy and relaxed, with your chosen birth partner and staff you know around you in familiar surroundings.

Contractions and pushing

The second stage is the expulsive stage – you push your baby out. It lasts from the time your cervix is fully dilated until your baby is born and, for a first baby, generally takes less than two hours. The average second stage lasts about one hour and it may be as little as 15–20 minutes for subsequent babies. At this time contractions are 60–90 seconds long and come at two- to four-minute intervals.

You'll almost certainly feel the urge to push, known as bearing down. The urge is caused by your baby's head pressing down on your pelvic floor and rectum, and is quite involuntary. Keep your pushing as smooth and continuous as you can; make the muscular effort smooth and slow so that your vaginal and perineal tissues and muscles have enough time to stretch

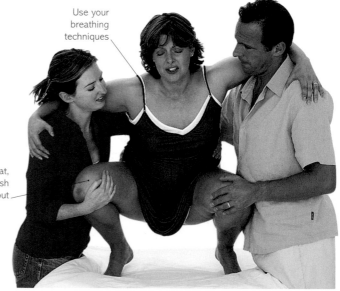

Use your breathing techniques

When you squat, gravity helps push your baby out

and will be able to accommodate your baby's head. The most efficient position to be in when you're pushing is upright, whether you sit on a birthing stool, stand with your arms around your partner's neck, or squat. This means that the downwards muscular force of your body and the downward force of gravity are working together to push your baby out.

As you push, it helps if your pelvic floor and anal area are fully relaxed, so make a conscious effort to let go of this part of your body. Don't be embarrassed if you urinate or lose a little stool – lots of women do. When you've finished a push, take two slow, deep breaths, but don't relax too quickly at the end of a contraction. Your baby will continue to maintain her forwards progress if you relax slowly.

Normal delivery

The first sign that your baby is coming is the bulging of your anus and perineum. With each contraction, more and more of your baby's head appears at your vaginal opening, until it doesn't slip back at all between contractions. This is known as crowning. Midwives can use hand manoeuvres to protect your perineum as your baby's head is born, but more often than not these days, they'll let nature take its course (the HOOP study – HOOP stands for hands on, or poised).

You'll probably feel a stinging sensation as your baby stretches your vaginal opening. As soon as you feel this, try to stop bearing down, pant, and allow the contractions of your uterus to push your baby. This may be difficult as you'll probably still feel like pushing, but if you continue to push you run a greater risk of tearing or needing an episiotomy (see p.110).

As you stop pushing, lean back and try to go limp. Make a conscious effort to relax the muscles of your perineal floor. The stinging sensation only lasts for a short time and is followed by a numb feeling as your baby's head stretches your vaginal tissues so thinly that the nerves are blocked, having a naturally anaesthetic effect.

When her head has been delivered, your baby will be face down, but almost immediately she will twist her head so that she's facing your left or right thigh. Your midwife will wipe your baby's eyes, nose, and mouth, and clear any fluid from her nose and upper air passages. The midwife will also check that the umbilical cord is not round your baby's neck – if it is, she will gently lift it over the head or make a loop through which the baby can be delivered. If the cord is very tight, she may clamp and cut it.

After delivery of your baby's head, your contractions will stop for a minute or so. When they start again, the first will usually deliver one shoulder and the next the other. Once both shoulders are delivered, the rest of your baby will slide out quickly and easily. Your attendants will hold her firmly as she'll be slippery with blood, amniotic fluid, and vernix.

What your baby does

Her body goes through several twists and turns as she comes down through the birth canal, all of which are aimed towards having a smooth, safe birth.

Your baby has a pliable body but a fairly firm, oval head. Both these parts have to adapt themselves to passing through a curved lower birth canal. This is made up of the lower part of your uterus inside your pelvis, your dilated cervix, and stretched vagina. There are various adjustments that your baby makes as labour progresses.

- She'll bring her chin down on to her chest as she descends through your pelvis.

- She'll turn her head

- She'll extend her head backwards so that the back of her head almost touches her back as she emerges from the birth canal and vagina.

- She'll make a little sideways wriggle so that her head turns to one side or the other; the shoulder of that side can then be delivered through your vagina.

- She'll make another little wriggle to swing her head all the way round so that the other shoulder is delivered. (If you imagine this in quick succession, it's like a shrug of one shoulder after the other – so fast that you hardly notice it.)

- Her trunk, buttocks, and legs follow her head out through your birth canal.

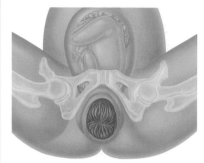

▲ THE HEAD CROWNS Your baby's head appears at the vaginal opening. Your midwife will tell you when this happens.

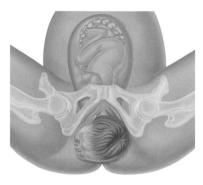

▲ THE HEAD EMERGES Once your baby's head is born, she turns it immediately so that she's facing the inside of one of your thighs.

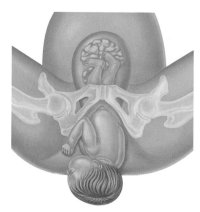

▲ YOUR BABY IS BORN With a couple of almost imperceptible shrugs, her shoulders are born and she slithers out into the hands waiting to catch her.

Giving birth

Your baby's journey down the birth canal lasts about an hour on average. You'll probably feel swept along by an unbelievably strong urge to bear down and push your baby out of your uterus. Listen to your midwife; she'll tell you when to push and when to relax. If you've had an epidural your urge to bear down may be reduced.

Pushing

As each contraction builds until it reaches its peak, you'll experience powerful urges to bear down and push out your baby as she descends. Bearing down is not something you decide to do; it's an instinctive reaction that you won't be able to resist.

The head crowns

There comes a point when your baby's head doesn't slip back between contractions, but remains visible at the vaginal outlet. This is when the baby's head is said to crown, and you'll feel a burning or stinging sensation as her head stretches your vagina. You'll need to stop pushing at this point so that you give the tissues of your perineum a chance to thin and stretch. This may be difficult as you may still want to bear down, but you must try to resist. If you continue to push at this stage, you'll put too much stress on your perineal area and you're more likely to tear or need an episiotomy. Quick shallow breathing is a good way to try and control your desire to bear down.

The head emerges

As her head is born, she'll immediately turn her head sideways. Your contractions will probably pause for a few moments at this point, and your caregivers will quickly feel around your baby's neck to make sure that the cord's not there. If it is, they'll either lift it up over her head or make a loop through which she can be born. Her shoulders will be delivered in the next contraction.

Your baby is born

As soon as her shoulders are free, the rest of her body will be born right away. As she slithers out of your vagina, she'll usually be followed by a great gush of amniotic fluid. Your caregivers will hold her very carefully as she'll be slippery. She may be breathing and crying already.

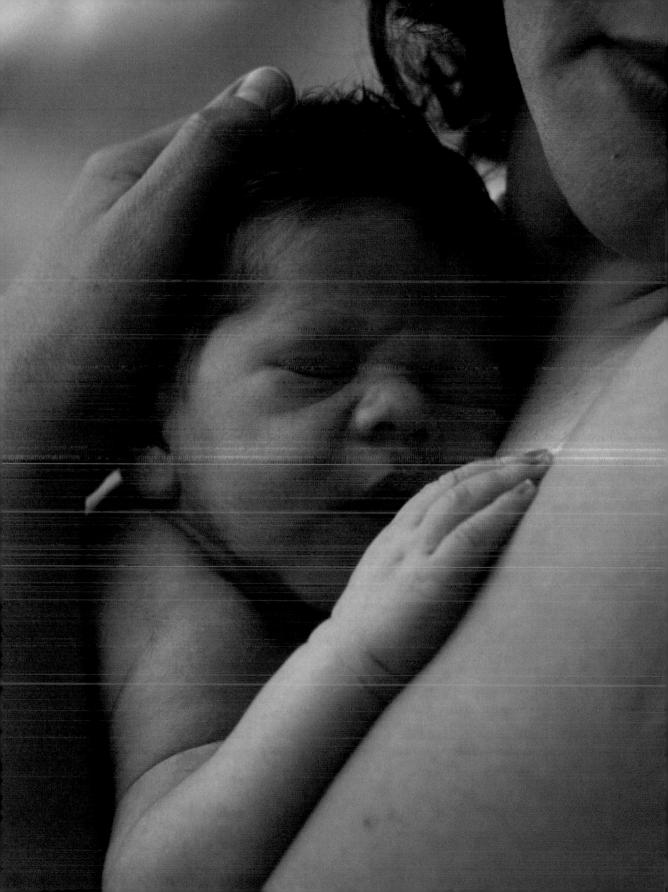

Pictures of your baby's birth

Everyone wants to take photographs – or even make a video – of their baby's first moments and all your family and friends will want to see pictures. There are a few points you need to bear in mind, though.

■ Before labour begins, check with your midwife and doctor that they're happy for you to take pictures.

■ If you want to take more than a few photos, or if you want to video the event, it may be better to ask a friend or relative to do it for you. Your partner will need you to be sensitive to her every need, not rushing around clicking the camera or focusing on the best image. You risk alienating yourself from her and the doctor and midwife, if you're constantly behind a lens.

■ Your partner will want soft, dim lighting in the delivery room to help her feel relaxed, so take account of this when assembling your camera equipment. Also, many hospitals don't like you to use direct flash as it can be irritating for the mother, distracting for the midwife, and damaging for your baby's eyes.

Partner's role at the birth

By this second stage of labour, your role in providing loving support for your partner will be well established. You've now passed through the most painful phase and have reached the climactic stage of delivery.

Second stage jobs

You'll need to continue doing many of the jobs you did during the first stage – making your partner comfortable, supporting her in different positions, providing drinks and sweets, and giving moral support. But you'll also now have to encourage her to push. All this will make the mother's job easier and help her feel emotionally secure and relaxed.

In the unlikely event of a medical emergency, staff have to move quickly and you might be in the way, so be sensitive to any situation that arises. You probably won't be asked to leave the delivery room, but be prepared to do so if necessary.

Helping with the delivery position Now your partner has been through the first stage of labour, she'll probably know which position she finds most comfortable. Your support is very important to help her through the pushing stage, but always ask the midwife's advice if you're not certain what to do. If your partner doesn't want to be held, suggest other positions that she might find comfortable, and place pillows or cushions under and behind her for support. It's a good idea to practise different ways of sitting or squatting before labour so that you're both familiar with them; if you feel unsure or uncomfortable about what you're doing it can make your partner nervous.

If your partner is happy sitting on the bed or on the floor, she might like to try the knee-chest position, which many women find comfortable in the second stage. For this, she should drop her chin on to her chest while holding on to her knees. Between contractions, suggest that she relaxes against the pillow to conserve her energy.

Helping her with breathing and pushing To help her through these last few contractions, tap out a rhythm for the different kinds of breathing, using words such as: breathe, breathe, pant, pant, blow. As she's pushing, gently remind her to relax her pelvic floor. At the peak of contractions,

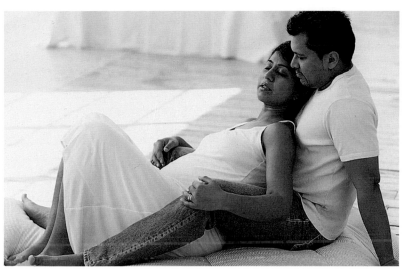

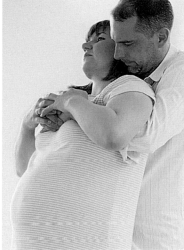

▲ **SUPPORTED SQUAT** If your partner wants to deliver standing up, you can help support her by standing behind her and taking her weight on your arms. Supported in this way, her pelvis will be completely open and she'll be able to take full advantage of gravity. Her legs should be apart.

◄ **SEMI-UPRIGHT POSITION** If she's happy for you to be as near as possible during labour, your partner can lean back against you for support. You'll be able to guide her through the contractions. Keeping close to her may help to make her feel more relaxed during the delivery.

suggest that she takes two or three deep breaths and pushes as hard as she can. She should push in a strong and steady way, and you can remind her that each push brings the birth of your baby nearer.

Encouraging her to relax Between contractions, help your partner to relax as she needs to save her strength for pushing her baby through the birth canal. Massage her back (see p.283) if she has backache or needs comforting and reassuring. If she's hot and bothered, mop her brow with a cool flannel or spray her face with a water spray.

Standing by Once your baby's head has crowned, your role may become more passive for a while as you watch the midwife guiding your partner through this pushing stage. Don't be disappointed if your partner doesn't take any notice of you during the birth and relies more on the midwife. She'll be fully preoccupied and involved with what's happening.

Showing her the baby When your baby's head is emerging, hold a mirror nearby so that your partner can see his head crowning and then his whole body slithering out. Help her to reach down and touch your baby's head as he is born.

Loving reception Ask the midwife if you can catch your baby in your arms as his body emerges. After you've greeted your baby for the first time, place him on your partner's stomach, and then cuddle them both. You and your partner will have a range of reactions – relief, tears, awed silence, exhausted collapse, whoops of joy. You may even feel squeamish at the sight of his bloodied, greasy, tiny body. Whatever your feelings, this moment marks a new phase in your family's history.

The placenta

Most first-time mothers are keen to have a look at their placenta.

The placenta measures about 20–25cm (8–10in) in diameter and weighs about 450g (1lb). It's shaped like a disc and its two surfaces look very different from each other.

The baby's side was adjoining the wall of your uterus and covered with membranes. It's flat and smooth, with blood vessels radiating out from the umbilical cord. Your side of the placenta was embedded in the wall of your uterus, and is made up of wedges (cotyledons) to make a larger surface area for the exchange of gases. This side of the placenta is dark red and looks like several pieces of raw liver joined together.

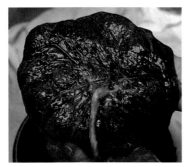

▲ **THE BABY'S SIDE** The side of the placenta that was facing towards your baby is flat and smooth. The umbilical cord emerges from its centre and there are prominent blood vessels.

The third stage

Once your baby's been born, your uterus rests for about 15 minutes, but it soon starts to contract again to deliver the placenta. This is the third stage and you'll be so absorbed in your baby you'll probably hardly notice it.

The third stage

During the third stage of labour the placenta becomes detached from the wall of your uterus and is delivered down the birth canal. The large blood vessels running to and from the placenta, which are about the thickness of a pencil, are simply torn across. Despite this, bleeding is rare because the muscle fibres of the uterus are arranged in a criss-cross fashion so that when the uterus contracts down, the muscles tighten around the blood vessels and prevent them from bleeding. This is why it's absolutely essential that your uterus contracts down into a hard ball once the placenta has been expelled. Massaging every now and then for an hour or so after the third stage is complete can help keep your uterus tightly contracted. Normally the third stage lasts about ten to 20 minutes but with active management it can be much shorter.

The placenta is delivered

Usually your midwife won't try to deliver the placenta until there are clear signs that it's separating from the wall of your uterus and moving down into your vagina. The signs your attendants will look out for are contractions starting up again a few minutes after the birth of your baby, which shows that the placenta is about to separate, and your desire to bear down – this also shows that the placenta has separated from the wall of your uterus and is pressing down on your pelvic floor.

Once these signs have appeared, your midwife may encourage the delivery of the placenta by pulling gently on the cord, at the same time pressing above the rim of the pelvis to control descent. The placenta is expelled from your vagina, followed by the membranes. Rarely, a blood clot will also be expelled.

Delivery The placenta may pass through your vulva in two different ways. In the first, the centre of the placenta comes out first, dragging the membranes behind it. In the second, an edge of the placenta presents first, then it slips out of the vulva sideways. Most women want to see the placenta – it's an amazing organ that's been the life-support system for your baby for nine months (see column, left).

After delivery Once the placenta is delivered, the midwifery staff will check it carefully to make sure it's complete and none of it has been left behind. If any of the placenta has been left in the uterus it can cause haemorrhaging later on, so must be removed as soon as possible. If there's any doubt, you may have a small procedure (ERPC, see p.219) to ensure the uterus is completely empty. The membranes should form a complete bag except for the hole through which your baby has passed. Your midwife will also check the cut end of the cord to make sure that the umbilical blood vessels are normal. After the placenta is delivered, the whole of your vulval outlet will be examined carefully for tears. Anything other than a minute one will be stitched immediately.

Active management of the third stage

Since the use of ergometrine began in 1935, the third stage of labour has been more actively managed by doctors and midwives. Giving ergometrine at the time of birth was soon found to reduce the number of cases of excessive bleeding, defined as loss of more than 500ml (18floz) of blood (postpartum haemorrhage).

Ergometrine causes the prolonged contraction of the uterus without a period of relaxation – while the uterus is contracted there's not likely to be any bleeding. The placenta separates very quickly from the uterine wall once the uterus starts to contract, so shortening the third stage.

Syntometrine Most midwives now use a combination of ergometrine and syntocinon known as syntometrine. Ergometrine on its own is rather slow to start to work and can cause nausea, but using it with syntocinon, which acts quickly to stimulate uterine contractions, gives a better result.

Syntometrine is given by injection just as your baby's head is crowning, or when her first shoulder is delivered. It's used automatically in most hospital births to reduce the risk of postpartum haemorrhage (see column, right). The hormone oxytocin is naturally produced by your body when you see and touch your baby and put her to your breast. It does the same job as syntometrine, but is less reliable.

How you'll feel

You may find yourself shivering with cold after the placenta's delivered. My own explanation of this is that your body has suddenly been deprived of the baby's heat inside you and your temperature drops. The only way the body can raise its temperature is to generate heat through muscular work and that's what shivering does – rapid contraction and relaxation of muscles produces body heat. The shivering usually passes in about half an hour, by which time your body temperature is back up to normal.

Postpartum haemorrhage

This is rare, largely because your uterus has a self-protecting device to stop it from bleeding.

Once your uterus is completely empty, it contracts down to about the size of a tennis ball. The contraction of the uterine muscles nips the uterine arteries so that they can't bleed. Under normal circumstances there's little bleeding after the delivery. What little bleeding there is appears as the lochia – the usual vaginal discharge after delivery. The lochia is red for two to three days, then turns brown, and disappears within two to six weeks.

If part of the placenta is retained in the uterus it may bleed and this bleeding is called postpartum haemorrhage. This is why the placenta is checked so if any part is missing it can be removed. If this is necessary, the mother is given a general or regional anaesthetic and any remaining placental tissue is gently taken out.

If there's any bleeding more than 24 hours after delivery, your lochia may become bright red again. This can happen if you're too energetic. Check with your doctor, who'll probably suggest that you rest for several days. If the bleeding starts again or becomes heavy, it can be the sign of infection or that a small piece of placenta has been retained. Call your doctor at once. If you pass large clots of blood, call an ambulance to take you to the nearest maternity unit.

Apgar score

Within a minute of your baby's birth, five simple assessments on her condition are carried out to check that she is fit and healthy. These are recorded on the Apgar score (named after Dr Virginia Apgar, who devised it). The Apgar score includes the following checks.

Activity (movement) Gives an indication of your baby's muscle tone. Active movements score 2, some movements 1, limp scores 0.

Pulse/heart rate This measures the strength and regularity of your baby's heartbeat: 100 beats per minute scores 2, below 100 scores 1, no pulse scores 0.

Grimace (crying) Crying and grimacing can show that your baby responds to stimuli. Crying scores 2, whimpering 1, silence 0.

Appearance (skin colour) This shows how well your baby's lungs are working to oxygenate her blood. Pink skin scores 2, bluish extremities 1, totally blue skin scores 0.

Respiration (breathing) This checks the maturity and health of your baby's lungs. Regular breathing scores 2, irregular 1, none 0.

Most babies score between seven and 10. A second test is done about five minutes after the first.

Baby's first hours

Once your baby is delivered, all the attention will be given to her and rightly so. She may cry when delivered and will cry lustily a few seconds after birth. She'll probably be a bluish-white colour and may be covered with vernix – a white, cheesy substance that protects her skin in the womb. She'll have streaks of blood on her and, depending on your delivery, her head may look slightly pointed after her journey down the birth canal.

Her first moments

If her breathing is normal, there's absolutely no reason why you shouldn't hold her immediately. If there's a danger of her being cold, you can be covered with a towel or blanket. Your gentle stroking movements and the sound of your heartbeat and voice will reassure your baby. Her eyes will almost certainly fasten on your face and she may scrabble as if trying to swim towards you.

Cutting the cord The first procedure is the clamping of the cord. Some doctors believe that a baby benefits from the return of placental blood through the umbilical cord, and that the cord should not be clamped until it stops pulsating. Others believe that this could cause the baby to develop anaemia. At the appropriate time, two clamps are applied to the cord, one a short distance from the navel, the other about 2.5cm (1in) away from the first clamp. These clamps prevent the cord from bleeding, the one closest to your baby being the most important. The cord is then cut between the clamps. It may have been clamped and cut during delivery if it was looped tightly around your baby's neck.

Her general condition The midwife will check your baby's general condition. She'll remove any fluid remaining in your baby's mouth, nose, or air passages by sucking it out with disposable plastic tubing. If your baby doesn't start to breathe immediately, the midwife will take her and give her oxygen.

Welcoming your baby

Once the midwifery and medical staff have checked that both you and your baby are well, by all means ask them to leave if you want to be left alone in the warmth of your house or hospital birthing room with your partner and your baby. If you've had an episiotomy you may have to wait until after you've been stitched; your midwife or doctor will be able to make a much neater repair if you're stitched as soon as possible after the birth before the tissues swell. Once this is done, you can relax after your hard work and enjoy this amazing new experience together. It's a good idea to put your baby to your breast immediately because it stimulates delivery of the placenta, even if your baby isn't hungry at first.

Spend these first few moments concentrating on your baby, getting to know her, learning to recognize her face, and cooing at her so that she can hear the sound of your voice. Ideally, hold her about 20–25cm (8–10in) away from your face – at this distance she can make out your face quite clearly. Smile and talk gently in a sing-song voice, because newborn babies are attuned to high vocal pitches.

Encourage your partner to hold his baby for the first time within half an hour of the birth. Men can bond as deeply and as quickly with their newborn children as women do.

After this initial bonding process, you'll be washed down and asked to pass urine to make sure that everything's in working order. You can then change and the midwives will check your baby more thoroughly.

A more thorough check

Shortly after birth (in addition to the Apgar score, see column, opposite), the doctor or midwife will make some specific checks on your baby. The doctor will check that her facial features and her body proportions are normal. She'll be turned over to check that her back is normal and there are no indications of spina bifida. Her anus is checked, as are her fingers and toes. The number of blood vessels in the umbilical cord is recorded – there are usually two arteries and one vein. Your baby will then be weighed, and her head circumference, and possibly her body length measured. All this takes only a few minutes in the hands of an experienced doctor or midwife.

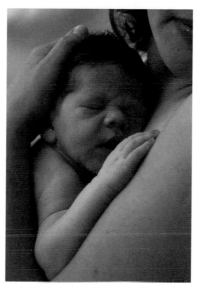

▲ **YOUR BRAND NEW BABY** As you hold your newborn baby you'll feel the glow of motherhood – a mixture of love, pride, awe, and wonder, mixed with the all-consuming tiredness that comes with a hard job well done.

Your baby's identification

Before your baby leaves the delivery room, she'll have some identification fastened to her, so that all the staff know she's yours.

Plastic bracelets will usually be sealed around both your baby's wrist and her ankle. The identifying bracelets must remain on your baby at all times while she's in hospital. These bracelets are usually marked with:

■ your surname (she'll be referred to by the staff as "baby Brown" for example)

■ her date of birth

■ an identification number (an identification number is used by most hospitals for both you and your baby).

In addition to the above:
■ her footprints may be taken

■ her cot may be marked with her name and number.

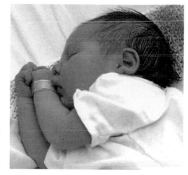

▲ **KEEPING HER BRACELETS** Like many parents, you may want to keep your baby's identity bracelets as souvenirs. As your child grows, it'll soon amaze you that her wrists and ankles could ever have been quite so tiny.

Special deliveries

Most babies are delivered without a hitch and are fit and healthy. But no two labours are alike, even for the same woman. Some need a special approach or even intervention. Don't worry – they can turn out just as well for mum and baby.

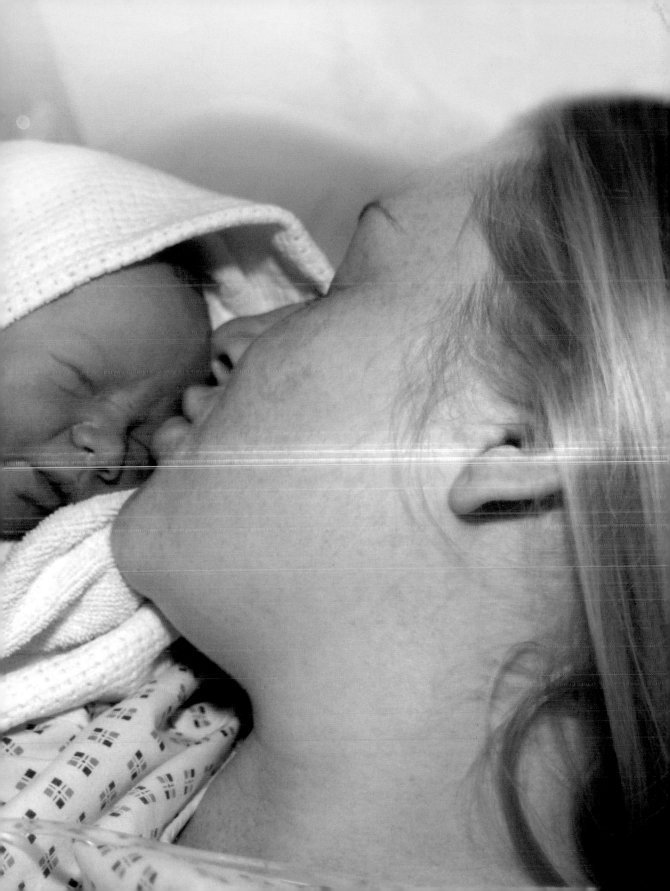

Your baby's presentation

The way your baby is presenting (her position in your uterus) can affect your labour and birth.

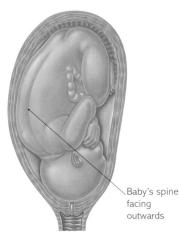

▲ **NORMAL PRESENTATION** The usual presentation is when your baby's spine faces outwards.

Baby's spine facing outwards

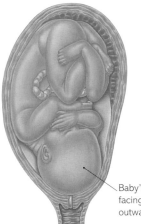

Baby's head facing outwards

▲ **HEAD OUTWARDS** If your baby's head is facing outwards, labour might possibly be delayed. But most babies do rotate into the correct position before passing down the birth canal.

Special labours

Don't worry – most labours are quite straightforward, but just occasionally there may be a complication that needs a special approach. With good antenatal care, any potential difficulties are usually spotted well in advance and avoided. Now and then, though, the first stage is underway before a problem becomes apparent.

Backache labour

Occasionally, a woman may feel the discomfort of uterine contractions mainly as low back pain. This is usually due to stretching of the cervix as it dilates. It may also happen if your baby lies in the posterior position with the back of his head up against your spine (this is not abnormal – one in ten babies lie this way). In this position, your baby's neck may not be properly flexed and a larger proportion of the head than normal presents, which may mean that labour takes longer. Usually, your baby will rotate the 180 degrees into the anterior position and labour will go ahead smoothly. If, as sometimes happens, the baby fails to turn, there's still no cause for alarm, although your doctor may deliver him using forceps or, more commonly, vacuum extraction. This kind of labour may start slowly and take a while, so it can be tiring. There are various ways in which you and your birth assistant can relieve your backache.

Counterpressure This is the most effective way of relieving backache (see p.283). But if you find being touched by someone else irritating, for example during transition, you may like to use your own knuckles by placing a hand underneath each buttock.

Change in position When you're lying flat on your back, your baby is pressing down hardest on your spine and its nerves. Try to stay upright and walk around as much as you can. You can also relieve the pressure of your baby on your spine by sitting tailor-fashion (see p.150), leaning forwards, or by rocking your pelvis. If you feel more comfortable lying down, lie on the side that your baby is turning towards (your midwife will be able to tell you which side that is).

Application of heat A heating pad or hot-water bottle placed against your lower back may help between contractions. A hot shower, directed on to your back, may also give some relief.

Prolonged labour

Labour is said to be prolonged when contractions fail to bring about the expected progress. This may be because the cervix hasn't dilated, or the baby hasn't descended through the birth canal. Doctors and midwives keep a very careful eye on the length of each stage of labour. If labour appears to be going more slowly than normal, your attendants may suspect delay and take an early decision to intervene – with an assisted delivery if it's suitable, or even a Caesarean section.

No woman is allowed to go on with a difficult birth for much over the accepted times (see p.273) as this may lead to maternal exhaustion and/or fetal distress. Your midwife will be monitoring your general condition throughout labour, and she'll be alerted to possible delay if your condition appears to get worse and you look tired and anxious.

If your labour is very long and you're going without food and rest, you might become too tired or upset to push enough. Your midwife will try not to let this happen.

Failure to dilate When contractions are weak and infrequent and your cervix is dilating slowly, the uterus may be failing to coordinate muscular activity. If this is the only reason for the lack of progress in your labour, your attendants may suggest speeding up dilatation. The membranes may be artificially ruptured and then a drug called syntocinon may be administered intravenously with a drip or with a pump. The dosage will be carefully increased until strong contractions are coming regularly about every three minutes.

Your midwife and doctor will keep a close check on you throughout to make sure there are no excessive increases in the strength or frequency of your contractions.

Failure to descend I've mentioned breech and posterior presentation as causes of delay. One other reason for a slow labour is disproportion. This means that the size of your baby's head and the size of your pelvis are failing to match up – for example, if your pelvis is too small relative to your baby's head. It's easy to understand how your baby might fail to descend in such circumstances (see also p.176).

If you're a first-time mother and your baby is still high and not engaged during the last few weeks of your pregnancy (see column, p.261), your doctor may suspect disproportion. This will also be taken into account if your baby's head remains high during labour even though you're having strong contractions.

If the disproportion is quite slight, your doctor may let you try to have a trial of labour (bear in mind that it's your uterus on trial, not you),

Causes of fetal delay

There are certain fetal conditions that cause delayed labour. Fortunately, most problems are discovered beforehand so everybody is well prepared. Conditions that can cause fetal delay include:

■ your baby is too large

■ your baby is lying in a transverse or oblique position

■ your baby is in a breech, face, or brow presentation

■ your baby is lying in the posterior position

■ your twin babies are entwined

■ your baby has a congenital abnormality such as hydrocephalus

■ your pelvis is particularly small or an unusual shape.

Maternal causes of delay

If your labour isn't progressing normally, there may be reasons why your pelvis or uterus is obstructing the descent of your baby. Causes include:

■ deformity or disproportion of the bony pelvis

■ pelvic tumours such as fibroids or an ovarian cyst

■ abnormalities of the uterus, cervix, or vagina

■ a contraction ring of the uterus, which is when the uterus pulls in excessively and a band of tight muscle occurs. This can stop contractions passing all the way down and may cause constriction of the uterus or cervix. Fortunately, this condition is very rare, unless the uterus has been overstimulated by oxytocin or prostaglandin, for example, during induction (see p.300). A Caesarean section is almost always needed.

provided there are no other irregularities, and the baby's head is felt to be descending. Once the baby's head has entered the pelvic cavity, there can usually be a vaginal delivery. If the disproportion is major, your baby will need to be delivered by Caesarean section.

Don't worry – most of the abnormalities that cause obstruction and a prolonged labour (see column, left, and p.297) will be picked up during your pregnancy so that early treatment is possible, and a plan of action can be made by the doctors and midwives before your labour begins.

Premature labour

This is a labour that starts at less than 37 weeks of gestation. The cause is a mystery in about 40 per cent of cases, but it's known to happen in the following circumstances: premature rupture of the membranes; multiple pregnancy; pre-eclampsia; cervical incompetence; and uterine abnormalities. Overwork, stress, and some maternal diseases, such as anaemia or malnutrition, may also have an effect.

Knowing whether you've actually gone into premature labour is almost as difficult for your doctors as it is for you (see column, opposite). The diagnosis is not easy, and criteria differ at different centres – showing that often it's quite arbitrary.

Testing for premature labour A new test called the fetal fibronectin test may be used to predict the likelihood of premature labour establishing. It is done by taking a swab from the upper vagina and is relatively painless. If the test is negative, there is a good chance you will not deliver early. Even if the test is positive, you might not go into established labour, but you will be encouraged to stay in hospital and possibly be given steroids to help the baby's lungs.

As a general rule, a premature labour begins without any warning; the first sign may be rupture of the membranes, the beginning of uterine contractions, or some vaginal bleeding. Labour can't be stopped if the contractions have started, your membranes have ruptured, and your cervix is dilating, but you or your doctor can take certain precautions while the membranes are intact or before labour really gets going.

What you can do If your membranes have ruptured (see p.273), but labour hasn't actually started, go straight to hospital. There is a small risk of infection and both you and your preterm baby will be vulnerable. The staff will monitor you closely for signs of infection, such as a fever, and may give you antibiotics, particularly if you are found to be carrying group B streptococcus bacteria. This does not usually cause problems for the mother but can be dangerous for her baby, particularly if he's premature. Labour is unlikely to be actively suppressed if the membranes have ruptured spontaneously. Nonetheless, if labour doesn't start spontaneously it won't usually be induced until after 37 weeks unless there are signs of infection.

What the hospital will do If labour starts between 24 and 34 weeks, you'll be given ritodrine or atosiban to delay your labour and allow time to mature the baby's lungs with steroids. A preterm baby (see also pp.344 and 345) has an increased risk of developing respiratory distress syndrome, and the shorter the gestation period, the greater the risk.

Being in hospital also allows your doctor to check for evidence of infection in cases of premature rupture of the membranes and to monitor your baby's condition carefully. It also means that your premature baby can be taken to the intensive care unit immediately after delivery and given all necessary care.

If the hospital where you've given birth does not have a neonatal intensive care unit that can handle very premature babies, you and your baby may need to be moved to another hospital that has these facilities. This may be farther away, which can make it harder for your partner, friends, and family to come and visit you, but be comforted by the thought that the unit will be able to give your tiny baby the best possible start in life after the birth (see p.344).

Drug treatments All of the drugs used cause some side effects and for that reason they're only suitable in certain cases of premature labour. The main criteria for drug treatment are that you are healthy, you have no heart disease, diabetes, high blood pressure, or an abnormally placed placenta. Another criteria, of course, is that your baby is alive, with no evidence of a congenital defect.

Managing labour Once the membranes have ruptured, labour may go on as normal (see p.270), although sometimes many weeks may pass before labour starts. As a general rule, a premature labour tends to be shorter and easier than full-term, mainly because a preterm baby's head is smaller and softer. However, an episiotomy may be given to protect the baby's head from pressure changes within the birth canal. You may prefer to have an epidural anaesthetic for pain relief instead of analgesic drugs, which can depress your baby's respiratory system.

Your medical team will take special care to avoid hypoxia (lack of oxygen to the tissues) throughout your labour and delivery. It may be necessary to deliver some premature babies by Caesarean section, particularly if there is fetal distress.

Premature labour?

Here are some useful pointers for diagnosing whether or not you're in premature labour:

■ you're less than 37 weeks into your pregnancy

■ you've had uterine contractions for at least an hour

■ you're having contractions every five to ten minutes

■ the contractions last for 30 seconds and persist over the period of an hour

■ vaginal examination by your doctor or midwife shows that your cervix is more than 2.5cm (1in) dilated and more than three-quarters effaced.

According to these criteria, two-thirds of all women who are thought to be in premature labour will actually be found not to be in real labour, and no treatment will be needed. This can be quickly confirmed if you go straight to hospital so that staff can observe uterine activity very carefully.

If you're overdue

Towards the end of pregnancy doctors are always on the look-out for any signs of placental insufficiency as the baby outgrows its food supply.

Whether to induce or not if you're overdue is a controversial issue, so it's worth talking to your midwife about this at one of your antenatal checks. Of course, induction isn't always necessary. A mother who reaches her estimated date of delivery, given that she and the baby are perfectly normal, should be allowed to go into spontaneous labour.

Once the EDD has been passed, though, I do think it's very important to have your own and your baby's condition monitored frequently. If there's any sign of fetal distress, I'd advise you to agree to medical intervention.

Induction of labour

Induction is a way of starting labour artificially by rupturing the membranes and giving oxytocin or prostaglandins to stimulate contractions. The same techniques are used to accelerate labour if contractions are weak and progress slow. If you're in any doubt about why your doctor is suggesting induction of labour, ask for a detailed explanation – this should cover all of the alternatives. In the end, the decision is up to you.

Reasons for induction

Only five per cent of babies actually come on their due date, but in general, induction is not considered until you are ten days or more past your EDD. Don't worry if you do have to be induced. Induction is fine provided it's done strictly for medical reasons and either for your well-being or the baby's. And please don't feel angry with yourself if your birth doesn't turn out just the way that you'd planned.

Anything that makes the uterine environment unhealthy is a reason for induction. Your labour may be induced if:

■ You have hypertension, pre-eclampsia, heart disease, diabetes, or antepartum bleeding.
■ There are signs of placental insufficiency (so your baby's in danger of not getting enough nutrients and oxygen from the placenta).
■ Your membranes have ruptured (see p.273) but labour hasn't started within 24–48 hours.
■ Your pregnancy goes beyond 42 weeks.

How it's done

Most obstetric units will normally use a combination of three different methods to induce labour.

Prostaglandin pessaries The most common method of induction uses prostaglandin pessaries, which soften the cervix and start it dilating. They can be inserted at any time of day, although most units put the first one in at night, particularly in first pregnancies. They usually start to take effect in six hours, although several may need to be used over 24–48 hours. This is a good method of induction as you are free to move around.

Artificial rupture of the membranes (ARM) This is also known as amniotomy and involves the use of an instrument not unlike a crochet hook. It is inserted through the cervix into the uterus to make a small opening in the membrane so that the waters escape. It can only be performed if the cervix is already partially open. Amniotomy is usually followed in a few hours by contractions, but if there are no contractions you'll need to have an oxytocin drip. If you have a drip, doctors usually advise fetal monitoring so that they can check the effect of the induced contractions on the fetus. Labour usually reaches full intensity quickly after ARM because the baby's head is no longer cushioned and it presses down hard against your cervix, which encourages the uterus to contract and the cervix to dilate. If left alone, the waters don't usually break until late in the first stage.

Amniotomy is not just a method of induction. It will be performed if an electrode needs to be attached to the baby's scalp to monitor his heartbeat (see p.275). It will also be performed if the baby's heart rate goes down because of distress. In this case, traces of meconium, the baby's first bowel movement, may be seen in the amniotic fluid.

Oxytocin-induced labour Oxytocin is the natural hormone from the posterior pituitary gland in the brain that stimulates labour. The synthetic form is used for inducing labour.

Oxytocin is given through a drip or syringe drive with careful regulation of the dose. Ask for the drip to be inserted in your left arm if you're right-handed, and check that you can have a long tube connecting you to the drip so you have more room to move around. Some drip stands are on wheels so that you can still move around the room and change position if you wish, which will help you control the more intense labour pains. The oxytocin drip can be turned down if you go into strong labour quickly. The drip won't be removed from your arm until after the baby is born because the uterine contractions help to expel the placenta.

Contractions brought on by an oxytocin drip are often stronger, longer, and more painful than normal contractions, with shorter breaks between them, so there's an increased need for painkilling drugs.

Expectations of induced labour

If properly handled, induced labour needn't be more difficult than natural labour and, using oxytocin, your midwife should be able to get you to the stage where you'll have a normal labour. You can still do all your breathing exercises and push the baby out at your own pace if you prefer to have a natural childbirth. If the induced labour does become too painful, you can ask for epidural anaesthetic or other pain relief (see p.280).

Rupture of membranes

The membranes usually rupture naturally towards the end of the first stage of labour.

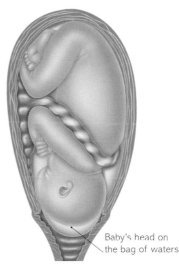

Baby's head on the bag of waters

▲ **INTACT MEMBRANES** The bag of waters provides a cushion for your baby's head as it presses your cervix.

Baby's head pressing on cervix

▲ **RUPTURED MEMBRANES**
Contractions get stronger, pressing your baby's head against your cervix and helping it to open.

Miriam's casebook

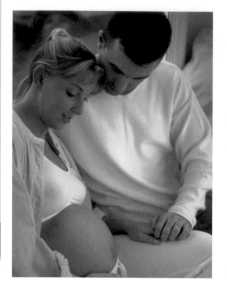

An induced birth

Rebecca and David's first baby was born in hospital, six days after term. Rebecca had no complications during her pregnancy and had decided to have her baby at a private natural birthing centre. However, things didn't go to plan and their baby was born in their local hospital after induction. The birth was induced because Rebecca's waters had broken and, after 48 hours, labour had not started.

Why is a baby induced?

Induction is a standard hospital procedure and is quite common (see pp.300–1). Births are induced if labour hasn't begun 14 days after the woman's expected delivery date (known as post-maturity) or a maximum of 48 hours after the waters break. Other reasons include complications in late pregnancy such as maternal high blood pressure, pre-eclampsia, and suspected placental insufficiency, though in emergencies a Caesarean is likely to be done.

Wednesday and Thursday

Rebecca's waters broke on a Wednesday morning about two days after her due date, before any signs of labour had appeared. It's quite normal for this to happen, and can be caused by pressure of the baby's head on the membranes of the amniotic sac. It's also quite normal not to go into labour immediately after the waters break. Once the waters have broken, there's a small risk of infection for the baby and most doctors advise an induction within about 24 to 48 hours.

Rebecca and David went straight to the private birthing centre they'd booked into. Their baby's heartbeat was monitored and the baby showed no signs of distress. But, no signs of labour had appeared by Thursday morning, and the

medical staff recommended that if labour hadn't begun by Friday morning, 48 hours after Rebecca's waters had broken, they should go to hospital.

Friday and Saturday

Friday morning came without any signs of labour starting, so at 8am David and Rebecca went to their local hospital, where the senior registrar in the maternity unit decided that Rebecca should have an induction.

Rebecca was given a prostaglandin pessary at 9am. Prostaglandin can be very effective in inducing labour, though many women need more than one pessary. In Rebecca's case, the first pessary didn't work, nor did a second pessary given about six hours later. Rebecca had to spend the night in hospital.

On Saturday morning the hospital staff decided that a syntocinon drip was needed to start Rebecca's labour. Syntocinon is a synthetic form of oxytocin, and because it's given intravenously, it works very quickly. However, the labour ward was very busy that day and although the drip hadn't been given, Rebecca's labour finally started spontaneously at about 6pm.

Progressing labour

Rebecca's labour progressed very slowly. She had gas and air, and then pethidine as her contractions were proving painful. By about 4am on Sunday, Rebecca's labour had progressed enough for her to be taken to a delivery suite.

Contractions were beginning to be very painful indeed, so a mobile epidural was given, which helped Rebecca manage the pain and meant that she could rest for a while in between each contraction. A "mobile" epidural is so called because it numbs feeling from the chest to the knees, but still allows some movement, standing, and even walking. A stronger full epidural means that a woman can't move her legs much at all, and makes it harder to push.

After several hours of contractions, a vacuum extraction was needed at the end to deliver the baby's head. Rebecca gave birth to a beautiful baby boy at midday on Sunday. He weighed in at 4.3kg (9lb 10oz) and was perfectly healthy.

After the birth

Not surprisingly, Rebecca was absolutely exhausted after being on the verge of giving birth for so long, and David was pretty shattered too by all the anxiety. Unforeseen eventualities can play havoc with the most carefully prepared birth plan, and induction is one of them. With the benefit of hindsight, Rebecca and David now feel that they'd have been better off letting nature take its course from the beginning. They've learned a lot from the experience, though, and feel that next time, if appropriate, they'd like to take a long, slow labour in their stride, relaxing at home during the early stages. Then they might be able to have their baby at their preferred birthing centre, although theirs is staffed by midwives and tends to refer special cases like Rebecca's to hospitals anyway.

However, they also understand that the hospital was following standard procedures to ensure the safety of Rebecca and her baby son and that everyone was doing their best to help. And of course, they were completely thrilled with their new arrival, who's more than made up for all the trials of the past four days!

Miriam's top tips

Induction is a standard procedure and quite common, especially in older mothers. My advice is to:

■ rest as much as possible towards the end of the last trimester, so you have reserves of strength to cope, if need be, with a long labour

■ write a birth plan while also bearing in mind that unforeseen circumstances may mean you'll need to be flexible about the kind of birth you have

■ remember your health and that of your baby are the prime concerns of your carers.

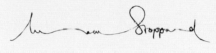

Why labour is sometimes long

Induction should always be done for good medical reasons but it can affect your labour. It can mean that labour is rather long and drawn out, which is why I always advise pregnant mothers to rest as much as possible in the last weeks of pregnancy. Rebecca's baby was a big boy and his size made his passage through the birth canal very slow. Vacuum extraction was needed at the end because he was so big he got stuck, even though Rebecca was fully dilated.

Prostaglandin pessaries, which work by softening the cervix, don't always "take". On average, two or three pessaries are given, with some women needing up to four – though this is unusual. It's necessary to wait for several hours between each one, which meant that Rebecca had to spend a long time in hospital rather than relaxing at home.

Induced labour can be more painful than natural labour. The prostaglandin means that the onset of labour is speeded up, and the contractions are more severe, and tend to be closer together. This makes it harder for the woman to use "natural" forms of pain relief such as massage or breathing. Statistics show that women who have induction are more likely to need pain relief such as epidurals.

On your way to the hospital

If the urge to bear down comes as you're driving to the hospital, use your breathing techniques to avoid pushing; do your best to stay calm.

If the urge becomes too strong for you to control, ask your partner to pull the car over and stop. Cover the back seat and car floor with a thick layer of newspapers or towels if you have them available and get as comfortable as possible. You can then deliver the baby into your partner's hands.

Follow the procedure for the birth in the main text. Once your baby is born, it's important that he's kept warm, so wrap him in a blanket or towel (or in your partner's shirt, jumper, or coat, if there's nothing else) and hold him close against your skin. If the placenta arrives before you reach hospital, wrap it up with your baby as this provides him with much-needed extra warmth. Do not cut the umbilical cord.

Sudden birth

Sometimes labour is so quick that your baby is born before you can get medical assistance. The following information is not intended to be used as a guide for an out-of-hospital birth without a professional attendant, as this can be very risky. It's reassuring, though, that there are rarely complications in emergency births of this sort.

What to do

When you get the urge to push, try to pant or blow for as long as you can to delay your baby's birth. The contractions alone are usually enough to push your baby out when he's coming this fast, so this won't delay things for long, although it may be long enough for your midwife or the ambulance to arrive. Never try to hold your legs together to delay delivery, or allow anyone else to do so: this may cause your baby to suffer brain damage. If you cannot comfortably delay your baby's birth, don't try to interfere. Deliver the head slowly. There's more chance that your vagina and perineum will tear if you push along with the force of your uterus, so pant lightly with each contraction.

Prolapsed cord If a loop of the umbilical cord washes out when the membranes rupture and your partner says he can see a piece of grey-blue shiny cord bulging out of your vagina, this means that you have a prolapsed cord. You must get help as soon as possible as your baby's oxygen supply is in danger of being cut off. Don't panic; you have time. Get on to the floor on your knees, with your chest to your knees, your head on the floor, and your buttocks in the air. This helps to take the pressure of your baby's head off your cervix. If the cord is still protruding, ask your partner to cover it with a wet, warm, very clean towel before he rings the hospital or goes for help. Don't touch or put any pressure on the cord. Stay in the knee-chest position even on the way to hospital, because it reduces pressure on the cord. A prolapsed cord means you'll have to have a Caesarean delivery, unless the cervix is fully dilated, in which case forceps or ventouse will be used.

What the birth assistant should do

If it looks as if your partner's going to give birth at home without medical assistance, telephone the hospital or your midwife if you haven't done so already. If you haven't got a telephone, on no account leave the mother alone. However anxious and overwhelmed you feel, it's vital for you to stay calm and reassure your partner – she needs to feel confident and relaxed. Encourage her to take up any position she finds comfortable.

Wash your hands thoroughly in soap and water, then fetch lots of clean bath towels. Fold one and put it on the floor to lay your baby on. Then fill several bowls with hand-warm water, and find plenty of clean hand towels, face flannels, and tea towels. They can be soaked in the water and used as wipes during and after delivery.

The birth Your partner will know when her baby's coming because she'll feel a stinging or burning sensation as the baby stretches her vagina. See if the top of the baby's head is visible in the vaginal outlet. Remind your partner to pant or blow, so that her vagina and perineum have time to thin and stretch, which might help to avoid tearing.

Your baby's head will probably be born in one contraction and the rest of his body in the contraction afterwards. When the head is born, wipe each of your baby's eyes from inside to outside with separate pieces of moist cloth, and then feel round his neck to see if the cord is present. If it is, crook your little finger underneath it and pull it very gently over his head, or lift it so that his body can be born through the loop.

Do not interfere with the cord because it may go into a spasm and deprive your baby of oxygen. If the membranes are still present over your baby's face, gently tear them off with your fingernail so that your baby can breathe. Be careful to hold him firmly, as he'll be slippery with blood, mucus, and vernix. Never pull on his head, his body, or the cord.

Once the baby is born, he'll probably give a couple of gasps, a cry, and then start to cry properly. If he doesn't cry at once, place him across your partner's thigh or abdomen with his head lower than his feet, and then gently rub his back. This helps any mucus to drain away and usually causes a change in blood pressure, which brings about his first breath. Talking to your baby lovingly and calmly will also help.

After the birth Once your baby's breathing, pass him to your partner so she can put him to her breast and keep him warm against her skin. If the baby's interested in feeding, the nipple stimulation will also release oxytocin, which encourages your partner's uterus to contract again and expel the placenta.

Keep your partner and your baby warm with blankets or towels, especially your baby's head, as most heat is lost from here. Bear in mind that the normal colour of a baby at birth is a bluish-white. He'll gradually become pink in the first minutes as oxygen enters his body. Don't try to wash off the vernix, and never cut the umbilical cord.

The delivery of the placenta

If the placenta is delivered before an attendant arrives:

- never pull on the cord

- don't cut the cord

- after the placenta is delivered, massage the mother's uterus firmly, with a deep circular motion, gently pushing downwards 5–7cm (2–3in) below the navel and rubbing. This is important to make sure the uterus contracts and stays hard after the birth so there's no haemorrhage

- it's normal for a couple of cups of blood to be delivered when the placenta comes out

- getting your baby to nurse immediately will help the uterus contract and minimize blood loss

- if your baby won't suck, massage your partner's nipples as another way of releasing oxytocin.

Forceps delivery

Forceps look like large sugar tongs and are designed to fit snugly over the sides of a baby's head, covering the ears.

The decision to use forceps is a medical judgment on the part of your attendants. Forceps are applied only when the first stage is complete, the cervix is fully dilated, and the head is in the birth canal.

Why forceps are used Forceps are applied when your baby's head has descended into your pelvis, but fails to descend further; when a baby presents in a posterior position; in a breech delivery (see main text); when the uterus fails to maintain contractions; or when you lack the strength to push. Occasionally, forceps may be used for a quick delivery early in the second stage if your baby shows signs of lacking oxygen, even if the birth is not imminent.

How it's done If you're going to have a forceps delivery, your legs will be put up in stirrups. Usually you will have had a spinal anaesthetic. Then the forceps will be inserted into your vagina one at a time. A few gentle pulls on the forceps, 30–40 seconds at a time, will bring your baby's head down on to your perineum. You should feel no pain. At this point you'll have an episiotomy (see p.110). Once your baby's head has been delivered, the forceps are removed and the rest of his body will be delivered as normal.

Complications at delivery

Delivery usually goes smoothly. Occasionally, though, there may be complications. Something unforeseen may happen once labour has started, meaning that forceps or a vacuum extractor have to be used. Other special deliveries, such as multiple and breech births, are usually diagnosed well in advance.

Assisted delivery

If, as sometimes happens, labour and delivery don't go quite as smoothly as expected, your obstetrician may need to give you some help to complete a vaginal delivery. Forceps (see column, left) can be used to protect your baby's head or, along with vacuum extraction, may be used to speed your baby's progress through the birth canal.

Vacuum extraction The vacuum extractor, or ventouse, is a gentler alternative to forceps, and is widely used throughout Europe. It's made up of a metal plate or cone-shaped cup of synthetic material. This plate or cup is placed over the baby's scalp. An attached pump is then used to create a vacuum that makes the plate or cup hold fast to the baby's head. This instrument then becomes a "handle", which the obstetrician can use to rotate the baby's head and apply traction.

Multiple deliveries

If you're having twins, their delivery will always be treated as though you're having two single babies: if one has a vaginal delivery it doesn't always follow that the other will. Your doctor and midwives will probably suggest you have the babies in hospital in case they aren't presenting properly. If all goes well, twins usually present head down, the second one arriving half an hour or so after the first. Twin labours can be long, so an epidural anaesthetic (see p.281) might help. Also the second baby may have to be turned – this is done by rupturing the second baby's membrane and moving him by hand and again an epidural is recommended.

Twin deliveries are much safer than they used to be because the exact position of the second baby, and his condition, can be determined by ultrasound and fetal monitors. If you're carrying three or more babies, you'll have a Caesarean section for their safety.

Breech birth

Four out of every 100 babies are born in the breech position so this isn't that unusual. A breech baby is usually born buttocks first, followed by his legs and body. Recent studies have suggested that it is safer for all full-term breech babies to be born by Caesarean section. But in some circumstances – for example, if you are already progressing well in labour – your doctors may encourage you to have a vaginal delivery. Before your baby's head can be delivered, you'll almost certainly need an episiotomy. The head is the widest part and your baby's rump will not necessarily have stretched your birth canal enough for his head to pass through it. Once your baby's body is born, his weight will start to pull his head down to your vagina. His body will then be lifted upwards and slightly backwards by the midwife, and one push is usually enough to deliver him. Forceps may be used to protect your baby's head.

It's now fairly common practice to have an epidural if you're having a breech birth. This is to prevent you pushing against an incompletely dilated cervix, but it also means that if you do need a Caesarean section, it can be done quickly and simply without further anaesthesia.

Vacuum extractor

This device takes up less room in the vagina than forceps and is easier to apply. It has several other advantages over forceps.

■ It can be applied to the lowest part of the baby's head.

■ It doesn't affect the shape of a baby's head. It does, however, leave a bruise, but this will fade within a week or two of the birth.

■ An episiotomy isn't always necessary when a ventouse is used for delivery.

Delivering a breech baby vaginally

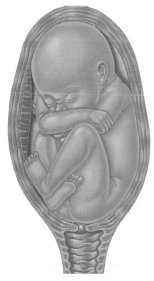

▲ **BABY IN BREECH POSITION**
Before the labour begins, the baby's breech (buttocks) has not engaged within his mother's pelvis and her cervix has not yet thinned.

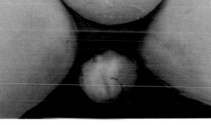

▲ **BUTTOCKS FIRST** In a breech birth the baby's buttocks (here still covered by the amniotic membranes) are delivered first.

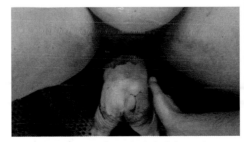

▲ **LEGS AND BODY** Once the baby's buttocks are clear of the birth opening, the membranes rupture and the baby's legs and body are delivered.

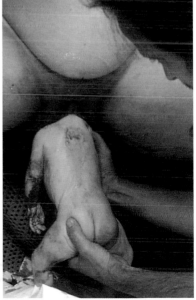

▲ **ARMS AND HEAD** In the final stages of a breech delivery, the baby's arms emerge. His body is gently supported by the midwife as his head is guided out.

What happens to you

A Caesarean operation usually takes 35–45 minutes, but the baby is delivered within the first five to ten minutes. The rest of the time is spent stitching you up.

Preparation Before the operation begins, a small amount of your pubic hair is shaved, you're given a spinal block, and an intravenous drip is set up to supply you with fluids during the operation. Then a catheter (a thin, flexible tube) is inserted up your urethra and into your bladder to drain it of urine. A small screen is placed in front of your face so you don't have to watch the operation. Your abdomen is cleaned down to prevent any infection. If the operation is urgent, for instance if your baby is in serious distress, you may need to have a general anaesthetic, but a spinal or epidural anaesthetic can usually be inserted very quickly.

The operation The obstetrician makes a short, horizontal incision along the "bikini line" at the base of your abdomen, then makes a similar incision in the lower segment of your uterus. The amniotic fluid is drained off by suction, and the baby is gently lifted out. Then the cord is cut, the placenta is removed, and your uterus and abdomen are stitched.

Caesarean section

If a normal vaginal delivery could be dangerous or even impossible for you, your baby will be delivered by Caesarean section. Small horizontal incisions are made in your abdomen and uterus, and your baby is delivered through them. The number of babies delivered by Caesarean section has increased rapidly and is now about one in four in the United Kingdom, of which two-thirds are emergency.

The need for a Caesarean section may be apparent well before labour begins, so you, your partner, and your obstetrician have time to talk through what will happen – this is an elective Caesarean. In emergencies, the need only becomes evident once labour is under way.

Elective Caesarean section

The most common medical reasons for choosing to have a Caesarean include your baby's head being too large to pass through your pelvis; your baby being in a breech position (see p.307) or lying across your pelvis; placenta praevia (see p.222); and certain medical conditions such as active herpes type II infection. Some women also ask for Caesareans as they believe they are easier and they feel more in control. But the more Caesarean sections a woman has, the greater the risk of bleeding during the delivery, and therefore of needing a hysterectomy.

A Caesarean section may be necessary if you've had one for a previous baby – the worry used to be that the previous scar would very often open up again. Experience has shown that this does not happen with the horizontal cut now generally used instead of the vertical cut. So hospitals often allow a trial vaginal delivery to begin; if there are no problems, labour goes on as normal – called a "trial of labour" or vaginal birth after Caesarean section (VBAC).

Elective Caesareans are often carried out under a spinal anaesthetic (see p.281). This has several advantages over a general anaesthetic: it's safer for your baby; you have no post-operative nausea or vomiting; and because you are conscious, you can hold your baby as soon as he's born. It's usually possible for your partner to be with you during the operation.

When you've had a Caesarean, you may feel disappointed or even cheated that you didn't have a vaginal delivery. It's natural to feel like this, and the best thing you can do is talk it all through with your partner. It also helps, of course, to prepare yourself in advance for this type of birth. Go and see the obstetrician with your partner and find out what the operation involves. If you can, talk to other women who've had Caesarean sections and get their advice.

Emergency Caesarean section

This may be needed when something goes wrong during labour, such as a prolapsed umbilical cord, placental haemorrhage, fetal distress, or serious failure to progress in labour.

After a Caesarean section

As is the case with any major surgery, it takes time to recover from a Caesarean, but even so you'll be encouraged to get up and walk around a few hours afterwards to stimulate your circulation. You'll be given pain relief if you need it, and the dressings will be removed after three or four days. Your internal stitches will be made with absorbable sutures, which will dissolve away naturally. Skin stitches may also be absorbable, but if not they will be removed within about a week.

The effects on your baby

Not having to pass through the birth canal is both a benefit and a drawback for the baby.

A baby born by vaginal delivery has a rather squashed look at first, while a Caesarean baby has smooth features and a rounded head. But often the Caesarean baby needs more time to adjust to the world – first, because of her sudden entry into it, and second, because she's missed the journey through the birth canal that helps to clear amniotic fluid from her lungs and stimulates her circulation.

Caesarean under epidural anaesthetic

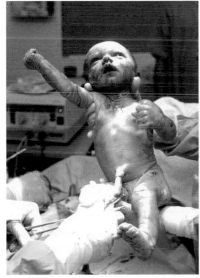

▲ **CAESAREAN DELIVERY** When the incisions have been made, the obstetrician begins to ease the baby out. Within five to ten minutes of the incisions, the baby is delivered (above) and the cord clamped and cut.

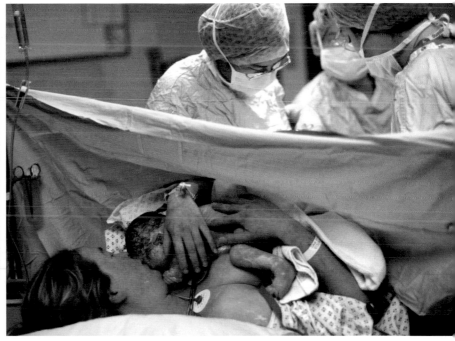

▲ **AFTER DELIVERY** If you've had a spinal anaesthetic you remain conscious, so while the placenta is delivered and the incisions stitched up you can hold your baby.

Miriam's casebook

An emergency Caesarean

Fran's first child is now three years old. Both the pregnancy and birth went smoothly. Her second pregnancy was also healthy and she and her baby were both doing well. Three days before her expected date of delivery, she went into labour, which progressed perfectly normally until the end of the first stage, when Fran was suddenly told she would have to have an emergency Caesarean section.

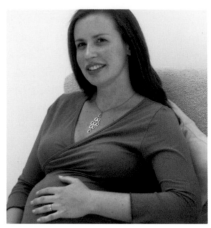

Being well-informed parents

Fran was glad she'd taken the trouble to find out about Caesarean sections in advance. About 25 per cent of babies in the UK are born by Caesarean section. A Caesarean is either planned, known as an "elective" Caesarean, or may need to be carried out as an emergency because the baby has to be delivered quickly.

Fran's waters broke halfway through the first stage of labour, when her cervix was only 4cm (1½in) dilated. Following the rule that every mother must have an internal examination as soon as her membranes have ruptured, the midwife examined Fran at once. She discovered a prolapsed cord – a loop of the umbilical cord coming through the cervix into the vagina in advance of the baby. This is an extremely dangerous situation because, as the baby's head presses down on the undilated cervix, the prolapsed section of the cord is squeezed tighter and tighter, cutting off the baby's blood and oxygen supply.

During the examination, the midwife touched the cord and could feel that it was pulsating. This was reassuring as it meant that Fran's baby was still receiving enough blood. However, within a couple of minutes the sonicaid (see p.275) picked up that the baby's heartbeat was starting to dip and the baby was showing signs of considerable fetal distress. Fran's obstetrician told her she needed an emergency Caesarean section to protect her baby's wellbeing.

Preparing for birth

While the operating theatre was prepared, Fran was asked to lie on her front with her buttocks in the air, relieving the pressure on the cord. Meanwhile, the midwife kept her fingers in Fran's vagina in order to keep the baby's head pushed up away from the cervix.

Fortunately, Fran had chosen to have an epidural anaesthetic early in labour, so she didn't need to have a general anaesthetic. And there was the bonus that she'd be awake during the birth.

The surgeon made a standard transverse incision (see column, p.308) through which Fran's baby was gently lifted out. As soon as the baby's head was delivered, the anaesthetist gave Fran an injection of syntometrine. This stimulates uterine contractions, making it easier for the placenta to separate from the uterine wall and follow the baby out through the incision. Once the baby was safely delivered and Fran was being sewn up, her partner Jonathan was able to hold their baby before taking her for her mother to see for the first time. Although Fran was disappointed about not having a normal vaginal delivery, she and Jonathan had shared the experience of Eleanor's birth and Fran had held Eleanor in the first few minutes after her birth.

After the operation, Fran returned to the postnatal ward with Eleanor where she could concentrate on feeding her and getting to know her better.

Going home from hospital

Fran found getting back to normal after the Caesarean was almost the hardest part. I suggested she join a self-help group for post-Caesarean mothers, where she'd get useful advice on how to handle the postnatal period. Fran also worried that her next baby would have to be delivered by Caesarean, too. I reassured her that most mothers can have normal deliveries following Caesareans, although there may be good reasons for having another one.

I reminded Fran that she had undergone serious abdominal surgery, so she needed plenty of rest and time for her scar to heal. When her stitches were removed, five days after the operation, she was told that the scar would heal in three weeks and would fade after six months. Fran was surprised to find herself losing blood from her vagina, just as she did after her first child, which was a vaginal delivery, but I explained that this is quite normal.

Starting to breastfeed

I explained to Fran that if she was going to breastfeed sitting up, she must sit up straight. Her abdominal wall was tender so she used pillows to prop Eleanor up level with her breasts. She also found it comfortable to breastfeed lying on her side, resting on one elbow, with Eleanor on a pillow next to her.

Taking things gently

Fran found standing up quite difficult because her stomach hurt, but I encouraged her to try and stand up perfectly straight as soon as she got out of bed, and to place her hands over her incision, supporting it, whenever she wanted

Miriam's top tips

Up to 25 per cent of all babies born in the UK are delivered by Caesarean section. My advice is to:

- read up on Caesarean sections as part of your information-gathering about pregnancy and birth

- ask questions about Caesarean birth at your antenatal classes and when you visit your labour ward so you are aware of what's involved

- be sure to allow yourself plenty of time to recover fully if you do have a Caesarean section – it's a major operation and it takes time for your body to heal.

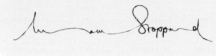

to laugh or cough. I told her that the more she managed to move around, the speedier her recovery would be.

After her stitches were removed, she was allowed home, but was told to rest and to be very careful when lifting anything. She had to avoid any strenuous exercise and driving for at least six weeks, and was advised not to drive until she felt fully recovered.

Delivering Fran's baby

Some aspects of Eleanor's birth were of course very different from that of a baby who is pushed down the birth canal. Once the incision was made in her mother's abdomen, the surgeon slipped a hand under her head and applied forceps in order to pull her head out gently. Next, her shoulders were manoeuvred carefully through the incision and her body was then gently pulled out. In the first moments after delivery, she was held with her head downwards while her mouth and pharynx were cleansed of fluid with a soft catheter attached to suction apparatus. Once she had taken her first breath, the cord was cut and she was checked to make sure that all her systems were functioning properly (see Apgar score, p.292). Once she was breathing normally, she was handed to her father for a cuddle.

A father's reaction

When a baby dies, both parents grieve. But a father may express his grief very differently from his partner, and this can lead to tension in the relationship.

If a father grieves in a different way to his partner, it doesn't mean his grief is any less intense. Some men try to hide their grief and throw themselves into work in order to find some relief from the pain they're feeling. Fortunately, all of us are learning that it's better for us to be open to feelings and express them. Hopefully, men will be more encouraged to let their true feelings show, especially to their partners.

Support groups for bereaved parents can put fathers in contact with other men who have lost their babies. Being with other men who've been through the same experiences may help a bereaved father express his grief, anger, and all the other possible emotions he may feel, in whatever way is best for him. What's important is that he's allowed and able to express his grief in his own way.

If a baby dies

The death of any child is always a tragic event, but the death of a baby before, during, or very soon after birth can be especially distressing. Today, in the Western world, the number of babies who are stillborn after 24 weeks or who die within the first few weeks of life has fallen to about one per cent, largely thanks to improved obstetric and paediatric care.

Why babies die

There are three main groups of perinatal deaths: stillbirths – babies who die before labour begins; intrapartum deaths – babies who die during labour; and neonatal deaths – babies who die within four weeks of birth.

Stillbirth About 45 per cent of perinatal deaths are stillbirths, and in about one-third of these cases the precise cause is not known. Of the rest, the most important causes are severe fetal defects (see also p.196) and a placenta that's not entirely healthy. Less common causes of stillbirth include Rhesus incompatibility (see p.202), and maternal diabetes that is not carefully controlled.

The first thing that happens when a baby dies in the uterus is the almost complete disappearance from the mother's blood of pregnancy hormones – oestrogen and progesterone. As a result, many of the signs and sensations of being pregnant fade quite quickly. Another early sign may be lack of fetal movement. If doctors or midwives suspect that a mother's baby may have died, an ultrasound scan will be done in order to look for the baby's heartbeat.

Labour usually starts within two to three days of a baby's death, although many women want to have their babies delivered as soon as they find out that they have died. If you find yourself in this unhappy situation, your wishes should be respected; usually doctors will suggest induction. It may seem very hard, but it is less risky than a Caesarean section and less likely to affect any subsequent pregnancies.

Babies who die in labour This is exceptionally rare, but the death of a baby during labour is usually caused by a lack of oxygen as a result of a problem with the placenta. Another possible cause is injury to the baby during labour and delivery. This is far less common than it was in the past, thanks to high levels of modern care.

Neonatal death Death of the newborn may be caused by breathing difficulties, especially in babies born preterm (see pp.344 and 348) or who are suffering from severe fetal defects. Fatal neonatal infections, once a significant cause of the deaths of newborn babies, are now very rare because of improved hygiene standards and modern antibiotics.

Coping with a death

It's very important for both partners to come to terms with their grief, to be open about the death of their baby, to accept it, and to go through the grieving process together.

It's absolutely normal for bereaved parents to feel isolated, angry with themselves, each other, the staff, or the unfairness of life, and often guilty about something they did or didn't do. However, accepting that everyone involved did everything possible and that nobody is to blame, while also acknowledging how you feel, will help the healing process.

Parents are encouraged to hold their stillborn baby for a while after the birth, and most are very glad of this later. Having a photograph of the baby can also be a great comfort in the future. It helps to give the baby a name, to bury the baby formally, and to be present at the burial.

Another important form of solace is to get in touch with other parents who have had stillbirths or neonatal deaths (see Addresses, p.370). Details of support groups are usually available from your hospital and you can also try sharing your experiences with other parents on Internet forums. Don't be afraid to ask for help from a counsellor if you need it.

Emotional effects The emotional and physical effects on the mother are due not only to the shock and grief of losing her baby but also to the sudden withdrawal of pregnancy hormones. This can affect her mood, bringing on tearfulness, depression, insomnia, appetite loss, and withdrawal, as well as loss of milk from the breasts. The milk can be suppressed with drugs. The comfort and support of her partner, family, and friends is vital. It helps if both partners are open with each other and share their grief so that they can give each other support and comfort.

Getting pregnant again

Parents need to allow plenty of time to grieve before another pregnancy is contemplated. Many women, however, find the key to normality and a return to happiness is through conceiving again. Once partners have decided to try for another baby, they may find that worry about losing this baby will be hard to shake off. The risk of a recurrence is very slight, but where there has been a predisposing cause, subsequent pregnancies are carefully managed.

Losing a twin

The death of one twin (or triplet) is just as tragic for the parents as the death of a singleton, and carries additional problems.

The loss of one baby in a multiple birth leaves parents with a complex emotional situation – they are mourning the death of the lost baby, while celebrating the life of the surviving twin or triplet(s). Faced with this impossible mix of emotions, many parents postpone their mourning. Others find they cannot attend to the needs of their living baby or babies properly because of the intensity of grief for the dead baby.

The loss of one baby may also cast a shadow over the life of the surviving twin or triplet(s), and birthdays may be particularly difficult for the first few years.

It must be stressed that a mother who's had a multiple pregnancy continues to think of herself as the mother of twins or triplets, regardless of whether any of the babies have died.

Parents who have lost a twin or a triplet may be told that they are "lucky" because they've still got their other child(ren). No other parent is expected to find comfort for the death of a child in the survival of its siblings.

Getting to know your newborn baby

Nurturing a relationship with your baby begins the second she's born. As you learn how to care for her and meet her needs, your love will deepen and grow, and what she's able to do from the earliest days will amaze you.

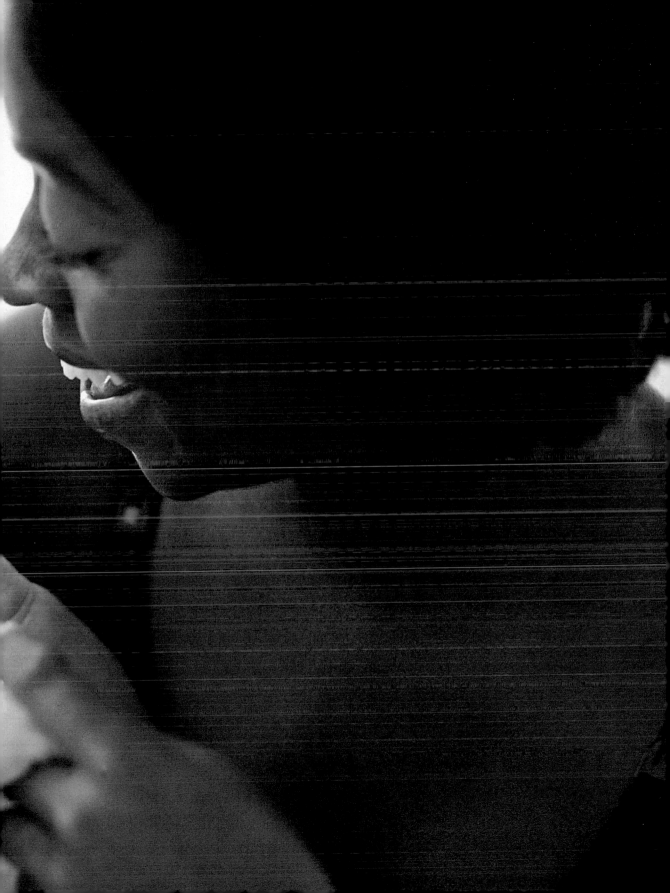

Your first reaction

Your newborn baby's appearance may surprise you when you first see him. He'll have wrinkly skin and you may think he looks more like an old man than a baby.

Some parents worry about how they feel when their baby actually arrives: he doesn't seem to be quite what they'd expected.

Unless you've had a Caesarean, his head may be slightly squashed with some bruising and his eyelids may be puffy, because of the pressure of passing through the birth canal.

He may look quite messy as he'll be coated in a greasy substance (see right), possibly mixed with some of your blood, and he may have patches of body hair. His limbs may be a bluish colour, and his genitals will look huge.

Don't be disappointed if you don't immediately feel love and tenderness when you first look at your baby. These feelings will develop as you get to know each other.

Your new baby

Take your baby in your arms and hold him as soon as possible after birth so that you can start to bond. Your baby will begin to learn about you, and how much you love him, as he hears your voice, smells and feels your skin, and is cuddled and suckled by you.

You're likely to feel many new emotions when you see your newborn baby's tiny, vulnerable body and realize his complete dependence on you. The way you react and what you do in these first moments are probably the most important interactions there'll ever be between you and your child.

Research shows that parents who can cuddle and be with their babies immediately after delivery tend to be more sympathetic to their children's needs later. Parents whose babies are taken away at birth may feel alienated for a while, but if this does happen to you, don't worry – just start bonding with your baby as soon as you're able to.

What your baby will look like

Newborn babies vary greatly in how much they weigh and how long they are. Average weights for a baby are generally from 2.5 to 4.5kg (5lb 8oz to 9lb 12oz), and average lengths are from 48 to 51cm (19 to 20in).

Head Your newborn baby's head will be one-quarter of his length and it'll look large compared with the rest of his body. The younger the baby, the larger his head is in proportion to his body. On average a newborn baby's head measures about 35cm (14in) round. His head will be measured after birth and this is an important check because the growth of his head is linked to the development of his brain.

A newborn baby's head usually looks pointed because it's been moulded as it came through the birth canal. Moulding is caused by the skull bones overriding each other. Sometimes this pressure also leaves one or both sides of the baby's head slightly swollen. This swelling doesn't affect your baby's brain and it goes down within a few weeks. If your baby was delivered by forceps or vacuum, he may have some slight bruising. You'll feel a soft spot on the top, called a fontanelle, where the skull bones haven't yet joined and won't until your baby is 18 months old.

Skin Some babies are born completely covered in a greasy, white substance called vernix caseosa. Others have vernix only on their face and hands. Vernix makes it easier for your baby to slide through the birth canal and helps protect him against minor skin infections. The vernix used to be cleaned off right away, but most hospitals now prefer to let it to rub off the skin naturally, which happens within two or three days.

Your baby's circulation takes a little while to settle down. While this is happening, the top half of his body may look paler than the bottom half, but this is nothing to worry about.

Your baby may have some downy hair on his body. This is called lanugo hair and it covered his body while he was in your womb (see p.80). Some babies only have lanugo hair on their head, but others may have hair on their shoulders. Both are quite normal and the hair usually rubs off within a couple of weeks.

More permanent hair will appear later. Some babies are born with a full head of hair but others are completely bald. If your baby is born with hair it might not be the colour he eventually ends up with.

Hands and feet These may have a slightly more bluish look than the rest of his body because his circulation hasn't quite got going. He may have dry patches with peeling skin, which will disappear in a few days. His fingernails may be long and sharp; gently nibble off the tips if he's scratching himself, but don't cut his nails.

Eyes Your baby's eyes may be puffy because of pressure on his head during the birth and he may not be able to open them at first. This pressure may also have broken some tiny blood vessels in his eyes, causing harmless red marks in the whites. These will soon disappear. Your baby can see clearly to a distance of 20–25cm (8–10in) or so, but

▼ YOUR BABY'S APPEARANCE Your newborn baby may not look at all as you expected and he'll have certain newborn characteristics that may surprise you

A beating pulse can often be seen under the fontanelle. Although it's quite tough, it should never be pressed hard

Your baby's legs may look bowed because he's been curled up in your womb

Your baby's stomach may look slightly bloated

His feet and hands may have dry, peeling skin as they've been immersed in liquid for so long

An identity bracelet will be attached to your baby's ankle

His genitals may look swollen and large

His umbilical cord is clamped and cut straight after delivery

His eyes may look puffy

His fingers are curled in towards his palms

Your baby's birthmarks

A group of small blood vessels under the surface of the skin may appear as a small blemish on your baby's body, but won't usually need any treatment.

Stork bites These are mild pink patches which usually appear on the nose, eyelids, and neck under the hair-line. They may take about a year to disappear.

Strawberry birthmarks These first appear as tiny red dots and may get bigger up to the end of the first year. They almost always disappear by five years of age.

Mongolian spots These are blue and are found on the lower back of babies with dark skin tones. They fade away naturally.

Port wine stains These large, flat red or purple marks are usually on the face and neck. These marks are permanent.

he cannot focus both eyes at the same time beyond that, so may squint or look cross-eyed. Both problems should gradually clear up as his eye muscles grow stronger (usually within a month). Check with your doctor if your baby still squints at six to eight months, or it gets any worse before then. All new babies have blue eyes and their adult eye colour may not develop until about six months.

Umbilicus Your baby's umbilical cord will be clamped with forceps and then cut with scissors. A short length of cord is left, which dries up and becomes almost black within two to four hours after the birth. The cord doesn't come away from the navel until about ten days after the birth. Some babies have umbilical hernias (small swellings near the navel), but these usually clear up within a year. If the hernia goes on longer than this or gets bigger, check with your doctor.

Breasts Pregnancy hormones may cause both boy and girl babies to have slightly enlarged breasts and leak a little milk. This is quite normal, and will adjust in a couple of days.

Your baby's care

Before you leave hospital your baby will be thoroughly examined by a paediatrician or midwife to make sure that everything's going well and there are no problems. They will also want to check that your baby is feeding well and that his stools are normal. On day seven a midwife will visit you at home and do a pinprick heel test on your baby for phenylketonuria (PKU), a rare metabolic disease, and a test for thyroid gland underactivity and/or cystic fibrosis. All babies are also tested for thalassaemia and sickle-cell disease. These can cause severe anaemia and are important to diagnose early.

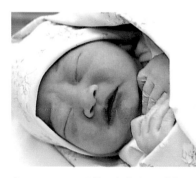

▲**PUFFY EYELIDS** Your baby's eyelids may be quite puffy because of pressure on the way through the birth canal. The swelling will go down in a couple of days.

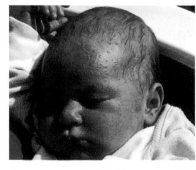

▲**SPOTTY SKIN** Small white spots, called milia, are caused by sebaceous glands that lubricate the skin becoming blocked. They're not serious and soon disappear.

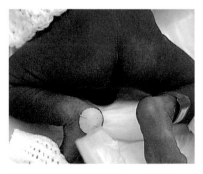

▲**BLOTCHY SKIN TONE** If your baby's circulation hasn't settled down, you may notice blotches on his body, and his legs may be a different colour.

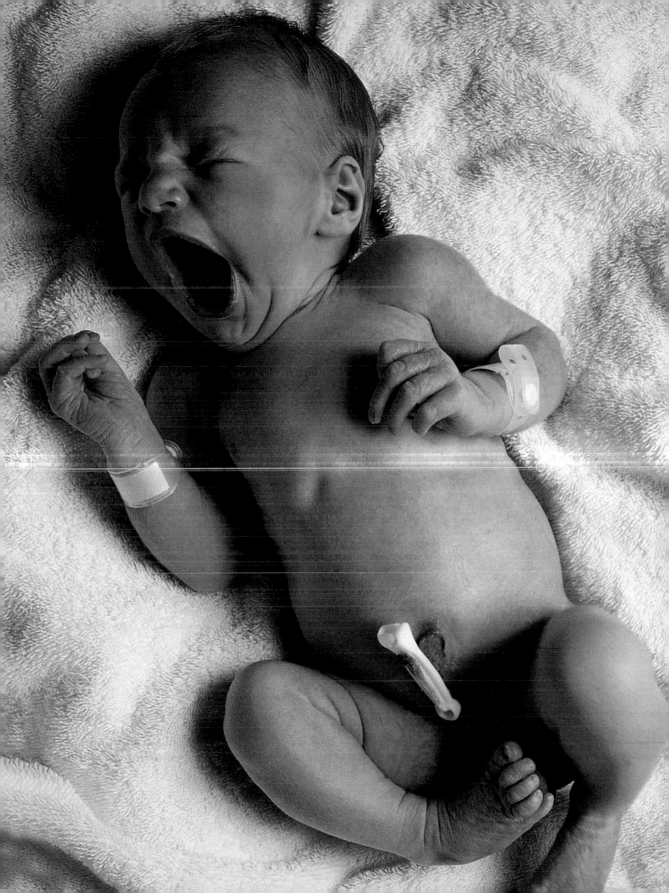

Get to know your baby

Spend as much time as you can playing with your baby – it's vital to her development.

Try to recognize her needs You will soon start to understand her different expressions. When she's content she'll look tranquil and quiet. When she's feeling miserable or uncomfortable she'll look rather red and flustered.

Playing together Don't worry about looking silly when you're playing with your baby. Pull funny faces and use a high-pitched voice, telling her how much you love her. She'll answer by nodding, moving her mouth, maybe sticking out her tongue, and jerking her body.

What your new baby can do

Your newborn baby has her own very special personality and she may surprise you with what she can do. Spend as much time as you can with her, and you'll soon get to know every little expression and sound she makes.

Posture and senses

At first, your baby's head is too heavy for her back and neck muscles to support. All her postures when not lying down are governed by her developing ability to control her head. If you put your baby on her back, she'll probably turn her head to one side, stretch out her arm on that side, and flex the opposite arm in towards her chest. When she's a week old, she'll raise her head in small jerks when she's supported on your shoulder. At six weeks she'll probably hold up her head for more than a minute.

From birth, she has fairly good senses of hearing, smell, and taste. At first, she mainly touches things with her mouth. She'll soon recognize you by smell, and by sight, too, within a couple of weeks. When you hold your baby close to you for the first time, she'll focus on your face, and look into your eyes. Babies like looking at faces more than anything else. Hearing high-pitched human voices gives her great pleasure, and she'll like yours, and your partner's deeper one, more than any others.

Reflex actions

◀ **STEP REFLEX** If you hold your baby under her arms and let her feet touch a firm surface, she'll make stepping movements.

▶ **GRASP REFLEX** Your baby's fingers will tightly grasp anything that's placed in her palm. Her grasp is so strong that her whole body weight can be supported if she grabs your fingers with both her hands. The soles of her feet will also curl over if they're touched or tickled.

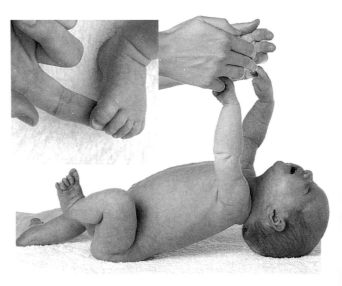

Sounds your baby will make

Breathing

Your baby's breathing may seem much lighter than yours. At times it may be irregular or fast and noisy, and she may snuffle as she tries to draw air through her small nasal passages. You might not always hear her breathing at first, but it'll get stronger every day.

Sneezes

Light stimulates the nerves to your baby's nose as well as her eyes, and bright lights may make her sneeze. A sneeze will clear out her nasal passages, and stop dust getting into her lungs. Don't worry when your baby sneezes – it's quite common and it doesn't mean she has a cold.

Hiccups

Your baby may hiccup often and this is perfectly normal. Hiccups can be caused when the diaphragm makes sudden, irregular contractions. They're a sign that the muscles used in breathing are getting stronger, and are trying to work together.

A newborn baby's reflexes

All babies have certain automatic movements – reflexes – which help them protect themselves. They usually last until about three months and are then lost. For example, your baby will close her eyes if you touch her eyelids. All babies have a strong sucking reflex if you press the palate in the mouth. Babies are born with the swallowing reflex – they've had to use it when swallowing fluids in the womb – and so they can swallow colostrum or milk the instant they are born.

▲ ROOTING REFLEX Your baby will search for your breast to feed. Gently stroke her cheek and she'll turn in that direction and open her mouth.

▶ MORO REFLEX If your baby's startled, she'll throw out her arms and legs as if to catch hold of something. Her limbs will then slowly curl inwards, with clenched fists.

Why your baby cries

Crying is your baby's only way of speaking to you. You'll soon learn to recognize her different cries, and what to do in response.

■ Your baby's first cry may sound more like a whimper, or splutter, before it turns into a full-blown cry. She'll take a deep breath, her body will tense, her face will grimace and become bright red, and she'll open her mouth wide and literally scream. Distressing as you might find this, it does show that your baby's perfectly healthy.

■ She'll cry when she's hungry, and usually won't stop until she's put to your nipple or given a bottle.

■ Tiredness, uncomfortable clothing, being too hot or too cold, or being undressed are all other reasons why babies cry.

■ Babies love being with you; if they feel abandoned they'll cry until picked up and cuddled.

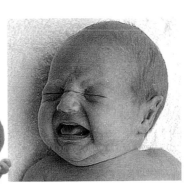

▲ A CRY FOR ATTENTION Sudden movements, very bright lights, loud noises, or feeling too hot or too cold – all these things may make your baby start to cry.

Going home

The routine for checking out varies from hospital to hospital – and from mother to mother. Usually, though, the following will happen before you're discharged.

■ A midwife or doctor will examine you. They'll check that your uterus is returning to its pre-pregnant size, that your stitches (if you've had any) are healing, and that your breasts are okay. They'll check your flow of lochia for colour and amount, and to see if you've passed any clots. Clotting with persistent bleeding may be a sign that there's still some placental tissue inside you.

■ If you've had a Caesarean, the doctor will check your incision and remove non-absorbable stitches.

■ Your midwife will talk to you about contraception, and give you a prescription for the contraceptive pill if necessary.

■ If you weren't immune to rubella (German measles) during your pregnancy, you'll be immunized.

■ You'll be shown how to clean your baby's umbilical cord.

■ You'll be given a date for your postnatal check-up, and advised to take your baby to the clinic for a six-week check-up.

When you leave, dress your baby warmly as he can't regulate his temperature very well yet. You'll need comfortable clothes, as your breasts will enlarge when your milk comes in and your stomach will still be bigger than before.

Your stay in hospital

What happens in hospital after your baby's been born will vary, depending on whether you've had a vaginal or Caesarean delivery (see p.306), which hospital you're in, how long you stay for, and the health of both you and your newborn baby.

Your care

Immediately after the birth, your midwife will take your temperature and note your pulse rate and blood pressure. These will be checked every four hours for the first day or so. The midwife will continue to check when she visits you at home. Your pulse rate may change slightly but this is normal, so nothing to worry about.

Medical staff will also check that any stitches or tears you have are healing properly and that you don't have any infection. They may suggest you apply ice packs to the area to prevent swelling and ease the pain, and you may be offered painkillers for afterpains during the first few days.

They'll also keep a close eye on the amount and appearance of your lochia in case there are any abnormal blood clots or excessive bleeding. Your uterus will be checked to make sure that it's starting to return to its pre-pregnant state and your legs will be examined for any signs of thrombosis. Your midwife may also ask a few questions to get an idea of your emotional state and make sure you're recovering from the birth.

Up and about It's best to start moving about as much as you can soon after delivery. This will help you get your strength back more quickly and helps your bowel and bladder to start working normally again (see p.354).

Unless you're very tired and simply want to sleep you can get up to go to the toilet, have a shower, or walk about any time after the birth. It's a good idea to have someone to help you at first in case you feel faint or weak. If you've lost a lot of blood at delivery, you'll probably have a blood test on about the fourth or fifth day after delivery to check that your haemoglobin is returning to normal.

Caesarean births About one in four women in the UK have Caesarean births. Many have regional anaesthesia but if you do have a general you may feel sick and wobbly. Your incision will be painful and the stitches will be covered by a soft dressing. You'll probably have a drip in your arm and may be given painkillers to help you sleep. If your baby is healthy and well, there's no reason why he can't be with you all the time.

If your stitches aren't self-absorbing, they'll be taken out about five days after delivery, which is only mildly uncomfortable. After a Caesarean, expect to stay in hospital for about five days if everything's normal (see also pp.306 and 308).

Hospital procedures

You may find hospital routines a little annoying, especially if you're woken for meals or routine checks by the midwives when you'd rather be asleep. But where breastfeeding is concerned, think about your own and your baby's needs above all else. Take the time you need to feed your baby and ask for help if you're finding it difficult. Start slowly, with short periods of two to three minutes on each breast, so that your nipples have a chance to harden up. That way they won't get sore and crack. Your baby may not seem very interested in feeding at first – he may be tired too – but after the first day, try putting him to your breast whenever he seems to want it. It's really important to eat properly yourself so you keep your strength up for breastfeeding. Hospital food can sometimes be bland and unappetizing so ask your partner to bring in some treats such as fresh fruit for you.

Visitors It's lovely to see your family and friends, but you'll find that visitors will tire you out more than you'd expect, so try to limit each visit to half an hour at the most. Ask everyone except your partner and your other children to stick to hospital visiting times so you can rest when you need to. Partners are usually allowed to come and see you whenever you want, but this policy does vary from hospital to hospital.

Social contact Being in hospital can be quite enjoyable. You'll have a chance to get to know the other mothers and to talk about your feelings and worries with them. You're all going through the same things and by sharing your experiences and working out plans together, you may find that you make friendships that last well after your stay in hospital.

Feeling unhappy If, on the other hand, you find that ward life doesn't suit you and you're feeling unhappy in hospital, you could ask if you can go home earlier than planned. Many maternity units are so busy that they're happy for mothers and babies to go home just six hours after the birth as long as all is well. You're unlikely to have to stay more than 48 hours in hospital, but even this can seem a long time if you're feeling homesick and anxious. Perhaps you could try talking to one of the midwives on the hospital staff or to another more experienced mother about your feelings. Comfort yourself by thinking about how you, your baby, and your partner will all be home together as a family very soon.

Registering the birth

By law, every birth must be notified to the Registrar within six weeks in England, Wales, and Northern Ireland, and within three weeks in Scotland.

The hospital will be able to give you the address of their nearest local registry office (which may not be near where you live). The Registrar will ask for your baby's name and place of birth, and the father's occupation. If partners are unmarried, both need to be present in order for both parents' names to appear on the baby's birth certificate.

In Scotland and Northern Ireland, the mother's maiden name will also be needed, and in Scotland, the date and place of the marriage as well, if applicable.

A short-form birth certificate, giving your child's name and sex, and the date and place of birth, will be issued free. A full certificate can be obtained later for a small fee. You'll need the birth certificate for claiming benefits for your baby.

Do register your baby as soon as you can because child benefit is only paid from the date of registration, not the date of birth.

The Registrar will also give you a form with your baby's National Health Service number on it. You need this form to register your baby with your doctor. Fill it in and take it to your doctor's surgery.

Benefits for your baby

Recent research has shown that the more physical contact babies have, the healthier and happier they become.

You can appeal to your baby's sense of rhythm by rocking and swaying him. Skin-to-skin contact stimulates his senses of touch and smell, and even helps him to grow. Human skin sends and receives warmth that has a positive effect on other human skins. Snuggling together will evoke a feeling of sensuous contentment.

Holding and handling

A newborn baby can appear very fragile and, at first, many parents are quite scared to pick up and handle their baby because of the feeling that he's so breakable. Your baby is actually very resilient and, as long as you support him firmly, there's no need to be afraid.

Firm support

Even if he's crying to be picked up, don't use jerky or quick movements when lifting him – do it as slowly, as gently, and as quietly as you can. Most babies like to be handled in a firm way; it makes them feel more secure. He won't be able to support his head for several weeks so you'll have to support it so that it doesn't loll. Always hold your baby close, keeping your arms close to your body, and bending over the place you're lifting from or putting down. To put him down, reverse the process of

Picking up your baby

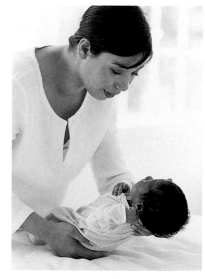

▲ **LIFTING YOUR BABY** Slide one hand under his neck and head, and the other behind his lower back. Lift him gently so that his head doesn't fall back.

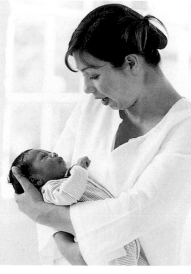

▲ **SUPPORT HIS HEAD** Always be sure to support your baby's head with your hand or in the crook of your arm so that it doesn't loll around.

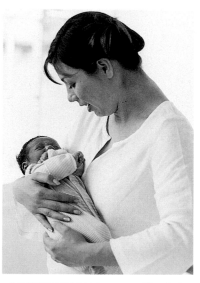

▲ **CRADLE HIM IN YOUR ARMS** Your baby will feel safe and secure cradled in the crook of your elbow, with his head and limbs well supported.

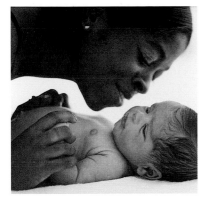

picking him up, always supporting his neck. When you lay your baby down, it's safest to put him on his back, or his side, if propped.

Loving support A mother often feels prime responsibility for her newborn baby, but most partners are keen to be fully involved as early as possible. Both your baby and his father will be able to develop a better understanding of each other through cuddling, handling, and carrying, and the more tactile their relationship, the more loving it will be.

All through the day, especially when changing him, you can discover ways to gently explore and caress his body. The best way to cuddle together is by lying naked in bed. In this way, he can smell your skin, feel its touch and warmth, and hear your heart beating clearly.

Benefits for you

From the moment your baby is born you can develop a special feeling of intimacy by holding him close to your bare skin.

Skin-to-skin contact enables you to become intimate with your baby. You will enjoy "skin bathing" with your baby – the feel of his soft, warm skin against yours, and the wonderful smell of newborn baby.

When you're feeding, whether by breast or bottle, don't let a barrier of clothing always come between you. You'll both benefit from holding him close against your bare skin (see column, opposite) – not least as he'll begin to recognize your smell (a key step in the bonding process, especially if you're not breastfeeding).

325

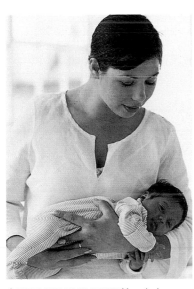

▲**HOLD HIM FACE DOWN** Your baby may like being held face down in your arms, his cheek resting on your forearm so he can feel your skin.

Your baby will be comforted by the familiar beat of your heart

◀ **HOLD HIM AGAINST YOUR SHOULDER** Held upright like this, your baby feels very secure. Put one hand under his bottom, and support his head with your other hand.

Producing milk

Your breasts change during pregnancy to prepare them for producing milk. Your milk will begin to come in a few days after you've given birth.

A female breast has 15–20 groups of milk-producing glands, connected to the nipple by the milk ducts. When you're pregnant, the placenta and ovaries make high levels of the hormones oestrogen and progesterone, which stimulate the glands to make colostrum. Colostrum gives your baby water, protein, sugar, vitamins, minerals, and antibodies to protect him against infection. Your body stops making colostrum and starts making milk three to five days after your baby is born.

Pituitary gland

Hypothalamus

Beginning to breastfeed

If you're planning to breastfeed for the first time, you might be worried that you won't be able to produce enough milk or that your milk won't be nourishing enough. Don't be anxious – you're not likely to have any problems. All women are equipped to feed a baby. No breast is too small and, in most cases, your supply of milk will automatically adjust to meet your baby's needs.

Feeding on demand

A baby can digest a full feed of breast milk in about an hour and a half to two hours (half the time it takes for a bottlefed baby to digest a full feed of infant formula). So breastfeeding on demand means frequent feeding, but this doesn't mean your milk supplies will run out. Research shows that mothers who breastfeed their babies on demand produce more milk than those who breastfeed at regular but less frequent intervals.

One study compared babies breastfed on demand with those fed only every three or four hours. The babies fed on demand got an average of nearly ten feeds a day, compared to an average for the others of just over seven. The more frequent feeding didn't mean that a daily amount of milk was being divided into more but smaller feeds – in fact, it was the opposite. The fed-on-demand babies got an average of just over 73ml (2½floz) at each feed (725ml/25floz a day), while those fed at fixed intervals got only 68.8ml (2⅖floz) each feed (502ml/17floz a day). As a result, after two weeks the babies who were fed on demand had gained more weight than the others – an average of 561g (20oz) compared to 347g (12oz).

Keeping up your milk supply

Milk production can be affected by many things, including how you're feeling, how healthy you are, and what you eat. The change from colostrum to breast milk is triggered by changes in your hormones after the birth, but continuing supplies of milk depend on the sucking action of your baby. When he sucks, nerve endings in your areolae are stimulated, sending

◀ **STIMULATING MILK** Your baby's sucking stimulates nerve endings in your areolae. These send messages to your hypothalamus, which in turn sends signals to the pituitary gland to release the hormones that stimulate milk production.

signals to a part of your brain called the hypothalamus. The hypothalamus in turn sends signals to your pituitary gland telling it to release prolactin, the hormone that stimulates milk production – this response to your baby's sucking is known as the prolactin reflex. Your pituitary gland also releases oxytocin, a hormone that causes the muscle fibres around the milk glands to contract, squeezing the milk from the glands into your milk ducts. This is called the milk ejection or "let-down" reflex. When your breasts are full, it can be triggered not only by sucking but also by your baby's hunger cries or even simply when he's near to you.

A good milk supply The best way to keep up your milk supply is to feed your baby often, so that the prolactin reflex and the milk ejection reflex are triggered frequently. This will also prevent engorgement – swelling of your milk-producing glands by milk.

If the glands do swell, they won't be able to make milk efficiently. And you won't feel like feeding because it'll be painful. For these reasons, the reflex that promotes the release of prolactin diminishes and so your milk production slows down. If this does happen, you can relieve engorged breasts by expressing milk (see column, right), and stop it happening again by feeding your baby often. It's also important to wait until your baby empties the first breast you give him before switching him to the other. This way he'll be sure to get not only the thirst-quenching, low-fat foremilk that comes from your breast first, but also the highly nourishing, fat-rich hindmilk that follows.

You'll need to eat well at this time, as your body has an even greater need for good nourishment than during pregnancy. You don't need to eat any special foods for breastfeeding, but it's best to have a balanced diet with plenty of protein, iron, and calcium, and lots of fluids, fresh fruit, and vegetables. Three good meals, with healthy snacks in between, will give you energy and keep you from getting too tired.

Refusal to feed

Occasionally, your baby won't want to breastfeed. This is most likely in the early days, when he may be too sleepy to be interested. If your baby refuses the breast, don't give up – express the milk he would have suckled and wait for him to want food. Babies feed better when they're hungry.

If you find that your baby tends to fall asleep soon after you've started feeding, try lying on your side, with him lying beside you. This way he'll find feeding less tiring. Your baby may also refuse to feed because he has difficulty latching on (see p.329). This is usually because your breasts are engorged – the swelling makes it difficult for your baby to latch on. If you express some milk before feeding, he'll be able to latch on more easily.

Expressing your milk

You may sometimes need to express milk from your breasts – perhaps so that your baby can be fed from a bottle if you have to go out for a while, you're returning to work, or if your breasts have become engorged (see p.356).

You can express milk by hand, but it's quicker to use a pump. When you've expressed your milk, put the cap tightly on the bottle. Refrigerate the milk until needed; it will keep for up to 24 hours in the fridge at a temperature of between 2°C and 4°C, or can be stored for up to six months in the freezer.

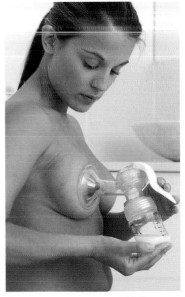

▲ **USING A MANUAL PUMP** Fit the funnel over your areola to form an airtight seal, then operate the lever to express the milk. You can buy electric pumps that are quicker to use.

The sucking effect

A baby stimulates milk to flow as he latches on to your breast. Then he presses the back of his tongue up towards his palate to squeeze the milk from your nipple into his throat.

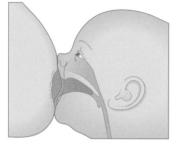

▲**STARTING THE FLOW** Your baby presses the tip of his tongue against the areola at the base of your nipple.

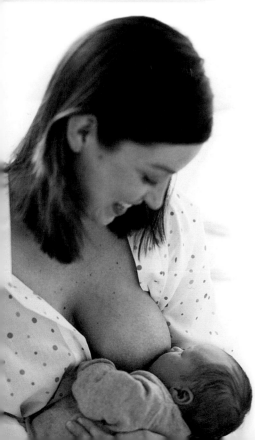

Breastfeeding your baby

Breastfeeding your baby is a loving, nurturing experience that strengthens the bond between you. It carries on the physiological relationship that began when your baby was developing in your womb. Your baby knows your milk will be there when he needs it and trusts it to be pure and good. Because of this, some people say that breastfeeding is the first way to tell the truth to a baby and to keep a promise.

Latching on

The key to happy, trouble-free breastfeeding is knowing how to get your baby's mouth correctly fixed or latched on to your breast. If your baby's latched on properly he'll get enough milk and you'll avoid breast and lactation problems. When your baby is feeding properly, his jaws will be clamped on your breast tissue rather than just on to your nipple, which will be completely inside his mouth.

To encourage your baby to latch on as easily as possible, give yourself plenty of time to feed and make sure you're comfortable and relaxed. Hold your baby high enough so he can reach your nipple without effort. Cradle his head in the crook of your arm, and support his back and bottom with your lower arm and hand. Express a little milk to soften the areola and ensure that his mouth contains the entire nipple.

Correct latching on is important to both you and your baby for two reasons. First, it prevents your baby from sucking on the nipple itself, which can cause soreness and cracking. Second, it allows him to stimulate a good flow of milk and makes sure that he gets the rich hindmilk as well as the less nourishing but thirst-quenching foremilk (see p.327). A good flow of milk also prevents your breast from becoming engorged (see p.356) because it hasn't been emptied.

◀ **GETTING STARTED** Hold your baby close to your own body, with his head a little higher than his body. If you're sitting, keep your back straight. You may find it more comfortable to rest your baby on a pillow on your lap so that you're not holding all his weight. Until your baby learns to seek out or "root" for the nipple, stimulate his rooting reflex by gently touching the cheek nearest you. He'll instinctively turn his head towards your touch, and so towards your nipple.

Breastfeeding positions

If you are sitting make sure you are well supported. Lying down is ideal for night feeds; when your baby is very small you may need to lay him on a pillow so that he can reach your nipple. You may find a lying position the most suitable if you have had an episiotomy and sitting is uncomfortable. If you've had a Caesarean section and your stomach is still tender, try lying with your baby's feet tucked under your arm.

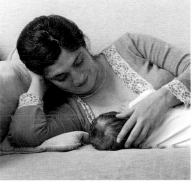

▲ **LYING POSITION** Breastfeeding positions that allow you to lie down are a restful alternative, especially at night. It can also keep a wriggling baby off a tender Caesarean incision.

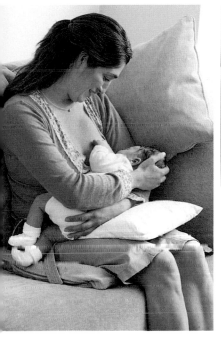

◄ **SITTING POSITION** Make sure that your arms and back are supported and you are comfortable and relaxed. Raise your baby to the right height with a cushion.

Supply and demand

Milk is produced in glands that are deeply buried in the breast, not in the fatty tissue, so breast size is no indication of how much milk you can produce; even small breasts are perfectly adequate milk producers.

Milk is produced according to demand – you supply what your baby needs, so don't worry that you'll run out of milk if your baby feeds very often. Your breasts are stimulated to produce milk by your baby's sucking, so the more eagerly he feeds, the more milk they will produce, and vice versa. Feeding makes you thirsty so keep a bottle of water by you.

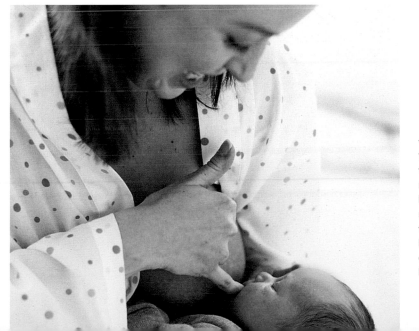

◄ **RELEASING THE BREAST** When he's feeding properly, his mouth will be wide open and, as his tongue and jaw muscles work to suck milk from your breast, you'll see his ears and temples moving. When he's finished feeding, or when all the milk has gone from the breast and you want to put him to the other, slip your little finger gently in between his jaws.

Breastfeeding tips

Breastfeeding is simple – if it weren't, so many millions of infants and mothers wouldn't have managed it successfully. Some mothers do have problems getting started, though, so do ask for help from friends, nurses, midwives, or the La Lêche League if you need to.

■ Establishing breastfeeding is always easier if you're able to put your baby to your breast within a few minutes of delivery. Once you've achieved successful suckling in the celebratory atmosphere that surrounds birth, you'll feel more confident about future feeding.

■ If your nipple is soft and small and your baby has trouble finding it, put a cold, wet cloth on it for a moment – your nipple will firm up and protrude.

■ Milk flows in both breasts at every nursing and it's better to use both at each feed. Start with the heavier breast.

■ Once feeding is going well and your nipples have toughened up, let your baby suck for as long as she likes on the first side so she gets both the foremilk and the hindmilk. (Foremilk is the dilute, thirst-quenching part; the hindmilk is the richer, creamier part.) Then switch to the other breast and let your baby stay there as long as she likes, too.

Preparing your nipples for breastfeeding

When you first start breastfeeding your nipples will feel delicate. They need time to toughen up, so increase the length of time on each breast gradually. Two minutes on each breast will give your baby sufficient colostrum at first. Build up the time on each breast to ten minutes each side by the time the milk has come in on about the third or fourth day.

All babies suck most strongly in the first five minutes, and during this time they take about 80 per cent of the feed. When she's had enough she'll lose interest and play with your breast or fall asleep. Alternate the breast you begin feeding with each time.

Taking care of your breasts

Your breasts need special care when you start breastfeeding. Buy at least two maternity bras and be very careful about the daily hygiene of your breasts. Bathe them every day with water; don't use soap because it defats the skin and can encourage a sore or cracked nipple to develop. Always handle your breasts with care. Never rub them dry; always pat them.

If you can, leave your nipples open to the air for a short time when you've finished feeding. Wear pads inside your bra to soak up any milk that may leak, and change these pads often. To avoid cracked nipples, apply a drop of olive oil or hypericum and calendula cream to the pad.

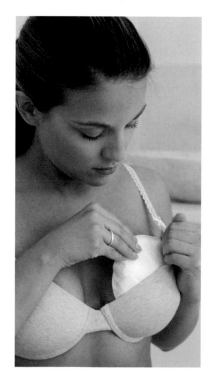

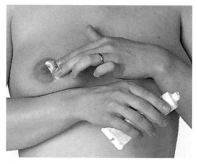

▲ **SORE NIPPLES** Use lotion to relieve cracked or sore nipples. Apply often, especially after each feed.

◀ **BREAST PADS** Leaking breasts can be embarrassing and uncomfortable, causing cracked nipples, and staining your clothes. Breast pads are easy to use so tuck them into the cups of your bra to soak up leaking milk. Don't leave a wet pad in for too long. Both washable and disposable pads are available, but avoid any backed with plastic.

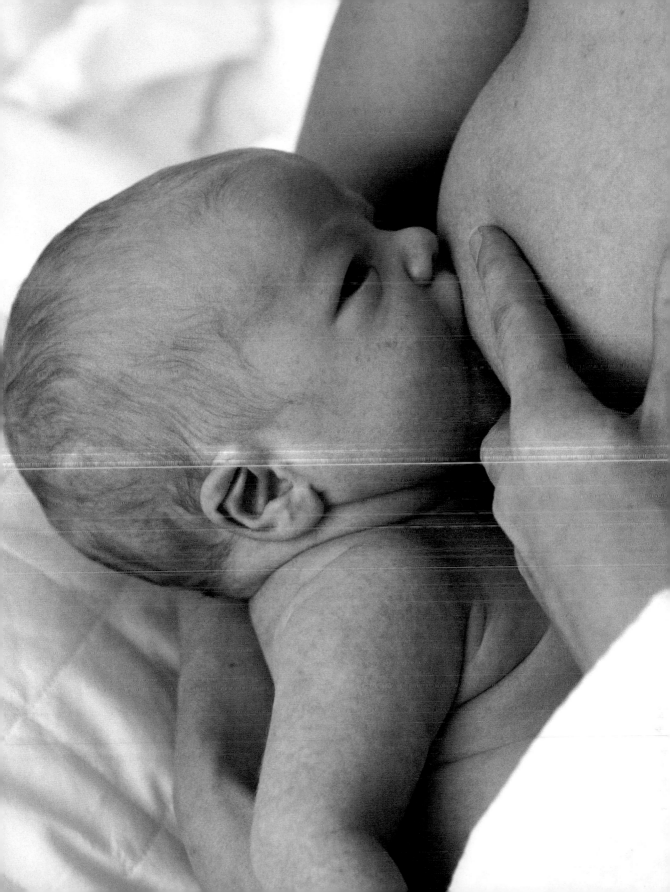

Take care

To reduce the risk of your baby contracting any kind of gastro-intestinal infection, make sure that everything that comes in contact with your baby's milk is thoroughly cleaned and sterilized before use.

Always make sure that you wash your hands before handling any formula or equipment. Your baby's dummies and teething rings should also be thoroughly cleaned each time they are used.

It's best to make up your baby's bottle when you need it, not in advance. Making up formula feeds in advance increases the risk of your baby becoming ill. If your baby doesn't finish a bottle or if you warm up a bottle for him but he doesn't want it, throw it away – reheated feeds are prime sources of infection.

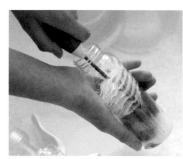

▲ WASHING BOTTLES AND TEATS
All equipment should be washed in hot, soapy water. Scrub the insides of the bottles with a bottle brush and rub the teats thoroughly to remove any traces of milk. Rinse everything well under warm, running water to remove any soap.

Bottlefeeding

It's perfectly safe and healthy to bottlefeed your baby with an infant formula, instead of breastfeeding, but you must follow the manufacturer's instructions very carefully. When you feed, give your baby plenty of warm, loving attention and eye contact.

Preparing formulas

Infant formula products range from relatively inexpensive dried-milk-based powders to ready-to-use, but expensive, liquid milk products. Infant formulas are enriched with vitamins and iron, and are carefully formulated to make them as close as possible to human milk. They're usually based on cow's milk, but there are soya-based formulas for babies who cannot digest, or who have an allergy to, cow's milk. If you're unsure which product to choose, ask your doctor or health visitor to recommend one.

Whichever formula you use, it's essential to keep all the bottles, spoons, mixing jugs, and teats absolutely clean, because a newborn baby is very vulnerable to infection. It's very important to make sure your work surface is clean and wash your hands thoroughly before making up formula or bottlefeeding your baby.

Bottles and teats

There's a wide range of different feeding bottles and teats now available. You may need to try a few to find out what suits your baby best. Some examples are shown below.

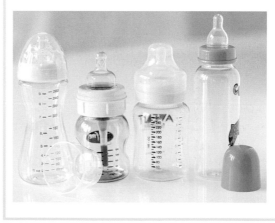

◄ BOTTLES (LEFT TO RIGHT)
Tapered bottle, waisted bottle, easy-grip bottle, disposable bottle

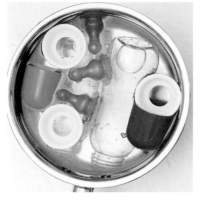

▲ **BOILING** To sterilize your baby's bottles by boiling, you need to boil them for at least ten minutes. Then remove them from the water and allow them to cool down before using.

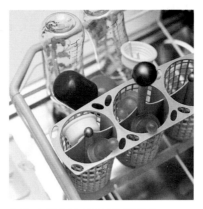

▲ **CLEANING IN A DISHWASHER** Once your baby is over 12 months you can wash feeding equipment in a dishwasher on the normal cycle. Clean teats before they go in (see column, left).

Keeping everything clean

You'll quickly develop your own routine for cleaning bottles. For sterilizing, use a sterilizing tank with a sterilizing chemical, or a steamer or microwave sterilizer. You can also sterilize equipment by boiling it in water. Sterilize all feeding equipment until your baby is 12 months old.

Before sterilizing, wash the feeding equipment in hot, soapy water or, if you have one, in a dishwasher. Scrub inside the bottles with a bottle brush. Clean the teats carefully, and rinse everything thoroughly (see column, opposite).

To use a sterilizing tank, half-fill the tank with cold water. Add a sterilizing tablet and wait for it to dissolve. Put in the equipment, filling the bottles with water to keep them submerged. Then fill the tank with cold water, and leave for the required time.

Measuring and mixing

Make up one bottle at a time, mixing it in the bottle according to the manufacturer's instructions. Never make feeds up in advance, as this increases the risk of contamination, which could make your baby ill. Never try to make the formula "more nourishing" by adding more powder than specified – your baby will get too much fat and protein and too little water. And if you add extra water to the powder, to make the formula more thirst-quenching, you run the risk of under-nourishing your baby.

Use only freshly boiled water that has been allowed to cool down slightly, and measure it out after it has cooled. If you measure it out before you boil it, the made-up formula will be too strong because of the water lost by evaporation.

Checking the temperature

While it's essential to give your baby a freshly made bottle of formula, its also important to make sure the milk's not too hot. So always check that the milk is at the correct temperature before you begin feeding.

■ **Testing milk temperature**
Try a few drops on your wrist: it should be neither hot nor cold to the touch.

■ **Cooling the milk** If the milk is too warm, place the bottle in a jug or bowl of cold water for a few minutes. You could also run it under the cold tap, shaking it all the time.

■ **Ready-made formula** This can be poured straight from the carton into a sterilized bottle, but it must be given to your baby straight away. You can warm it by placing the bottle in a bowl of warm water.

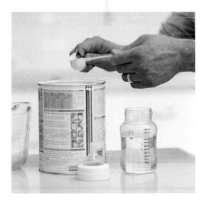

▲ **MEASURING OUT** Using the scoop provided, measure out the quantities accurately. Use a sterilized knife blade to level off the powder in the scoop exactly. Don't heap up the powder in the scoop, or pack it down tightly.

Breast to bottle

If you've been breastfeeding your baby and for any reason you want to change over to bottlefeeding with formula, it's best to do it gradually.

Make the switch from breast to bottle very slowly so that your baby has time to get used to bottlefeeding and to the taste of formula. Your milk supply will then slowly reduce as your baby's demand for it lessens.

Before starting the change to bottlefeeding, ask your health visitor for detailed advice.

Giving the bottle

When you feed your baby by bottle, whether with formula or with expressed breastmilk, be just as patient and loving as you would be if you were breastfeeding her. Allow her to take a break if she feels like it and to decide when she's had enough.

Getting comfortable

When you or your partner give your baby a feed, it's important to look at her, cuddle her close, and talk to her – just as you would when breastfeeding. Find a quiet, comfortable place to feed your baby. You may like to sit on the floor or in a low chair so you can support her on your lap. Rest her head in the crook of your elbow, with her back supported on your forearm, and hold her securely.

Never leave your baby with the bottle propped up on a cushion; it can be dangerous. She could become very uncomfortable if she swallows a lot of air with the feed, and she could choke. Moreover, she'll miss the cuddling and affection that she should be able to enjoy while she feeds.

Bottlefeeding

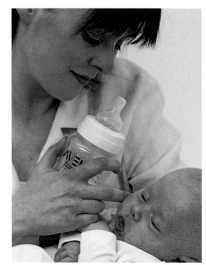

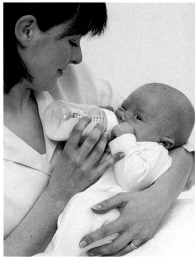

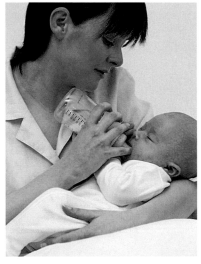

1 PREPARING FOR A FEED Hold your baby with her head slightly raised so she can breathe and swallow safely and there's no risk of choking. At first, you may need to trigger her sucking reflex by stroking the cheek nearest you.

2 GIVING THE BOTTLE When you gently put the teat into her mouth, be careful not to push it too far back. When she begins to suck, hold the bottle at an angle to keep the teat full of formula or milk, and free of air.

3 RELEASING THE TEAT Sometimes, your baby will want to keep sucking away at a bottle even though it's empty. If you want her to let go, gently slide your little finger between her gums. This will break the suction.

Before feeding, splash a few drops of milk on your wrist to check the temperature before starting to feed – the milk should feel tepid on your skin (see column, p.333). Unscrew the teat ring a little so that air can get into the bottle when your baby sucks out the formula. This will prevent the teat from closing up. Always hold the bottle at an angle so the teat is full of milk or your baby will swallow air with the feed. Your baby's appetite will vary, so if she seems satisfied, allow her to leave what she doesn't want. If your baby falls asleep during a feed, she may have wind that is making her feel full. Sit her up and burp her.

Burping your baby

The point of burping is to help your baby bring up any air she's swallowed during feeding, or when crying before feeding, so it doesn't cause her any discomfort. If your baby has wind, one of the best ways to burp her is to hold her against your shoulder and gently rub her back (below). Another way to help your baby to clear any wind is to sit her on your lap and lean her forwards, without bending her over at the waist. As you do this, support her head with your hand so it does not flop forwards.

Possetting

If your baby tends to bring food straight back up (some babies never do) you may wonder if she's keeping enough of her feed down. My youngest

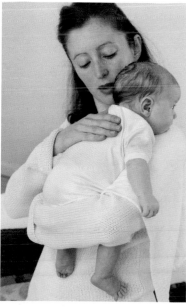

son had a tendency to posset, and I worried in case he wasn't getting enough to eat. I simply followed my own instinct, which was to offer him more food. If he didn't take it, I assumed that he had possetted an excess of milk that he didn't need. The most common cause of possetting in very young babies is overfeeding, and this is another reason why you should never insist that your baby finishes his bottle.

Forcible vomiting, especially if this happens after several feeds in a row, should be reported immediately to your doctor; vomiting is always very serious in a young baby as it can quickly lead to dehydration.

▲ **BURPING** To burp your baby, hold her against your shoulder and gently stroke or rub her back.

Wind and burping

Babies vary a great deal in how they react to wind. In my experience, most babies aren't noticeably more contented for having been burped.

Babies differ in the amount of air that they swallow during feeding. Some, including most breastfed babies, swallow very little. Once a baby is clamped on to the breast, it's virtually an airtight seal, so it's almost impossible for a baby to swallow air while on the breast.

Swallowing air is much more common in bottlefed babies, but even then it doesn't really seem to be a problem.

One thing in favour of burping is that it makes you relax, take things slowly, hold your baby gently, and stroke her in a firm and reassuring way and this can help both of you. My feeling about burping is that by all means do it, but don't become fanatical.

Don't rub or pat your baby too hard as you may jerk her and she'll bring up some of her feed. A gently upward, stroking movement is better than firm pats.

You don't need to stop halfway through a feed to burp your baby. Wait until she pauses naturally, and then put her on your shoulder. If she doesn't burp, don't worry; it's because she doesn't need to.

Range of nappies

There are range of different nappies available. Choose what's best for you and your baby.

Disposable
■ Disposable nappy, available in different sizes and sometimes in boy and girl styles.

Reusable
■ Traditional terry nappy for use with pins or clips, plastic pants, and biodegradable or reusable liners.

■ Shaped resuable nappy.

■ Shaped resuable nappy with built-in waterproof covering.

Choosing nappies

Your baby will need to wear nappies day and night for the next two to three years, until he's able to start using a potty. There are lots of different types available in pharmacies and supermarkets so choose whatever's best for your lifestyle and budget.

Types of nappy

The basic choice is between disposable and reusable fabric nappies. Think about which type will be most comfortable for your baby as well as cost-effective and manageable for you.

Disposable nappies These are convenient and easy to use. They come ready-shaped with elasticated legs to prevent leakage and there's no need for pins or plastic pants. Sizes range from newborn to toddler and some come in boy and girl styles. However, disposables are expensive and as millions are thrown away every day they are creating a huge waste problem.

Reusable nappies Fabric nappies may seem more expensive at first as you need to buy at least 24 of good quality. But they can work out cheaper in the long term as you can use them over and over again and for more than one child. Some parents also find that reusable nappies are better for older babies at night because they're more absorbent.

Reusables are more work as they need to be washed and dried after every use, although in some areas there are nappy-laundering services that will pick up dirty nappies from your home and return them clean and dry. Use reusable nappies with liners that allow urine to pass through and away from the baby's skin and lessen the risk of a sore bottom. You'll need a supply of plastic pants to stop leakage, unless the type you choose has a plastic outer layer (see below). Choose plastic pants with popper fasteners for a good fit. To keep them soft and pliable, wash them in warm water with a little washing-up liquid, pat dry, and leave them to air. Traditional square-shaped terry nappies can be fiddly to fold and put on. The latest shaped reusables fit your baby without being folded. They fasten with Velcro tabs too, so there's no need for pins or clips. Some have a plastic outer layer; for others you need plastic pants.

Resealable tapes let you check if the nappy is clean

Efficient leg elastication gives a good fit with less chance of leaks

Elasticated leakage barriers provide extra protection

Absorbent inner layer has a plastic covering

▲ DISPOSABLE NAPPIES Easy to put on and take off, disposable nappies are also convenient when you're travelling because used nappies can be discarded in a nappy sack and put in a dustbin.

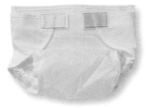

Plastic pants

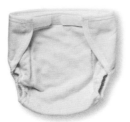

Shaped reusable nappy
with Velcro fastener

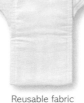

Reusable fabric
nappy liner

▲ **FABRIC NAPPIES AND ACCESSORIES** If you choose fabric nappies, you'll need separate liners (biodegradable or reusable). You may need plastic pants too.

Benefits of different nappies

DISPOSABLES	REUSABLES
Advantages No washing, drying, pins, or plastic pants. No risk of hurting your baby with a pin. More practical when travelling as you need fewer accessories and you don't have to carry a bag of dirty nappies home.	**Advantages** Only need one set so don't need to keep buying new supplies. Work out cheaper in the long run and can be used for another child.
Disadvantages Can only be used once. More expensive in the long run. Create mountains of rubbish – never flush them down the toilet.	**Disadvantages** Washing and drying is a lot of work. Can be more difficult to put on, unless you use shaped reusables.

Nappy contents

After your baby is born, you'll notice some changes in the colour and consistency of his stools. During the first couple of days your baby will pass meconium, a sticky, greenish-black substance. This contains bile and mucus and comes from the amniotic fluid he swallowed in your uterus. Once he starts feeding, the stools will become greenish-brown, with a looser consistency, and then a yellowish-brown. The colour, smell, and consistency of the stools varies, depending on whether you're breastfeeding or bottlefeeding your baby. The stools of breastfed babies are looser and bright yellow. Bottlefed babies pass a firmer, pale brown stool, with a more pungent smell.

The number of motions also varies. Some babies fill their nappies after every meal, while others are less frequent. Sometimes, a couple of days may pass without a bowel movement – unless there are other problems (see column, right), this is nothing to worry about.

Signs to watch for

As long as your baby is healthy, don't worry too much about the contents of his nappy.

A baby's bowel motions may vary, but there are a few signs to look out for (see Newborn health, p.342). For example, streaks of blood in stools aren't normal, so you if you spot these, call your doctor right away.

Immediately after birth, your baby's urine contains substances called urates that may stain his nappy a dark pink or red, but this is normal, so don't be alarmed. He'll urinate often, maybe every half hour because his bladder can't hold urine for even a few minutes. Don't worry unless he stops urinating for several hours. If this happens, check with your doctor in case there is an abnormality in his urinary tract or he's dehydrated.

After every feed you'll probably need to change your baby's nappy

▲ **FREQUENT CHANGES** Young babies can't hold urine for long and it's quite normal to need to change his nappy several times a day.

Nappy rash

Bacteria on the skin break down urine to form ammonia which burns and causes nappy rash.

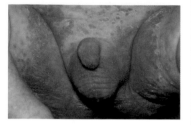

▲ **SORE BOTTOM** To prevent nappy rash, don't wash your baby's skin with soap and water: use baby lotion. You can also buy a special cream from a chemist. Avoid plastic pants.

Changing a nappy

You'll need to change your baby's nappy when it's wet or dirty, which will be very often – especially with a new baby. To prevent your baby having nappy rash, change her nappy when she wakes up in the morning, after every feed, and when she goes to bed at night. Make sure you have somewhere safe to change your baby with all the equipment you'll need close at hand. As often as you can, leave her nappy off for a while to air her bottom.

Cleaning your baby

1 **CLEAN HER NAPPY AREA** Holding both her ankles in one hand, clean her genital area. Wipe off any faeces with a tissue. With cotton wool moistened with water or baby lotion, wipe from her vagina toward her rectum. Never pull back the labia to clean inside.

Wipe from front to back to prevent soiling her vulva

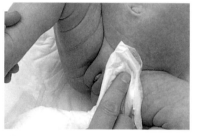

2 **CLEAN HER LEG CREASES** Holding one leg at a time, use moistened cotton wool to clean inside all the creases at the tops of her legs. Wipe downward and away from her body. Clean her thighs and buttocks, wiping inward toward the rectum. Remove the dirty nappy.

Cleaning a boy

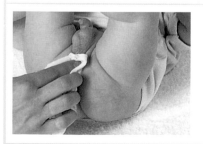

◀ **WIPE HIM CLEAN** Holding his ankles with one hand and lifting him up, clean his bottom using cotton wool moistened with water or baby lotion. Gently wipe his testicles and under his penis (don't pull the foreskin back). Clean his leg creases as above. Use petroleum jelly to protect his penis.

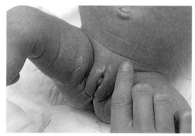

3 **DRY HER BOTTOM** If you've used water, dry the area with a tissue, then let her kick her legs for a while, so that air reaches her bottom. Apply barrier cream to prevent nappy rash.

Changing a shaped reusable nappy

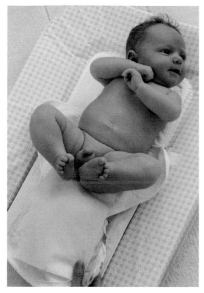

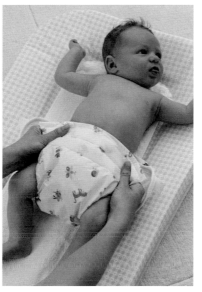

1 **POSITIONING THE NAPPY** Begin by sliding the reusable nappy under your baby so his waist aligns with the top edge of the nappy.

2 **MAKING IT FIT SNUGLY** Bring the nappy up between his legs and hold it in place while you fold the sides in to the centre and fasten with Velcro tabs.

Nappy washing

It's important to wash fabric nappies thoroughly, as any traces of ammonia can irritate your baby's skin and faecal bacteria can cause infection.

It's best to use pure soap flakes or a non-biological washing powder because biological washing powder can be too harsh for a baby's delicate skin and cause rashes and skin reactions. If you use fabric conditioner, always make sure that it is completely rinsed away.

An outdoor washing line is ideal for drying nappies, but you might find you also need a tumble drier when the weather is not so good.

Changing a disposable nappy

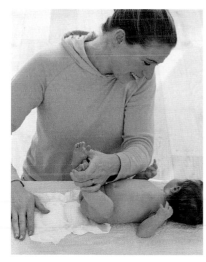

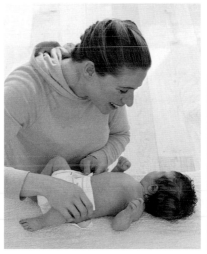

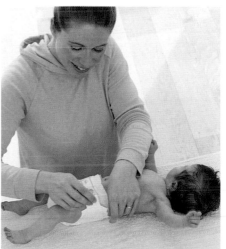

1 **POSITIONING YOUR BABY** Lay the nappy flat, with the tabs at the back. Slide the nappy under your baby so that the top aligns with her waist.

2 **FASTENING THE FRONT** Bring the front up between the legs and tuck it around her tummy. Unpeel the sticky tabs at each side of the nappy.

3 **A COMFORTABLE FIT** Pull the tabs firmly over the front flap of the nappy and fasten securely. The nappy should fit snugly around your baby.

Tips for bath time

You might feel a bit nervous the first time you give your baby a bath. But once you get used to it, you'll both relax and enjoy the time of extra closeness.

■ Keep the room warm – at least 20°C (68°F) – and don't leave your baby undressed for too long.

■ Make sure the bath is at a comfortable height for you.

■ Check that everything you need for washing, drying, and dressing is within easy reach.

■ Always test the water first and don't add hot water while your baby is in the bath. Add baby bath liquid to the water; it's easier to use than soap.

■ Chat and smile to your baby at bath time, and take the chance to have lots of body contact.

Washing your baby

You don't need to give your newborn baby a bath every day – once a week on a regular day is often enough. You can bathe him more often if you both enjoy it – lots of babies do like having a splash in the bath once they get used to it. You can bathe him in any room in the house as long as it is warm enough. Always check the temperature of the water first to make sure it's not too hot by dipping in your elbow, or the inside of your wrist.

Wash the parts that matter

A young baby doesn't need bathing very often as only his face, neck, bottom, and skin creases get dirty. Topping and tailing is a quick way of washing the parts that really need cleaning with the minimum of disturbance and distress to him. Many young babies don't like having their skin exposed to the air and this way you don't have to completely undress your baby. For a newborn, use pieces of cotton wool dipped in cooled, boiled water and squeezed dry, but when your baby is a little older you can use warm water straight from the tap.

Wipe his eyes carefully, using a clean piece of cotton wool for each eye to avoid spreading any infection that may be present. Don't try to poke around in your baby's nose and ears; they are self-cleaning.

Topping and tailing

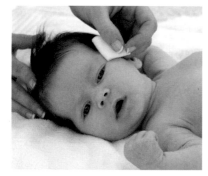

◀ **CLEAN HER FACE, NECK, AND EYES** Wipe her face and chin and the creases in her neck with moist cotton wool to remove any traces of milk or spittle. Use a clean piece of cotton wool for each eye and wipe from the inside outward.

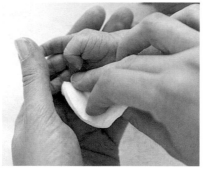

▲ **CLEAN HER HANDS** Gently uncurl her fingers. Using a moistened piece of cotton wool, wipe over the fronts and backs of her hands, and in between her fingers. Take a new piece of cotton wool and wipe her arms. Dry with a soft towel.

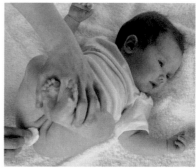

▲ **CLEAN HER BOTTOM** Undo any lower garments and remove her nappy. Using a new piece of cotton wool, wipe around her genital area (see p.338). If she's soiled, moisten the cotton wool with some baby lotion.

Bathing

1 **BEFORE THE BATH** Undress
your baby down to his vest
and nappy. Before you put him in
the bath, wipe his eyes and face
with some moist cotton wool.
Then undress him completely and
wrap him in a soft, clean towel.

2 **WASH HIS HEAD** Hold him just
above the bath in a football
carry, so that he lies along your
arm and his head is supported by
your hand. With your other hand,
carefully wash his hair with the
bath water. Then gently dry his
hair with a soft towel.

Support your
baby's head
with your hand

Cleaning his cord stump

Your baby's umbilical cord stump
dries and drops off within a week
after the birth.

Every day gently wipe the skin
creases around the stump with a
surgical baby wipe containing pure
alcohol. Continue after the stump
has separated so it heals quickly. If
you notice any redness, discharge,
or other signs of infection, check
with your midwife or health visitor.

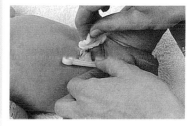

▲ **AVOID INFECTION** Dry the umbilical
area carefully every time you bathe
your baby. Leave the area open to the
air as often as you can in order to
avoid infection.

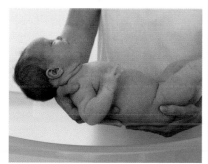

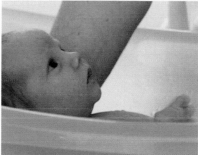

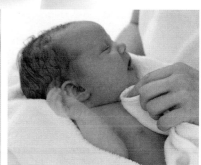

3 **PUT HIM INTO BATH** Support your
baby's shoulders with one hand,
tucking your fingers under his armpits,
and support his legs or bottom with the
other hand. Always hold him securely and
keep smiling and talking to your baby as
you place him in the bath.

4 **WASH HIM ALL OVER** Keep him
semi-upright and slowly splash
water over his body with your free hand.
Talk and smile to him all the time. When
you're finished, lift him out, with your
free hand held firmly under his bottom,
and wrap him gently in the towel.

5 **DRY HIM CAREFULLY** Pat your baby
dry after the bath and be very careful
to dry his skin creases well. It's best
not to use baby powder, particularly in
the nappy area. It can be drying to your
baby's skin and tends to cake in the
creases and cause irritation.

When to call the doctor

As your baby gets older you'll learn how to deal with minor ailments, but there are times when you'll need the doctor.

Sometimes when your baby is ill you'll be torn between not wanting to bother the doctor unnecessarily and feeling more and more worried about your baby's wellbeing. Don't take any chances with your baby's health – call the doctor promptly, especially if your baby is showing one or more of the symptoms listed below or if you have any other reason to worry.

Call your doctor if your baby:

- is having convulsions

- is hard to rouse

- is having trouble breathing, is wheezing, or has a loud, dry cough

- has a very high temperature, or an abnormally low one

- has stools that are frequent, loose, green, and watery

- is vomiting a significant amount (not just the usual after-feed possetting)

- has refused several of his feeds in a row

- is showing the symptoms of dehydration (see right)

- is listless and crying for no apparent reason

- seems to be bothered by his ears, head, or neck

- has an unusual rash.

Newborn health

Newborn babies, especially breastfed babies, are generally healthy during their first weeks of life. But their immune systems and internal organs are not yet fully developed, so there are some ailments that can affect them at this early age.

Jaundice of the newborn

This is a yellowish discoloration of the skin and whites of the eyes caused by too much bilirubin in the blood. Bilirubin is a yellow pigment that's produced when primitive red blood cells are destroyed – something that often happens after birth.

Infant jaundice usually appears by the second or third day after birth, and lasts for about seven to ten days. By this time, the surplus red blood cells have died off and the baby's liver has matured enough to mop up the excess bilirubin in the body. The jaundice usually clears up by itself, but if the bilirubin levels are particularly high, a baby may need phototherapy. In this treatment a baby is exposed to carefully controlled amounts of ultraviolet light, which breaks down the bilirubin pigment in the skin.

Haemolytic disease of the newborn This is a more serious condition caused by too much bilirubin in a baby's blood. It can result from the breakdown of large numbers of red blood cells due to the action of antibodies from a Rhesus-incompatible mother (see p.202). The main symptoms are jaundice, pallor, enlargement of the liver and spleen, and blood abnormalities. It's usually treated by blood transfusion.

Diarrhoea and vomiting

Mild cases of upset stomach or diarrhoea will soon pass but a young baby's digestive system is extremely vulnerable. Breastfed babies are less prone to these gastro-intestinal infections than bottlefed babies, because of the protective antibodies that are contained in breastmilk.

Contact your doctor immediately if your baby vomits up all his feeds over a six-hour period or is passing frequent, loose, green, watery stools.

Dehydration The major danger to babies who are suffering from vomiting and diarrhoea is dehydration because of the loss of fluids. Symptoms of dehydration include a dry mouth, sunken eyes, the fontanelles looking or feeling unusually low, irritability, lethargy, and refusal to feed. Never ignore these symptoms; call your doctor at once.

Bowel and bladder problems

Breastfed babies don't get constipated – the ideal composition and digestibility of breastmilk keeps everything moving. Bottlefed babies can get constipated and this is usually because they're not getting enough fluid. If your bottlefed baby passes no stools for a day or two, then produces a hard one, give him drinks of water between feeds to increase his fluid intake. If this doesn't make his stools softer and more frequent, ask your doctor or health visitor for advice.

Urinary problems If your baby starts to urinate infrequently it might be a sign of a fever, or of a blockage or infection in his urinary system. If he goes for a couple of hours without wetting his nappy, give him plenty of water to drink. If his nappy is still dry two hours later, call your doctor.

If your baby's urine becomes strong-smelling and deepens in colour, he may not be having enough to drink. This makes the urine more concentrated. Increase his liquid intake by giving him several drinks of water between feeds. If this doesn't make any difference, he could have a urinary infection and might need treatment, so call your doctor.

Fever

A fever is a sign that your baby's body is fighting an infection – the rise in temperature acts to make the body's own defence system work harder. If you think your baby may have a fever, take his temperature. Check it again in 20 minutes to see if it's changed and note each reading. If his temperature rises slightly, but he seems his usual self and shows no other signs of illness, it's probably a minor infection and will usually pass within a day or two, but tell your doctor just in case. Call your doctor at once if your baby's temperature rises by a degree or more, if he gets hot and distressed, or shows symptoms such as lethargy, vomiting, or diarrhoea.

Ear infections

Babies often get colds, and these can lead to an ear infection called otitis media. This happens when the bacteria travel along one, or both, of the Eustachian tubes (which link the middle ear to the back of the throat and equalize pressure in the ears) into the middle ear. Babies spend most of their time lying down, which allows the bacteria to pass along more easily. When the mucous membrane of the Eustachian tube gets inflamed, bacteria are trapped in the middle ear, where they multiply.

Symptoms include a high temperature, diarrhoea, crying for no apparent reason, and any kind of discharge from the ear. Call your doctor right away. Your baby will need to be seen to confirm the diagnosis and to rule out meningitis, which has similar symptoms.

Colicky baby

Colic is more common in male babies. The exact causes of this exasperating blend of indigestion and inconsolable crying are still not known.

Some medical researchers looking into the cause of colic suspect that it happens because the baby's digestive system is immature. Other research suggests that babies whose mothers have been particularly anxious while pregnant are more prone to being colicky (see p.193).

In a typical colicky baby, the problem begins at about two weeks and disappears at about three months. The attacks usually happen in the evening. The baby draws up his legs to his stomach or sticks them out straight in an attempt to relieve the stomach cramps and wind, and cries loudly.

There's really not much you can do about colic, except wait for him to grow out of it. Stomach massage can often ease the discomfort, as does lying him face down across your lap with a warm towel placed under his belly. Other ideas include taking your baby for a ride in a car, putting him face down across your knees and stroking his back, and giving him a dummy to suck on.

Colic doesn't damage your baby's health (although it can be very frustrating for you), but when it first starts to happen, check with your doctor to make sure that it's nothing more serious.

How to help your baby

Your baby will receive lots of care and attention from specialist staff, but there are things you and your partner can do to help him thrive.

■ Spend as much time with him as you can; he needs the same love and attention as a full-term baby.

■ Touch and fondle your baby, both in and out of the incubator, whenever and as soon as you can. Cuddling and stroking help him to grow and thrive.

■ Express your breast milk at regular feeding times for your baby. You'll be giving him the best possible food and at the same time you'll build up your milk supply for when he's able to suck on his own.

■ Research shows that the colostrum and milk of a mother whose child is preterm contain more of certain nutrients than those of mothers whose babies are born at term. This makes up for a preterm baby's missing out on nutrients he would have received in the uterus. A preterm baby fed on his mother's breast milk develops at almost exactly the same rate as he would if he were still in her uterus.

■ Get involved with your baby's care. Ask the nurses to show you how to help with feeding, washing, and changing him. This will help you bond with your baby and give you confidence in caring for him.

■ Don't struggle with feelings of anxiety, ignorance, or worry – ask the medical team for information.

Special care baby

About one in ten newborn babies needs to spend some time in a special care baby unit. Most have been born too soon or have not grown as much as they should have before birth. A small number may be ill. The aim of the unit is to protect your baby from any risks to his health and to care for him until he's outgrown them.

Low birthweight babies

In general, any baby weighing less than 2kg (4½lb) at birth is probably smaller than he should be and may need special care. About four to eight per cent of all babies have low birthweights. Of these, two-thirds are preterm – born before their due date – and one-third are small for dates.

Preterm babies The pace of an unborn baby's development is geared to his being born at full term (40 weeks from your LMP). If, for any reason, he is born a few weeks or more before full term, he may not yet be ready for life in the outside world. A baby born before week 37 is said to be preterm or premature. Depending on how premature he is, he'll need the help of a special care baby unit or a neonatal intensive care unit.

Small-for-dates babies A baby is "small for dates" if he weighs less than expected for the number of weeks that have passed since he was conceived. A small-for-dates baby is usually a full-term baby who's very small at birth. These babies may present different problems of care after the birth from a premature baby. Babies who are only three or four weeks premature and low birthweight full-term babies, who are otherwise well and feeding properly, can usually stay on the postnatal ward with their mothers, or in a so-called "transitional care" nursery where their progress will be more closely monitored than normal.

Health risks A premature baby born before 37 weeks faces a number of health risks that don't usually affect a full-term infant, as well as more common ones such as jaundice. If his internal organs are underdeveloped, for example, he may have difficulty breathing, regulating his body temperature, and feeding; he'll also be very vulnerable to infection. He may also have a low blood-sugar level (hypoglycaemia), which can cause brain damage if untreated, and he may need iron or calcium supplements if he lacks these essential minerals.

Caring for babies with special needs

Today, a baby who's born preterm or small for dates, or with an illness or disability, has a far better chance than he would have had 20 or even ten years ago. This is because so much more is known about how to care for newborn babies and this knowledge is applied in special care baby units. If a baby is simply too weak or young to be able to suck, and needs tube feeding, or has jaundice and so needs phototherapy treatment, he'll probably be looked after in the special care baby unit (SCBU) attached to the local maternity unit. If he's very premature or ill, he'll need specialist, "high-tech" care in the neonatal intensive care part of the unit (NICU).

An NICU is dedicated to looking after babies who need highly specialized nursing attention. In modern NICUs the tiniest premature babies – even ones born at only 24 or 25 weeks' gestation and weighing barely 450g (1lb) – can be helped to thrive.

If you go into labour very prematurely you may be taken to a hospital with an NICU, even if it's not the hospital into which you were booked, or your baby may be taken there by ambulance in a special incubator immediately after the birth. If this should happen to you, ask the consultant paediatrician in charge to explain all about your baby's particular needs and how you can help.

Most NICUs encourage parents to stay with their baby and play an active part in his everyday care by helping with tasks such as feeding, washing, and nappy changing. Parents are encouraged to cuddle their babies skin to skin, as this helps them develop more quickly (see also p.349). But with a very premature baby it may be some time before he's strong enough to be handled outside the incubator, and parents may have to wait until their baby's condition has improved.

(see also p.349)

Reasons for special care

Every baby born prematurely or small for dates is assessed individually, but your baby will definitely be taken to a neonatal intensive care unit if any of the following applies:

■ birthweight less than 1.5kg (3lb)

■ less than 34 weeks in the womb

■ severe respiratory problems, known as respiratory distress syndrome

■ severe birth asphyxia (lack of oxygen or fetal distress)

■ severe infection

■ convulsions (seizures)

■ jaundice that requires an exchange transfusion

■ drug withdrawal, if the mother has been addicted to narcotics.

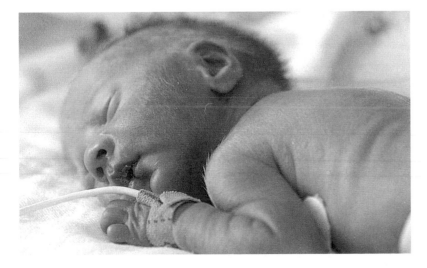

◀ **A SPECIAL CARE BABY** Most special care babies, like this premature baby, spend some time in an incubator. This keeps their temperature steady and monitors their breathing.

Your experience

If your baby needs special care you'll probably be concerned about the bonding process. Don't worry – the staff will encourage you both to be as involved as possible with your baby and his daily care.

■ You'll be encouraged to watch the nurses care for your baby and to help with the practical care and nursing.

■ Don't be afraid to touch your baby as often as possible. As well as helping you to feel closer to him, this loving attention also has huge benefits for your baby, helping him to thrive and grow.

■ Keep talking and singing to your baby. He'll get to know your voice and be soothed and comforted by the familiar sound.

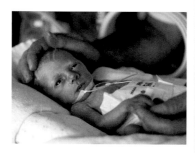

▲ **PHYSICAL CONTACT** An incubator has circular doors in the plastic top so the nurses can attend to your baby and attach any monitor leads, feeding tubes, or intravenous drips he might need. The doors also allow you to reach in and touch your baby, helping you to bond with him and feel close.

Special care unit

In the special care unit your baby is cared for 24 hours a day by specially trained staff with a wide range of technology to help them. The main concerns for a special care baby are temperature control, breathing, brain and immune system, and feeding. There'll be a lot of tubes, electrodes, monitors, and drips, but they're there to help your baby so try not to be alarmed.

Why your baby needs care

Your baby needs special care to help him to grow and thrive once he's outside your womb. The following key areas are closely monitored.

Temperature control All babies are at risk of getting cold – a premature or small-for-dates baby is even more at risk, because he has little or no body fat for insulation. A premature baby is usually placed in an incubator, in which he can be kept warm and supplied with warmed, humidified air (or oxygen, if he needs it).

Breathing Under 30 weeks, and certainly before 27 weeks, a baby's lungs are not mature enough to allow the transfer of oxygen to the bloodstream. If you go into premature labour, you'll probably be given an injection of

Monitoring your baby

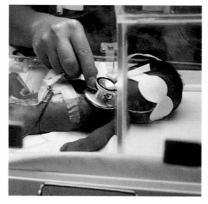

▲ **CHECKING HEART RATE** A stethoscope is used to monitor and record a premature baby's heart rate so doctors are alerted to any change.

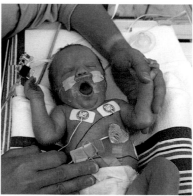

▲ **CENTRAL NERVOUS SYSTEM** The baby's nervous system needs careful monitoring with electrodes that feed information into a visual display unit.

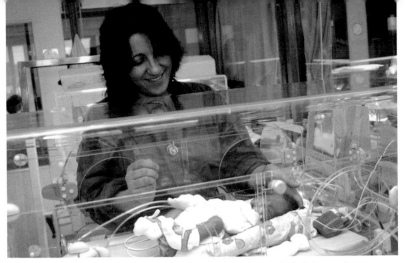

▲ **YOUR BABY'S ENVIRONMENT** A preterm or small-for-dates baby's internal organs may not be completely developed and he'll need help so he can breathe and grow. Inside the incubator the temperature, oxygen levels, and humidity are all carefully controlled to provide the best possible conditions for your baby to develop and thrive. Always ask questions if there's anything you don't understand about your baby's care.

corticosteroids to help mature your baby's lungs. Because the nervous system is immature, this can affect a baby's breathing, and may cause pauses in breathing, known as apnoea, sometimes accompanied by a slowing of the heart rate, known as bradycardia.

Feeding Initially, your baby will have small feeds once an hour, progressing to one every three hours. A very premature or sick baby may be unable to digest milk and will be given a solution of sugar, salts, and potassium. When he's able to take milk, he'll have a special formula or your own expressed milk. Breastmilk is the ideal food for a special care baby.

Your baby's needs

A special care baby needs his mother and father as well as specialist medical care.

Although a special care baby receives 24-hour medical care, he also needs to feel his parents' love. Physical contact with you and your partner will reassure and comfort him, and help you to develop a warm, close, and loving relationship.

Hold him close whenever you can so that he gets to know your smells and can feel close to you. When your baby is stronger, you may be able to give him kangaroo care. This means holding him against your bare skin, which can help his development.

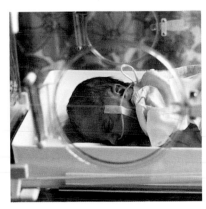

▲ **FEEDING** Most premature babies have to be fed through a soft, thin tube which is inserted through the nose. Expressed breast milk is best.

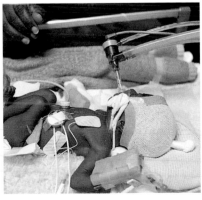

▲ **DETECTING THE HEARTBEAT** Electrodes placed on the baby's chest monitor his heartbeat so the medical team can keep a constant check.

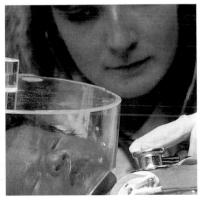

▲ **ASSISTED BREATHING** A premature baby's lungs are likely to be under-developed, so he may need help with his breathing through a special ventilator.

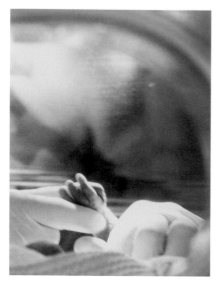

Premature baby

At 28 weeks of pregnancy, Carol noticed that her fingers, hands, and feet were swollen. Two weeks later she had raised blood pressure, so her blood pressure, blood, and urine were monitored. Her baby was checked too, with electronic fetal monitoring (see p.275) and ultrasound scans. There was albumin in Carol's urine, which is a symptom of pre-eclampsia, along with high blood pressure and swelling.

Monitoring Carol's baby

After a week of careful monitoring, Carol's blood pressure hadn't gone back to normal and there was still albumin in her urine. At the beginning of the 32nd week of pregnancy, the baby was showing signs of fetal distress. Her obstetrician decided that labour would have to be induced. After a straightforward induced labour, Carol delivered her baby, Alice, who weighed in at 1.4kg (3lb).

Carol's obstetrician thought that her placenta had begun to fail at the beginning of the third trimester and so her baby's nutrition had been inadequate for some time. When this happens late in pregnancy, the baby's head is disproportionally large because of the relatively normal growth of the brain at the expense of the rest of the body.

He explained that low-birthweight premature babies like Alice are born with insufficient energy stores and don't have enough fat to maintain their body temperature. Premature babies are more likely to suffer from hypothermia, hypoxia (lack of oxygen to the tissues), and hypoglycaemia (abnormally low blood sugar), so it's crucial that they are kept warm. Alice was put straight into an incubator and her immature lungs were helped by a ventilator. Carol was given a room next door so she could be with Alice as much as

possible. Carol and Mark were quite taken aback by the first sight of Alice even though they'd had time to get used to the idea that she would be premature. When they looked at Alice inside the incubator, attached to a ventilator and taped with wires and tubes for monitoring and feeding, she seemed very tiny, and very far away and isolated.

Appearance of Carol's baby

Alice didn't look like they had expected her to. Born eight weeks early, she had none of the fat that a baby normally puts on in the last few weeks and her movements tended to be jerky because of her immature nervous system. She looked too small for her skin, which was red, wrinkled, loose-fitting, and dry, and her head looked large in comparison to her body. She had lanugo (fine downy hair) on her back and the sides of her face.

Her bottom looked bony and pointed due to lack of fat, and her chest, which looked small with prominent ribs, rose and fell dramatically as she breathed. She seemed to have to make a huge effort to take every breath and sometimes her breathing would stop for a few seconds, but this is not abnormal in a preterm baby.

Seeking reassurance

Understandably, Carol found herself bursting into tears at the sight of her tiny daughter, so alone and shut away. At the same time, she realized she was having considerable difficulty relating to her baby in the incubator even though she knew this was her longed-for child. Mark encouraged Carol to explain her difficulties to the counsellor on the ward, who comforted Carol and said that her feelings were common and normal. The staff of the special care unit were understanding; they encouraged Carol and Mark to touch and stroke Alice through the portholes of the incubator. Research shows that this helps a premature baby to establish breathing more readily. The staff explained to Carol that her love was more important for the baby's survival than all the technology they could offer.

Getting to know their baby

As Carol became involved in caring for Alice, she realized that she loved her and desperately wanted her to survive. The nurses showed her how to express her colostrum (see p.327) so that it could be fed to Alice via the tube. The colostrum of the mothers of premature babies is extra rich in trace minerals – those minerals the baby would be getting if she were still in the uterus – and their milk contains extra protein to help their babies grow.

Meanwhile, Mark became interested in the machines in the unit and what each one was doing for his daughter. Busy as they were, the staff found time to answer his questions.

Skin-to-skin contact

Once Alice had gained weight and her breathing had improved, she was taken off the ventilator and feeding tube. The staff of the postnatal unit then encouraged Carol to tuck Alice under her blouse and hold her in an upright position between her breasts. Alice was naked except for a nappy and this meant that mother and baby were in skin-to-skin contact for long periods of time.

Premature babies thrive on this treatment. A mother's body is better than an incubator for keeping a baby warm

Miriam's top tips

When a baby is born earlier than expected, it can take time for parents to adjust to the shock of premature delivery. My advice is to:

- ask for as much information as possible so you know what's happening with your baby and why

- give yourselves time to adjust to your baby's early arrival and don't be surprised if it takes longer to bond with your newborn than you'd expected

- touch, stroke, and hold your baby as much as you are able, even while she's in her incubator.

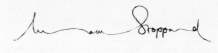

because her temperature rises automatically if her baby is cold, then falls again once the baby has warmed up. The nurses called it kangaroo care, because it's similar to the way in which kangaroos keep their infants in a warm, protective pouch. This skin-to-skin contact strengthens the mother-and-baby bond. Alice began to suckle spontaneously.

The unit staff were delighted with her progress and Carol and Mark were now eager to take Alice home. The paediatrician explained that it wasn't a question of Alice reaching any target weight; each baby was considered as an individual case and allowed home when her weight and general health were satisfactory given her circumstances. Generally, premature babies are usually kept in hospital until they reach 2.5kg (5lb).

Special baby clothes

Most newborn baby clothes were too big for Alice, but Carol's mother found a specialist mail order catalogue and Mark found one or two department stores had a stock of clothes for premature babies. Ordinary nappies were far too big, so Carol cut some disposables down to fit Alice and fastened them with tape. Alice thrived at home and soon began to catch up with full-term babies of the same age.

Adjusting to parenthood

You may find the responsibilities of parenthood take some getting used to, particularly if they mean dramatic changes to your lifestyles. But you'll soon find that watching your baby grow and develop will bring you great joy as you start to experience the closeness that only a family can bring.